Textbook of Pharmaceutical Chemistry-I (Inorganic)

(For First Year Dioploma and B Pharm)
Revised as per latest PCI syllabus

Mohammed Al
Faculty of Pharmacy
Jamia Hamdard (Hamdard University)
Hamdard Nagar, New Delhi

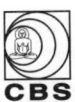

CBS

CBS Publishers & Distributors Pvt Ltd

New Delhi • Bengaluru • Chennai • Kochi • Kolkata • Lucknow • Mumbai
Hyderabad • Jharkhand • Nagpur • Patna • Pune • Uttarakhand

Textbook of Pharmaceutical Chemistry-I (Inorganic)

ISBN: 978-81-239-0415-3

Copyright © Publisher

First Edition: 1995

Reprint: 1999, 2000, 2001, 2002, 2003, 2004, 2005, 2006, 2007, 2008, 2009, 2010, 2012, 2013, 2014, 2015, 2016, 2017, 2018, 2019, 2020, 2022, 2023, 2024, **2025**

Published by **Satish Kumar Jain** and produced by **Varun Jain** for

CBS Publishers & Distributors Pvt Ltd

4819/XI Prahlad Street, 24 Ansari Road, Daryaganj, New Delhi 110 002, India.
Ph: 011-23266838, 23289259   Website: www.cbspd.com
                                  e-mail: delhi@cbspd.com
Corporate Office: 204 FIE, Industrial Area, Patparganj, Delhi 110 092
Ph: 011-4934 4934   Fax: 011-4934 4935
                              e-mail: publishing@cbspd.com; publicity@cbspd.com

Branches

- **Bengaluru:** Seema House 2975, 17th Cross, KR Road, Banasankari 2nd Stage, Bengaluru 560 070, Karnataka, India
  Ph: +91-80-26771678/79   Fax: +91-80-26771680   e-mail: bangalore@cbspd.com
- **Chennai:** 18/8B, Subbarayan Street, Shenoy Nagar, Chennai 600 030, Tamil Nadu, India
  Ph: +91-44-42032115, 26681266   e-mail: chennai@cbspd.com
- **Kochi:** 42/1325, 1326, Power House Road, Opp KSEB, Power House, Ernakulam Kochi 682 018, Kerala, India
  Ph: +91-484-4059061-65,67   Fax: +91-484-4059065   e-mail: kochi@cbspd.com
- **Kolkata:** 147, Hind Ceramics Compound, 1st Floor, Nilgunj Road, Belghoria, Kolkata-700056, West Bengal, India
  Ph: +033-25633055, 033-25633056
                                                           e-mail: kolkata@cbspd.com
- **Lucknow:** Basement, Khushnuma Complex, 7 Meerabai Marg (Behind Jawahar Bhawan), Lucknow-226001, UP, India
  Ph: +0522-4000032
                                                           e-mail: tiwari.lucknow@cbspd.com
- **Mumbai:** PWD Shed, Gala no 25/26, Ramchandra Bhatt Marg, Next to JJ Hospital Gate no. 2, Opp. Union Bank of India, Noorbaug, Mumbai-400009, Maharashtra, India
  Ph: 022-66661880/89
                                                           e-mail: mumbai@cbspd.com

Representatives

- Hyderabad   0-9885175004   • Jharkhand   0-9811541605   • Nagpur   0-8692091830
- Patna   0-9334159340   • Pune   0-9664372571   • Uttarakhand 0-9716462459

Printed at Glorious Printers, Jhilmil Industrial Area, Delhi, India

PREFACE

In every branch of science, whether basic or applied, chemistry plays a very significant role. Pharmaceutical inorganic chemistry is concerned with the chemistry, properties, assay methods and uses of inorganic products. The book is intended for use by the undergraduate students of pharmacy course according to the Education Regulation-1991 of the Pharmacy Council of India. This edition follows the general arrangement and classification of drugs as mentioned in the syllabus. The general format of presentation of each compound includes introduction, preparation, physical characters, chemical properties, identification tests, purity tests, assay methods and uses.

The author has received suport and encouragement from many people. First, I with to thank all readers of my previous books who appreciated the compliments. I also acknowledge a very pleasant and continuining association with Shri Satish Kumar Jain and Vinod Kumar Jain, CBS Publishers & Distributors. The project could not have been completed without their encouragement and assistance. Much of the book's final form and appearance are due to continuous efforts of Mr. Sunil Kumar Dhir, Super Computers who has typeset it on a laser printer. I also feel pleasure in expressing my sincere thanks to Professor (Dr.) C.I. Jolly, Department of Pharmacognosy and Phytochemistry, prin. K.M. Kundani College of Pharmacy, Worli Seaface, Bombay, Mrs. Sarita Gupta, Pharmacy College, Bangalore, Mr. Shamim Ahmed, Dehat Vikas College of Pharmcy, Taigaon, Faridabad, Mrs. Pratibha Nand and Mrs. Neelima Goel, Maharaja Surajmal Institute of Pharmacy and Technology, New Delhi, Mr. P.N. Raju, College of Pharmacy, New Delhi, and Mr. Shahid H. Ansari, Faculty of Pharmacy, Jamia Hamdard, New Delhi for providing examination question papers of their respective Institutions. I express my indebtedness to those authors of monographs, articles and books from which I have gained so much information for compiling the mamuscript. Finally, my greatest debt of gratitude is to my family members for being supportive in times of stress and for assisting with the tasks of manuscript preparation. No major professional project can be undertaken without a cooperation of one's family.

Being a scientist, I appreciate the value of criticism. The quality of science improves through critical decussions. Therefore, constructive suggestions, comments and criticism on the subject matter of the book will be gratefully acknowledged as they will certainly help to improve future editions of the books.

Dr. Mohammed Ali

CONTENTS

SYLLABUS

PHARMACEUTICAL CHEMISTRY-I

1. General discussion on the following inorganic compounds including important physical and chemical properties, medicinal and pharmaceutical uses, storage conditions and chemical incompatibility.

   A. Acids, bases and buffers – Boric acid, Hydrochloric acid, strong ammonium hydroxide, Calcium hydroxide, Sodium hydroxide and official buffers.

   B. Antioxidants – Hypophosphorous acid, Sulpher dioxide, Sodium bisulphite, Sodium meta-bisulphite, Sodium thiosulphate, Nitrogen and Sodium Nitrite.

   C. Gastrointestinal agents :

      (i) Acidifying agents – Dilute hydrochloric acid.

      (ii) Antacids – Sodium bicarbonate, Aluminium hydroxide gel, Aluminium Phosphate, Calcium carbonate, Magnesium carbonate, Magnesium trisilicate, Magnesium oxide, combinations of antacid preparations.

      (iii) Protectives and Adsorbents – Bismuth subcarbonate and Kaolin.

      (iv) Saline cathartics – Sodium Potassium tartrate and Magnesium sulphate.

   D. Topical Agents :

      (i) Protectives – Talc; Zinc oxide, Calamine, Zinc stearate, Titanium dioxide, Silicone polymers.

      (ii) Antimicrobials and Astringents – Hydrogen peroxide, Potassium permanganate, Chlorinated lime, Iodine, Solutions of iodine, Povidone-iodine, Boric acid, Borax, Silver nitrate, Mild silver protein, Mercury, Yellow mercuric oxide, Ammoniated mercury.

(iii) Sulphur and its compounds - Sublimed sulphurs, precipitated sulphur, Selenium sulphide.

(iv) Astringents : Alum and Zinc sulphate.

E. Dental products - Sodium fluoride, Stannous fluoride, Calcium carbonate, Sodium meta phosphate, Dicalcium phosphate, strontium chloride, Zinc chloride.

F. Inhalants - Oxygen, Carbon dioxide, Nitrous oxide.

G. Respiratory stimulants - Ammonium carbonate.

H. Expectorants and Emetics - Ammonium chloride, Potassium iodide, Antimony potassium tartrate.

I. Antidotes - Sodium nitrite.

2. Major Intra and Extracellular electrolytes :

A. Electrolytes used for replacement therapy - Sodium chloride and its preparations, Potassium chloride and its preparations.

B. Physiological acid-base balance and electrolytes used– Sodium acetate, Potassium acetate, Sodium bicarbonate injection, Sodium citrate, Potassium citrate, Sodium lactate injection, Ammonium chloride and its injection.

C. Combination of oral electrolyte powders and solutions.

3. Inorganic official compounds of Iron, Iodine, and Calcium Ferrous Sulfate and Calcium gluconate.

4. Radio pharmaceuticals and Contrast media-Radio activity-Alpha, Beta and Gamma Radiations, Biological effects of radiations, Measurement of radio-activity G.M. Counters-Radioisotopes-their uses, storage and precautions with special reference to the official preparations.

Radio Opaque Contrast Media - Barium Sulfate.

5. Quality control of Drugs and Pharmaceuticals–Importance of quality control, significant errors, methods used for quality control, sources of impurities in Pharmaceuticals. Limit tests for Arsenic, chloride, sulfate, Iron and Heavy metals.

6. Identification tests for cations and anions as per Indian Pharmacopoeia.

1

INTRODUCTION

Inorganic pharmaceutical chemistry deals with the preparation, assay methods and uses of inorganic agents used as pharmaceutical aids and as therapeutic and diagnostic agents. The acids, bases, buffer, antioxidants, water, etc. are the products used as pharmaceutical aids. The products containing fluid electrolytes and other ions, antacids, protectives, cathartics, topical agents, dental products, inhalants, antidotes, astringents, respiratory stimulants, expectorants and emetics are the important therapeutical agents. Radiopharmaceuticals are employed both as diagnostic and as therapeutic products. Inorganic compounds are also used as radiopaque contrast media, tablating aids and suspending agents.

Medicinal substances and pharmeceutical aids are included in monographs of the pharmacopoeia of each country and are considered as official records. An official substance is required to comply with certain standards of purity specified in the pharmacopoeia and may often contain some other substances for specific reasons. For example, all oxidants generally contain preservatives which reduce their oxidising action. Official chloroform contains 1-2%. of ethyl alcohol to retard the formation and to inactivate phosgene gas which is formed in contact with the air during storage.

Monograph

A pharmacepoeia includes introductory section which summarizes changes in the current editions, general notice, monographs of official drugs, preparations, appendices, etc. The monographs give information about titles, chemical formulae, description, solubilities, identification and purity tests, methods of assays, storage conditions, labelling, preparations, action and uses, and doses. The following points are considered for writing a monograph.

Titles : The names of the pharmacopoeial drugs, preparations, substances and process are given with capital initial letters in English.

Chemical Formulae : The graphic and molecular formulae and the molecular weight are given at the beginning of the monograph.

This information refers to the chemically pure substances and is not to be regarded as an indication of the purity of the drug.

Chemical Names : Chemical names of specified substances are given in the monographs as employed by the International Union of Pure and Applied Chemistry (IUPAC).

Molecular Weights : The molecular weights are given on the basis of atomic weights and of elements adopted by the IUPAC.

Category : It generally represents an application of the best known pharmacological action of the article or of its active ingredient.

Doses : Doses are mentioned for general guidance and represent the average of quantities as suitable for adults. The oral doses may be represented three to four times in 24 hours.

Usual Strength : It indicates the strength(s) normally marketed and which the pharmacist should dispense.

Description : It indicates properties of an article complying with the standards. They may help in the preliminary of the integrity of an article.

Odour and Taste : The terms 'odourless' or 'practically odourless' are descriptive only and are not to be regarded as standards of purity for a particular lot of an article. When there is an odour, it is mentioned in the monograph.

Statements on taste are provided only in cases where this property is a guide to the acceptability of the material.

Solubility : Defferent descriptive phrases used are: very soluble, freely soluble, soluble, sparingly soluble, stightly soluble, very slightly soluble and insoluble or practically insoluble.

The statements on solubility are not standards or tests for purity, but are provided primarily an information, and are applied at ambient temperature.

Official Standards : A substance is not of pharmacopoeial quality unless it complies with all the requirements stated under 'standards'.

Where the standard for a substance described in a monograph is expressed in terms of chemical formula for that substance and upper limit is not stated, the upper limit is not more than the equivalent 100.5 per cent.

Limits and Tolerances : Limits of contents are given in a monograph and they are determined by the method prescribed therein.

Where limits are expressed numerically, the upper and lower limits of a range are inclusive. The values are expressed as precentages or as absolute numbers.

The limits and tolerances stated in the definitions in the monograph allow for analytical error, for unavoidable variations in manufacture and compounding, and for deterioration.

Abbreviated Statements in Monographs : Incomplete sentences are employed in parts of the monographs for directness and brevity (for example, Iodine value.... or Arsenic-not more than.... parts per million). Where the tests are so abbreviated, it is to be understood that the page number shown designates the relevant procedure to be followed, and the values specified are the required limits.

General Monographs : These are monographs which describe dosage forms and include requirement of general application and requirements of tests which apply to all the monographs for the relevant dosage form.

Other Requirements : In the monographs on dosage forms under the sub-heading 'other requirements' are included the requirements of tests detailed in the general monographs on dosage forms such as Capsules, Injections, Tablets, etc.

Tests and Assays : A specification for a definite size or type of container or apparatus in tests or assay is given. Concentrations of solutions are mentioned. The term 'water bath' means a bath of boiling water. Sometimes specific temprature is indicated. The term 'desiccator' means a tightly-closed container of suitable size and design. The term 'vaccum desiccator' means a desiccator that maintains the low moisture atmosphere at a reduced pressure.

Expression of Strengths : In defining standards, the expression 'per cent' is used with one of four different meanings: per cent w/w (percentage weight in weight); per cent w/v(percentage weight in volume); per cent v/w (percentage volume in weight); per cent v/v (percentage volume in volume) express the number of grams or mililitres of active substance in 100 grams or mililitres of product.

Limits of Impurities : In certain tests, the concentration of impurity represented by the test is given in parts per million by weight (ppm) or as a percentage.

Percentage of Alcohol : All statements of percentage of alcohol refer to volume of C_2H_5-OH at 15.56°.

Reagents and Solutions : Their nature, degree of purity and the strengths of the solutions to be made from them are mentioned.

Reference Substances and Standard Preparations : These of antibiotics and other substances are authentic specimens that have been verified for suitability for use as comparison standards.

Solvents : The term 'solution' implies a solution in 95 per cent v/v of ethanol. The term 'ethyl alcohol' means absolute alcohol or dehydrated alcohol.

Procedure : Assay and test procedures are provided for determining compliance with pharmacopoeial standards of identity, strength, quality and purity. In assays and tests, the quantity to be taken is indicated. Assay and test procedures may be performed on the undried or unignited substances.

Dilution : When required a solution is accurately diluted by adding water or other solvent in one or more steps.

Filtration : When directed, the liquid is filtered through a suitable filter paper or equivalent device until the filtrate is clear.

Blank Determination : Any necessary correction is made by a blank determination using the same quantities and the same procedure, but omitting the substance being examined.

Identification Tests : The identification reactions of ions and groups of substances are mentioned.

Ignition to Constant Weight : The specification 'ignite to constant weight' means that ignition shall be continued at 800 ± 25°, unless otherwise indicated.

Indicators : Approximately 0.1 ml or three drops of indicators shall be added, unless otherwise directed.

Loss on Drying and Water : Absorbed water or water of hydration is determined by drying under specified conditions. Loss in weight also represents residual volatile constituents including organic solvents as well as water.

Negligible : The term 'negligible' indicates a quantity not exceeding 0.5 mg.

Temperature : All temperatures in a monographs are expresed in celsius (Centigrate) scale and all measurement are made at 25°.

Pressure Measurements : Pressure has been indicated in terms of 'mm of mercurry' or 'Torr'.

Normal Temperature and Pressure : This refers to an atmosphere pressure of 760 Torr and a temperature of 0°.

Time Limit : In conducting the tests and assays, five minutes shall be allowed for the reaction to take place, otherwise specified.

Vacuum : The term 'in vacuo' or 'in vacuum' denotes exposure to a pressure of less than 20 Torr.

Biological and Microbiological Tests and Assays : These are ascertained the purity of the material and to determine the total activity of the drug in a container.

Calculation of Results : The results of assays should be calculated to one decimal place more than indicated in the requirement.

Packaging, Storage and Labelling : The 'container' is the device that holds the article. The container should not interact physically or chemically with the article placed in it so as to alter the strength, quality, or purity of the article beyond the official requirements. A light-resistant container protects the contents from the effects of light. A well-closed container protects the contents from extraneous solids and from loss of the article. A tightly closed container protects the contents from contamination by exraneous liquids, solids or vapours, from loss of the article from effervescence, deliquescence or evaporation. A gas cylinder may be considered to be a metallic, tightly-closed container designed to hold gas under pressure. A single dose container is designed to hold a quantity of drug equivalent to a single dose. A multiple-dose container is designed to permit withdrawal of successive portion of the contents without changing the strength, quality or purity of the remaining portion.

Storage : The terms used under this sub-head are : 'cold' means any temperature in between 2 to 8°; 'cool' means any temperature between 8 to 25°; 'room temperature' means the temperature prevailing in a working area; 'excessive heat' is any temperature above 40°; 'warm' means any temperature between 30 and 40°.

Where no specific directions are indicated in the individual monograph, it is to be understood that the storage conditions include protection from moisture, freezing and excessive heat.

Labelling : In some cases, additional information which must be stated on the label is specified in the monograph.

2

ACIDS AND BASES

There are many concepts of acids and bases. An acid has a sour taste, turn blue litmus paper red and has pH lower than 7. A base has a bitter taste, turns litmus paper blue and has pH higher than 7. The mineral acids, hydrochloric, nitric and sulphuric acids, are wholly ionized in dilute solution and show apparent dissociation constants greater than one.

Arrhenius Theory (1887) : Acids are substances which on dissolution in water provide protons (H^+, hydrogen ions) and bases are substances which on dissolving in water yields hydroxyl ions (OH^-).

$$HCl \rightleftharpoons H^+ + Cl^- \text{ (Acidic)}$$
$$NaOH \rightleftharpoons Na^+ + {}^-OH \text{ (Basic)}$$

Acids and bases react each other to yield water and a salt. The reaction is known as neutralization.

$$HCl + NaOH \longrightarrow H_2O + NaCl$$

When an acid yields excess concentration of protons, it is known as strong acid and when a base gives large amount of hydroxyl ions it is termed a strong base. If the degree of ionization is less, then they are called as weak acids or weak bases. The ionization takes places only in aqueous solution and the theory is not applicable for solid substances; for basic substances like ammonia and sodium carbonate which do not contain hydroxyl group, for acidic compounds like carbon dioxide or sulphur dioxide which do not contain protons and for non-aqueous systems. The neutralization of an acid and a base in the absence of a solvent does not take place.

Brönsted-Lowry Theory (1923) : An acid is a substance that can donate a proton to any other substance and a base is a substance that accept a proton from any other substance. Thus, an acid is a proton donor and a base is a proton acceptor. They are conjugated to each other in a reaction.

$$HA \rightleftharpoons A^- \text{ (conjugate base)} + H^+ \text{ (proton)}$$

$$HCl \rightleftharpoons H^+ + Cl^- \text{ (conjugate base)}$$

$$H_2SO_4 \rightleftharpoons H^+ + SO_4^{2-} \text{ (conjugate base)}$$

$$CH_3COOH \rightleftharpoons H^+ + CH_3COO^- \text{ (conjugate base)}$$

$$NH_4^+ \rightleftharpoons H^+ + NH_3 \text{ (conjugate base)}$$

$$H_2PO_4 \rightleftharpoons H^+ + HPO_4^{2-} \text{ (conjugate base)}$$

$$H_3PO_4 \rightleftharpoons H^+ + H_2PO_4^- \text{ (conjugate base)}$$

A base (proton acceptor) could be an electrically neutral substance like ammonia (NH_3) or a negative ion such as OH^-, Cl^- CH_3COO^-, HPO_4^{2-}. The species formed on addition of a proton to a base is called as conjugate-acid of that base.

$$\underset{\text{Base}}{B} + H^+ \rightleftharpoons \underset{\text{Conjugated acid}}{BH^+}$$

$$OH^- + H^+ \rightleftharpoons H_2O \overset{H^+}{\rightleftharpoons} H_3O^+ \text{ (conjugate acid)}$$

$$SO_4^{2-} + H^+ \rightleftharpoons HSO_4^- \text{ (conjugate acid)}$$

$$NH_3 + H^+ \rightleftharpoons NH_4^+ \text{ (conjugate acid)}$$

$$H_2PO_4^- + H^+ \rightleftharpoons H_3PO_4 \text{ (conjugate acid)}$$

Water acts as a proton donor in the presence of a proton donor and as a proton acceptor in the presence of an acid. Some species like HSO_4^- and $H_2PO_4^-$ may react both as an acid or a base. An acid can exhibit its acidic property in the presence of a proton accepting species, e.g.

$$\underset{\text{Acid}}{HA} + \underset{\text{Base}}{B} \rightleftharpoons \underset{\substack{\text{Conjugate} \\ \text{acid}}}{HB} + \underset{\substack{\text{Conjugate} \\ \text{base}}}{A^-}$$

$$\underset{\text{Acid}}{HCl} + \underset{\text{Base}}{H_2O} \rightleftharpoons \underset{\text{Acid}}{H_3O^+} + \underset{\text{Base}}{Cl^-}$$

In this reaction HCl is a proton donor yielding hydronium ion (H_3O^+) and chloride ion (Cl^-) in water. It is a reversible reaction and Cl^- accepts a proton to form HCl (Brönsted acid). The hydronium ion (H_3O^+) loses a proton and form H_2O. According to Bronsted-Lowry theory the reaction of an acid and a base yields another acid and base. The acidic and basic properties of the species, e.g. water, ammonia, glacial acetic acid, formic acid, etc. are called as *amphoteric* and these solvents are termed as *amphoteric* solvents.

$$H_2SO_4 + H_2O \rightleftharpoons H_3O^+ + HSO_4^-$$

$$CH_3COOH + H_2O \rightleftharpoons H_3O^+ + CH_3COO^-$$

$$NH_4^+ + H_2O \rightleftharpoons H_3O^+ + NH_3$$

$$H_3PO_4 + HO^- \rightleftharpoons H_2O + H_2PO_4^-$$

$$H_2PO_4^- + HO^- \rightleftharpoons H_2O + HPO_4^{2-}$$

$$CO_3^{2-} + H_2O \rightleftharpoons HCO_3^- + HO^-$$

$$SO_2 + 2H_2O \rightleftharpoons HSO_3^- + H_3O^+$$

$$C_2H_5NH_2 + H_2O \rightleftharpoons C_2H_5NH^+_3 + OH^-$$

According to Bronsted-Lowry concept the strongest acids have the weakest conjugated bases and the strong bases have weak conjugated acids. The strong acids lose their proton as they are not attracted strongly and the proton is not expected to come back to the ion. The conjugated base of a weak acid would be a strong base (e.g., acetate ion) which has great tendency to accept a proton.

Lewis Acid-Base Theory (1923) : An acid is an electron pair acceptor and a base is an electron pair donor. All compounds or ions containing unshared electron pairs are Lewis bases, e.g. hydroxyl ion, ammonia, amines, ethers, alcohols, etc. All Brönsted acids are electron pair acceptor and are also Lewis acids. All Brönsted bases are also Lewis bases since they donate a pair of electrons. All Lewis bases do not react with a proton, they cannot be Brönsted bases.

The molecules BF_3, $ZnCl_2$, $AlCl_3$ and SO_3 have a deficient pair of electron in their sextet and they can accept a pair of electrons from a donor species to form a covalent bond to complete sextet.

The metal ions like Ag^+, Fe^{2+}, Na^+, and Zn^{2+} accept electron pairs from the donor species, e.g. NH_3, H_2O, Cl^-, CN^-, etc.

$$Ag^+ + :Cl^- \longrightarrow Ag:Cl$$

$$Cu^{2+} + 4NH_3 \longrightarrow Cu(NH_3)_4^{2+}$$

Copper ion, Cu^{2+}, accepts electrons from ammonia to form cupra-ammonium ion. Therefore, the copper ion acts as a Lewis acid and ammonia is a Lewis base. Transition metal complexes are formed when metal cations (Lewis acids) react with ligands (Lewis bases). There are some compounds, e.g. SiF_4, $Sn Cl_4$ and I_2, in which a central species expand the valence shell to accept a pair of electrons and act as Lewis acid. Some examples of Lewis acid base reactions are given hereunder :

$$BF_3 + : NH_3 \longrightarrow BF_3 : NH_3$$
$$BF_3 + : F^- \longrightarrow BF_4^-$$
$$ZnCl_2 + 2Cl^- \longrightarrow ZnCl_4$$
$$NH_3 + H^+ \longrightarrow NH_4^+$$
$$SiF_4 + 2F^- \longrightarrow [SiF_6]^{2-}$$
$$Fe^{3+} + 6H_2O \longrightarrow [Fe(H_2O)_6]^{3+}$$
$$Cu^{2+} + 4H_2O \longrightarrow [Cu(H_2O)_4]^{2+}$$

The acids and bases are used in the conversion of drugs to chemical forms convenient to their product formulations. Acids and bases are further categorized according to the properties of charge, size, polarizability, etc. Hard acids, H^+, Na^+, K^+, Mg^{+2}, Ca^{+2}, Al^{+3}, As^{+3}, Sn^{+4}, etc., are electron acceptors having high positive charges, relatively small sizes, and unfilled valence shell orbitals. Due to these properties, the hard acids are high electronegative and low polarizable. Soft acids, Cu^+, Ag^+, Hg^{+2}, I_2, Br_2, Br^+, etc., have the opposite properties, i.e. low positive charges, relatively large sizes and filled valence shell orbitals. These are properties which impart low electronegativities and high polarizabilities. Hard bases, H_2O, OH, CO_3^{-2}, ClO_4^-, NO_3^-, Cl^-, etc., have high electronegativities, are easily reduced, have stable valence shell structures, and low polarizabilities. Soft bases, I^-, CN^-, H^-, R_2S, RSH, etc., have low electronegativities, are easily oxidized, have empty low lying orbitals and high polarizabilities. The most stable adducts are formed between hard acids and hard bases and between soft acids and soft bases. The relative stabilities of various adducts are dependent upon the relative softness or hardness of the acids and bases involved. The harder acids have the higher oxidation states. Hardness and softness can be influenced by the attached groups in a complex ion.

The reactivity of acids and bases is a function of their strength. The strength of an acid is a measure of the ease of proton donation, and in a base, the ease of protonation. There are numerous acids and bases with specific therapeutic properties.

Strong and Weak Acids and Bases

The strength of an acid or base depends on the degree of its ionization in a solvent. In aqueous solution hydrochloric acid is a strong acid while in ammonia acetic acid shows strong acidic character. The acids like HCl, HNO_3, H_2SO_4, etc. dissociate or ionize completely in aqueous solutions and the amount of dissociation depends on the strength of the acid. They release excess amount of protons (H^+ ions). These acids are called as strong acids. The acids like HCOOH, CH_3COOH, H_2CO_3, etc. dissociate to a small extent in aqueous solution and release small amount of proton. Therefore, these acids are called a weak acids. In the same way, the bases like NaOH and KOH ionize to a greater extent in aqueous solutions and release excess amount of hydroxyl ions (OH^-). These bases are called strong bases. Some bases, e.g. $Ca(OH)_2$ and NH_4OH, ionize to a small extent in aqueous solutions and release small amount of hydroxyl ions. Therefore, these bases are called weak bases.

Hydrogen Ion Concentration, pH

The strength of an acid is determined by the degree of dissociation of proton from the conjugated base in aqueous solution.

$$HA + H_2O \rightleftharpoons H_3O^+ + A^-$$

The degree of ionization for the above reaction is expressed by the equilibrium constant (Keq) :

$$Keq = \frac{[H_3O^+]\,[A^-]}{[HA]\,H_2O]}$$

$$Ka + Keq\,[H_2O] = \frac{[H_2O^+]\,[A^-]}{[HA]}$$

Where Ka is ionization constant for an acid and is expressed as the product of the equilibrium constant and the concentration of the water. The Ka varies directly with the strength of the acid. All strong acids (e.g., HCl, HNO_3, H_2SO_4) have ionization constant more than 1 (Ka>1), while weaker acids (e.g., HCOOH, CH_3COOH) have smaller ionization constant less than 1 (Ka<1).

The strength of an acid can be expresed in terms of hydrogen ion concentration. In aqueous solution the concentration of proton is considered as the concentration of hydronium ion (H_3O^+). Pure water dissociates as :

$$H_2O \rightleftharpoons H^+ + OH^-; \qquad 2H_2O \rightleftharpoons H_3O^+ + OH^-$$

The ion product constant, Kw is represented as :

$$Kw = [H_3O^+] [OH^-] = 1 \times 10^{-14}$$

Kw is expressed by involving the concentration of ionic species on right-hand side of the reaction and has a constant value of 1×10^{-14} at 25°C. In pure water, the concentrations of both the ions are equal, each having the value 1×10^{-7} M, i.e. H^+ = OH^- = 1×10^{-7}.

When an acid is added to water, the concentration of protons increases more than that of hydroxyl ion concentration. In the same way, if a base is added to water, the hydroxyl concentration is greater than the concentration of hydrogen ion. To maintain the constant value of Kw, they are expressed by the expression.

$$[H_3O^+] [OH^-] = 10^{-14}$$

The hydrogen ion concentration is usually expressed in units of mole/litre or gram-equivalent litre.

In neutral solution the concentration of proton $[H^+]$ is equal to the concentration of hydroxyl group $[OH^-]$, in acidic medium $[H^+]$ is greater than $[OH^-]$ and in alkaline medium, $[H^+]$ is lesser than $[HO^-]$. When an acid is added to an aqueous solution to the extent that $[H]^+ = 1 \times 10^{-4}$ M; than the corresponding hydroxide ion concentration $[OH^-]$ is 1×10^{-10} M.

For expressing the hydrogen ion concentration, Sorenson expressed acidity as a negative logarithm to the base 10 of the hydrogen ion concentration, known as pH (p = power; H = hydrogen). The pH is defined as negative logarithm of the hydrogen ion concentration and is represented as :

pH = -log $[H^+]$ = log $1/[H^+]$

In pure water, $[H]^+$ = $[OH-]$ = 10^{-7}

pH = -log $[10^{-7}]$ = -log $1/10^{-7}$ = log 1 + log 10^7 = 7

Hence water is neutral, neither acidic, nor basic.

BORIC ACID

H_3BO_3; Mol. Weight = 61.83

Boric acid, occurs in nature as the mineral *sassolite*, contains not less than 99.5 per cent and not more than the equivalent of 100.5 per cent of H_3BO_3, calculated with reference to the dried substance.

Preparation

1. **From Natural Source :** It comes out with jets of steams, called *soffioni*, from the ground in certain parts of Tuscany. The condensed steam is concentrated by its own heat, cooled and the crystallized boric acid is separated.

2. **By Decomposition of Borax :** A mixture of concentrated sulphuric acid and water is added to a hot aqueous solution of borax. The hot solution is filtered, cooled and the crystallized boric acid is filtered off.

$$Na_2B_4O_7 + H_2SO_4 + 5H_2O \longrightarrow Na_2SO_4 + 4H_3BO_3$$
Borax

3. **From Colemanite :** By passing sulphur dioxide through colemanite suspended in water, crystals of boric acid separate out on cooling.

$$Ca_2B_6O_{11} + 4SO_2 + 11H_2O \longrightarrow 2Ca(HSO_3)_2 + 6H_3BO_3$$
Borax

Physical Characters : Boric acid occurs as odourless, colourless, transparent plates, crystals or white granules or powder; some what pearly lustrous scales. It is unctuous (greasy) to touch; m.p. 171°; with a sweetish after taste. When heated to 100° it loses water and is slowly converted into metaboric acid (HBO_2); tetraboric acid ($H_2B_4O_7$) is formed at 140° and boron trioxide (B_2O_3) at higher temperatures. It is volatiled with steam; pH 5.1; soluble 1 in 20 of water; 16 of alcohol and 4 of glycerol. Solubility in water is increased by HCl, citric, tartaric acids or by heat. Most solutions of boric acid contains only small amounts of tetraboric acid. When the solution is neutralized with an alkali, e.g. NaOH, and concentrated, the stable crystalline salts, tetraborates, are precipitated.

Boric acid is stored in well-closed containers.

Chemical Properties

1. It is a weak acid and in solution gives a slightly red colour with litmus.

2. Heating of boric acid to certain temperatures produces various dehydration products. For example, heating at 100° causes the loss of one molecule of water to produce metaboric acid. Heating to about 160° causes a further loss of water to produce tetraboric or pyroboric acid. Heating to still higher temperatures will yield the anhydride of boric acid, boron trioxide, a glassy appearing solid.

$$H_3BO_3 \xrightarrow[-H_2O]{100°} HBO_2 \xrightarrow[-H_2O]{160°} H_2B_4O_7 \xrightarrow[-H_2O]{\text{Red heart}} 2B_2O_3$$

| Ortho-boric acid | Meta-boric acid | Tetra-boric acid | Boric anhy-dride |

3. It changes turmeric paper brown which turns blackish when dipped in sodium hydroxide solution.

4. A mixture of ethyl alcohol and boric acid burns with a green flame due to formation of ethyl borate.

5. The reaction of boric acid with equimolar amounts of glycerin at 140°-150° produces a compound known as Boroglycerin glycerite $(C_3H_5BO_3)$ which is used as a suppository base.

Tests for Purity : Tests for arsenic; lead; heavy metals; sulphate; alcohol insoluble substances; acidity; clarity and colour of solution; organic matter.

For determining sulphate, an acidified solution is boiled and filtered. The filtrate complies with the limit test for sulphates.

Tests for Identification

1. Boric acid (0.1g) is dissolved in methanol (5 ml) by heating to which a few drops of sulphuric acid have been added. On ignition the solution, the flame has a green border.

2. An aqueous solution of boric acid is acidic in nature (pH between 3.8 and 4.8).

Incompatibility : Alkali carbonates and hydroxides.

Assay

Boric acid is a very weak acid and cannot be titrated accurately with alkali. However, it can be titrated acurately with a standard solution of a strong alkali if glycerol is first added to the boric acid before starting the titration.

1. **(I.P.) :** Accurately weighed sample (2g) is dissolved in a mixture of water (50 ml) and glycerin (100 ml), previously neutralized to phenolphthalein solution. The solution is titrated with 1N sodium hydroxide, using phenolphthalein solution as indicator. Each ml of 1N sodium hydroxide is equivalent to 0.06183 of H_3BO_3.

The presence of glycerin causes the acid to behave as a strong monoprotic acid which can be titrated to a phenolphthalein end point. The monoprotic character of boric acid in glycerin is thought to occur through esterification to a tetravalent boron ester known as glyceroboric acid, with the net release of one hydronium ion into the solution. The glyceroboric acid has an ionization constant 10,000 times greater than that of boric acid. Therefore, glyceroboric acid gives a satisfactory end point when it is titrated against a standard alkali.

$$2 \begin{array}{c} CH_2OH \\ | \\ OHOH \\ | \\ CH_2OH \end{array} + \begin{array}{c} OH \\ | \\ B \\ / \backslash \\ HO \quad OH \end{array} \longrightarrow \left[\begin{array}{c} CH_2-OH \qquad HO-CH_2 \\ | \qquad\qquad\qquad | \\ CH-O\diagdown_{\diagup}O-CH \\ \qquad B \\ | \diagup\qquad\diagdown | \\ CH_2-O \qquad O-CH_2 \end{array} \right] + H_3O^+ + 2H_2O$$

Similarly, boric acid can be esterified with other polyhydroxy compounds such as glycol, mannitol, and catechol.

2. **(B.P.)** : An aqueous solution of boric acid (1g) and mannitol (10g) is titrated with 1N sodium hydroxide, using phenolphthalein as indicator. Sodium metaborate is formed by neutralizing one equivalent of sodium hydroxide.

$$NaOH + H_3BO_3 \longrightarrow \underset{\substack{\text{Sodium}\\\text{metaborate}}}{NaBO_2} + 2H_2O$$

Mannitol forms a mannitylboric acid which helps for giving a sharp end-point. Each ml of 1N sodium hydroxide VS is equivalent to 61.8 mg of H_3BO_3.

$$\begin{array}{c} CH_2OH \\ | \\ (CHOH)_2 \\ | \\ CH-O\diagdown \\ \qquad\qquad B\diagdown \\ CH-O\diagup \\ | \\ CH_2OH \end{array} \qquad \begin{array}{c} CH_2OH \\ | \\ (CHOH)_2 \\ | \\ C-CH \\ \diagup \qquad | \\ O-CH \\ | \\ CH_2OH \end{array}$$

Mannitylboric acid

Uses : Boric acid possesses weak bacteriostatic, fungistatic, astringent and antiseptic properties. It is externally used as a buffer and antimicrobial in eye-drops, as insecticide for cockroaches and black carpet beetles.

It is also used as mouth washes, skin lotions for local anti-infective action, as douches for irrigating the bladder and vagina; in ointment for emollient and antiseptic action; and as an ingredient in dusting powder due to its smooth-unctious touch. Boroglycerin glycerite, formulated by combination of boric acid, water and glycerin, is used as a suppository base. Boric acid is used in buffer systems such as Ephinephrine bitartrate ophthalmic solution, Aluminium acetate and Aluminium subacetate solutions.

Side effects on ingestion include vomiting, diarrhoea, erythematous rash, abdominal cramps, circulatory collapse, coma, etc.

HYDROCHLORIC ACID

HCl; Mol. Weight = 36.46

Synonymes : Muriatic acid; Spirit of salt.

Hydrochloric acid is a solution of hydrogen chloride gas (HCl) in water.

Preparation

1. **From Sodium Chloride :** Hydrochloric acid is manufactured by treating concentrated sulphuric acid with sodium chloride (Leblanc Soda Process). Calculated amounts of sodium chloride and concentrated sulphuric acid are heated in the cast-iron pan of a salt-cake furnace. Hydrochloric acid gas is produced by slow heating which passes out through the exit at the top.

$$NaCl + H_2SO_4 \longrightarrow NaHSO_4 + HCl$$
Sodium
hydrogen
sulphate

The pasty mass of sodium hydrogen sulphate is mixed with more quantity of sodium chloride and heated to redness to yield a further supply of hydrogen chloride leaving behind anhydrous sodium sulphate (Salt-cake).

$$NaCl + NaHSO_4 \longrightarrow Na_2SO_4 + HCl$$
Sodium
sulphate

Hydrochloric acid gas is collected in a chamber where cold water is spread over the gas. The dilute acid is obtained at the bottom. The acid so obtained is spread down the tower to absorb more HCl gas for getting concentrated hydrochloric acid.

The acid so prepared contains impurities of sulphur dioxide, sulphuric acid, arsenic acid, ferric chloride and chlorine. Treatment of the acid with barium chloride removes sulphuric acid by formation of precipitate of barium sulphate. Volatile impurities (SO_4, Cl_2) come out first and are rejected. Ferric chloride is left behind as residue. Heating the commercial acid with stannous chloride removes arsenic.

$$2\ AsCl_3 + 3\ SnCl_2 \longrightarrow 2\ As + 3\ SnCl_4$$

2. **By Synthesis** : Large amount of hydrogen and chlorine gases are obtained as by-products by electrolysis of sodium chloride solution during the manufacture of caustic soda. These gases are dried and then combined to produce hydrogen chloride gas. The gas is cooled and water is spread over the gas. The solution of hydrochloric acid flows into storage tank.

Physical Characters : Hydrogen chloride is a colourless gas with an acrid irritating odour and an acid taste. It is about 25% heavier than air. The gas can be liquefied under pressure. It is very soluble in water. A 0.1 N aqueous solution is ionized at 18°C and conducts electricity. Muriatic acid is a technical grade of hydrochloric acid contaning 35 to 38% of HCl and a number of impurities including chloride, arsenous and sulphurous acids, and iron.

Hydrochloric acid is a clear colourless fuming aqueous solution of hydrogen chloride with a pungent odour and sour taste; specific gravity is about 1.18. It fumes in air and is heavier than air. It may be coloured yellow by traces of iron, chloride and organic matter. Reagent grade concentrated hydrochloric acid contains about 38.0% HCl. A nonfuming solution can be prepared by diluting hydrochloric acid with two volumes of water.

It gives constant boiling azotrope with water (b.p. 108.5°). Boiling aqueous solutions results in loss of either component until the constant boiling acid is obtained.

Storage : Hydrochloric acid should be kept in a stoppered container of glass or other inert material and stored at a temperature not exceeding 30°.

Chemical Properties

1. It turns moist blue litmus to red.

2. It reacts with metals and their salts like oxides, hydroxides and carbonates to form the chlorides of the metals.

$$Mg + 2HCl \longrightarrow MgCl_2 + H_2$$
$$KOH + HCl \longrightarrow KCl + H_2O$$
$$Na_2CO_3 + 2HCl \longrightarrow 2NaCl + CO_2 + H_2O$$

The hydrogen in the hydrochloric acid is displaced by metals yielding hydrogen gas.

With silver nitrate, hydrochloric acid gives a white precipitate soluble in ammonium hydroxide and insoluble in nitric acid.

$$HCl + AgNO_3 \longrightarrow AgCl + HNO_3$$
$$AgCl + 2NH_4OH \longrightarrow Ag\,(NH_3)_2\,Cl + 2H_2O$$
$$\text{Complex}$$
$$\text{compound}$$
$$\text{(soluble)}$$

With lead acetate, it gives a white precipitate soluble in hot water.

$$(CH_3COO)_2\,Pb + 2HCl \longrightarrow PbCl_2 + 2CH_3COOH$$
$$\text{White}$$
$$\text{precipitate}$$

3. Fluorine decomposes hydrochloric acid to form chloride.

$$2HCl + F_2 \longrightarrow 2HF + Cl_2$$

4. Hydrochloric acid gas forms dense white fumes of ammonium chloride with ammonia.

$$HCl + NH_3 \longrightarrow NH_4Cl$$

5. A mixture of concentrated hydrochloric acid (3 parts) and concentrated nitric acid (1 part) is called *aqua regia* which is used for dissolving noble metals, gold and platinum as their chlorides.

$$3HCl + HNO_3 \longrightarrow NOCl + 2H_2O + Cl_2$$

6. Hydrochloric acid decomposes salts of weaker acids such as carbonates, bicarbonates, sulphides, sulphites, nitrites and thiosulphates.

$$NaHCO_3 + HCl \longrightarrow NaCl + CO_2 + H_2O$$
$$Na_2SO_3 + 2HCl \longrightarrow 2NaCl + SO_2 + H_2O$$
$$2NaNO_2 + 2HCl \longrightarrow 2NaCl + NO + NO_2 + H_2O$$

Hydrochloric acid gives chlorine when warmed with oxidising agents, such as manganese dioxide or potassium permanganate.

$$MnO_2 + HCl \longrightarrow Mn + H_2O + Cl_2$$
$$2\ KMnO_4 + 16\ HCl \longrightarrow 2MnCl_2 + 5Cl_2 + 2KCl + 8H_2O$$

Tests for Purity : Weight per ml; tests for free chlorine; bromide; iodide; sulphate; heavy metals; arsenic; lead; oxidizable substances; clarity and colour; and non-volatile matter.

For determining bromide and iodide, chloroform and chlorinated lime solution are added with constant shaking. The chloroform layer does not become brown or violet.

The presence of sulphite is found out by treating the acid with barium chloride solution and 0.001 N iodine. The colour of the iodine is not completely discharged.

Sulphate as an impurity is detected by dissolving sodium bicarbonate in the acid and evaporating the solution to dryness. The residue complies with the limit test for sulphates.

Free chlorine is detected by treating the acid with potasium iodide solution and chloroform. The chloroform layer does not become violet within one minute.

$$CdI_2 + Cl_2 \longrightarrow CdCl_2 + I_2$$

For detection of bromide and iodide a neutralized solution of the acid is slightly acidified with sulphuric acid and treated with an oxidizing agent, chloramine, to form bromine and iodine from bromides or iodides. This is extracted with chloroform to remove bromine or iodine. The extract is shaken with an acetic acid solution of a dye, magenta. If bromine is present, magenta is converted into a blue-violet chloroform-soluble product. Iodine does not react with magenta and forms a violet solution in chloroform.

Incompatibility : The chloride ion is precipitated with silver, mercurous mercury and lead salts. It is oxidized by oxidizing agents; chlorine is liberated.

CONCENTRATED HYDROCHLORIC ACID

Concentrated hydrochloric acid is an aqueos solution of hydrogen chloride in water. It contains not less than 35 per cent w/w and not more than 38.0 per cent w/w of HCl.

Tests for Identification

1. When neutralized and diluted, it gives the reactions of chlorides.

2. When added to potassium permanganate, chlorine is evolved.

Assay : Hydrochloric acid is a strong monoprotic acid which can be assayed conveniently by titrating against sodium hydroxide solution using methyl red as an indicator.

Accurately weighed sample (4 g) is added to water (40 ml) in a stoppered flask and titrated with 1N sodium hydroxide, using methyl orange. Each ml of 1N sodium hydroxide is equivalent to 0.3646 g of HCl.

$$HCl + NaOH \longrightarrow NaCl + H_2O$$

Uses

Hydrochloric acid is an escharotic; used as a pharmaceutical aid or as acidifying agent. In dilute form it is used for the treatment of achlorhydria (absence of HCl from the stomach juice). It is given intravenously in the management of metabolic alkalosis (increase in alkalinity of the blood).

Weak basic compounds form water-soluble hydrochloride salts :

$$R\text{-}NH_2 + HCl \longrightarrow R\text{-}NH_3^+\ Cl^-$$

This type of reaction is used to convert water insoluble organic bases, e.g. alkaloids, into a water soluble form for extraction or other separations.

Concentrated solutions cause severe burns; permanent visual damage may occur. Dertmatitis and photosensitization may occur. Inhalation may cause cough, choking, inflammation and ulceration of respiratory tract.

AMMONIUM HYDROXIDE

NH_4OH; Mol. Weight = 35.0

Preparation

1. In laboratory ammonia is prepared by heating ammonium chloride with calcium hydroxide.

$$2NH_4Cl + Ca(OH)_2 \longrightarrow 2NH_3 + CaCl_2 + 2H_2O$$

2. Commercially ammonia is obtained from the 'ammonical liquor' which is a by-product during the production of coal-gas. Ammonical gas is obtained by passing the hot gas through cooling pipes. Lime water is added to the ammonical

liquor and steam is passed through the mixture. The mixture of steam and ammonia evolved is bubbled through sulphuric acid. From it, ammonium sulphate is produced which is the most important commercial ammonium salt and used as fertilizer.

$$2NH_3 + H_2SO_4 \longrightarrow (NH_4)_2 SO_4$$

3. Ammonia is also synthesized by Habers' process in which nitrogen and hydrogen are combined in the presence of a catalyst (iron and molybdenum) at 450-500°C at 200-900 atm ospheric pressure.

$$N_2 + 3H_2 \rightleftharpoons 2NH_3$$

The reaction is reversible and exothermic. The ammonia produced is stored in liquid form in metal cylinder or absorbed in water, or converted into ammonium salts by combination with acids.

4. Hydrolysis of cyanamide with superheated steam gives ammonia. Atmospheric nitrogen is passed over calcium carbide and heated to a high temperature in an electric furnace to yield calcium cyanamide which is used as a fertilizer.

$$CaC_2 + N_2 \longrightarrow CaN.CN + C$$
Calcium
cyanamide

$$CaN.CN + 3H_2O \longrightarrow CaCO_3 + 2NH_3$$

5. Ammonia is also obtained as a by-product in the purification of bauxite (Serpek's process). Bauxite and coke are heated in a current of nitrogen to form aluminium nitride which is hydrolyzed with water.

$$Al_2O_3 + 3C + N_2 \longrightarrow 2 AlN + 3CO\uparrow$$

$$AlN + 3H_2O \longrightarrow Al (OH)_3 + NH_3\uparrow$$

Physical Characters : Ammonia is a colourless gas; very pungent odour; lighter than air; specific gravity is 0.596; extremely soluble in water. One volume of water dissolves 1300 volumes of ammonia at 0°C and 760 mm to form ammonium hydroxide which is a base :

$$NH_3 + H_2O \longrightarrow NH_4OH \rightleftharpoons NH_4^+ + OH^-$$

Mixtures of ammonia and air explode when ignited under favourable conditions. The gas may be liquefied at atmospheric pressure by cooling to 60°C or by cooling to 10°C at pressures of

6.5 or 7 atmospheres. Liquid ammonia is a good solvent and ionizing medium.

In aqueons solution, ammonia exists in the form of NH_3; only a small amount reacts with water to form ammonium hydroxide.

Chemical Properties

Ammonia molecule possesses an unshared pair of electrons, therefore, it acts as a ligand in forming soluble complex ions with many metal cations, e.g. Cu, Ag, Au, Zn, Cd, Cr, Ni, Co, Mn and Pt. The hydroxides or insoluble salts of these metals dissolve in ammonia solution. It reacts with certain metallic salts and precipitates hydroxides of the metals.

$$3NH_4OH + FeCl_3 \longrightarrow \underset{\text{Brown PPt}}{Fe\,(OH)_3} + 3NH_4Cl$$

$$2NH_4OH + ZnSO_4 \longrightarrow \underset{\text{White ppt}}{Zn\,(OH)_2} + (NH_4)_2\,SO_4$$

Ammonia forms ammonia-basic salts by ammonolysis when reacts with mercuric chloride.

$$HgCl_2 + NH_3 \longrightarrow Hg\,(NH_2)\,Cl + HCl$$

Salts of ammonia react as acids in the presence of bases. Depending upon the particular salt, the pH of aqueous solutions of ammonia compounds will range from neutral to acidic.

$$NH_4Cl + NaOH \longrightarrow NH_3\uparrow + NaCl + H_2O$$

Ammonia is burnt in an atmosphere of oxygen :

$$4NH_3 + 3O_2 \longrightarrow 2N_2 + 6H_2O$$

Ammonia is a typical weak base. It turns red litmus blue, phenolphthalein solution pink and forms salts with acids.

$$NH_3 + HCl \longrightarrow NH_4Cl$$

Ammonia is decomposed into nitrogen and hydrogen at red heat.

$$2NH_3 \longrightarrow N_2 + 3H_2$$

Ammonia is oxidized when passed over heated copper oxide.

$$3CuO + 2NH_3 \longrightarrow 3Cu + N_2 + 3H_2O$$

Both chlorine and bromine oxidize ammonia to give nitrogen.

$$8NH_3 + 3Cl_2 \longrightarrow N_2 + 6NH_4Cl$$

When ammonia is passed over heated sodium or potassium at 300°C, amides are produced.

$$2NH_3 + 2Na \longrightarrow 2NaNH_2 + H_2$$
Sodamide

Liquid ammonia dissolves alkali and alkaline earth metals to form blue solutions which decomposes slowly in the presence of impurities, yielding hydrogen and amide of the metal, e.g. $NaNH_2$.

STRONG AMMONIA SOLUTION

It is a clear colourless liquid with a strongly pungent characteristic odour, containing 27 to 30% w/w of ammonia. It is not quite saturated with the gas at ordinary temperatures. The most concentrated commercial solution contains about 35% of NH_3, and has a specific gravity of 0.880. Upon exposure to air, it loses ammonia readily. The solution is clear, colourless liquid with a strong pungent, characteristic odour. It is stored at a temperature not exceeding 20° in airtight containers.

Tests for Identification

1. Strongly alkaline, even when freely diluted with water.
2. When the vapour is brought into contact with gaseous hydrochloric acid, dense white fumes are produced.

Tests for Purity : Weight per ml; tests for arsenic; heavy metals; pyridine and homologues; tarry matter; non-volatile matter.

Pyridine and homologues are determined by measuring absorbance at the maximum at 252 nm.

Tarry matter is detected by dissolving citric acid in a dilute ammonia solution. No tarry unpleasant odour is produced.

When evaporated on a water bath and dried to a constant weight at 105°, not more than 10 mg of residue is left.

Strong ammonia solution complies with the limit test for arsenic and heavy metals.

Strong ammonia solution is used carefully due to caustic nature of the solution and the irritating properties of its vapour.

Assay : Strong ammonia solution is assayed via residual titration. The solution (2 g) is added to 1M hydrochloric acid (50 ml), taking precautions during the addition to avoid loss of ammonia and the excess of acid titrated with 1M sodium hydroxide using methyl red solution as indicator. Each ml of 1M hydrochloric acid is equivalent to 17.03 mg of NH_3. The proton acceptor properties of ammonia are illustrated by its reaction with very weak acids, e.g., HCO_3^-, which are generally neutral in solution.

$$Ca(HCO_3)_2 + 2NH_3 \longrightarrow CaCO_3 \downarrow + (NH_4)_2 CO_3$$

DILUTE AMMONIA SOLUTION

It is prepared by diluting strong Ammonia solution with freshly boiled and cooled purified water. It contains 9.5 to 10.5 per cent of NH_3; stored at a temperature not exceeding 20° in well-closed containers.

Uses : Dilute solutions of ammonia have been used as reflex stimulants, rubefacients and counter-irritants and to neutralize insect stings. Strong ammonia solution is used in the preparation of Aromatic ammonia spirit and ammonical silver nitrate solution. Dilute ammonia solution may be used as reflux stimulant in fainted persons. It is inhaled from a smelling salt to cause vasoconstriction in the nose, reducing flow of nasal secretion in cold. It is also used in the manufacture of nitric acid; sodium bicarbonate and ammonium salts of acids, Aromatic spirit of ammonia and strong ammonium acetate solution.

Ingestion of strong solutions of ammonia causes severe pain in the mouth, throat, and gastrointestinal tract, with cough, vomiting, and shock.

CALCIUM HYDROXIDE
(Slaked Lime)

$Ca(OH)_2$, Mol. Weight = 74.09

Calcium hydroxide contains not less than 90% of $Ca(OH)_2$. It is manufactured by spraying water on to quicklime which is itself is prepared by heating limestone. The lumps of quicklime break into powder and heat is evolved. The process is known as *slaking*.

$$CaCO_3 \rightleftharpoons CaO + CO_2$$

$$CaO + H_2O \longrightarrow Ca(OH)_2$$

Water is absorbed by the oxide with the evolution of excess of heat; swelling of CaO lumps and finally disintegration into a fine powder take place.

Physical Characters

Calcium hydroxide occurs as crystals or soft, odourless, granules or powder with slightly bitter alkaline taste. It is almost entirely soluble in water (1 in 600); soluble in aqueous solutions of glycerol and of sugars. The aqueous solution is alkaline to phenolphthalein and readily absorbs CO_2 from air forming $CaCO_3$. The solubility of calcium hydroxide diminishes with increasing temperature.

It is preserved in air tight containers.

Chemical Properties

1. Calcium hydroxide absorbs carbon dioxide from air forming calcium carbonate. In the presence of excess of CO_2, soluble calcium bicarbonate is formed.

$$Ca(OH)_2 + CO_2 \xrightarrow{-H_2O} CaCO_3 \xrightarrow{+CO_2} Ca(HCO_3)_2$$

2. Calcium hydroxide loses water when ignited forming calcium oxide.

$$2Ca(OH)_2 \xrightarrow{heat} 2CaO + H_2O$$

   When calcium hydroxide is mixed with 3 to 4 times its weight of water, the suspension is called **Milk of lime.**

   A clear and saturated aqueous solution of calcium hydroxide is lime water which is used to neutralize acids and to absorb acid gases (e.g. CO_2, SO_2, H_2S).

$$Ca(OH)_2 + SO_2 \longrightarrow CaSO_3 + H_2O$$

   If calcium hydroxide is added to the solution of calcium bicarbonate, calcium carbonate is precipitated.

3. When H_2O_2 is added to a solution of calcium hydroxide, calcium peroxide is precipitated.

$$Ca(OH)_2 + H_2O_2 \longrightarrow CaO_2 \cdot 8H_2O \downarrow$$

4. Chlorine reacts with cold Milk of lime to form calcium hypochlorite.

$$2Ca(OH)_2 + 2Cl_2 \longrightarrow Ca(ClO)_2 + CaCl_2 + 2H_2O$$

   With hot Milk of lime chlorine yields calcium chlorate.

$$6Ca(OH)_2 + 6Cl_2 \longrightarrow Ca(ClO_3)_2 + 5CaCl_2 + 6H_2O$$

Calcium
chlorate

Chlorine reacts with cold dry calcium hydroxide to form a mixture of calcium hypochlorite and basic calcium chloride (bleaching powder).

$$3Ca(OH)_2 + 2Cl_2 \longrightarrow Ca(ClO)_2 + CaCl_2\ Ca(OH)_2 + 2H_2O$$

Bleaching
powder

Test for Purity : Tests for aluminium, iron, phosphate, and matter insoluble in hydrochloric acid; heavy metals; arsenic; lead; chloride; and sulphate.

The test for aluminium, iron, phosphate and HCl insoluble matter is carried out by boiling the substance with HCl to liberate carbon dioxide. The reaction mixture is made alkaline with ammonia to precipitate aluminium and iron. The precipitated ions and acid insoluble matter (silicates, etc.) are filtered off and washed with a solution of ammonium chloride. The precipitate of the hydroxides on the filter is dissolved in dilute HCl and reprecipitated with ammonia. It is filtered through the same filter which may contain undissolved acid insoluble residue. The residue, containing aluminium, iron, phosphate, and HCl insoluble matter, is finally ignited at a temperature not below 1000° and weighed.

For detecting the presence of heavy metals, the acidified solution of the substance is treated with hydrogen sulphide solution. The colour produced is compared with the colour obtained by treating standard lead solution with the hydrogen sulphide solution.

The substance dissolved in water with the addition of nitric acid complies with the limit test for chlorides.

The substance dissolved in water with the addition of dilute hydrochloric acid complies with the limits test for sulphates.

Test for Identification : A solution in acetic acid gives the reactions of calcium.

Assay : Calcium hydroxide solutions are basic, pH 12.3, and are neutralized by acids.

Accurately weighed sample (3g) is shaken with alcohol (10 ml), previously neutralized to phenolphthalein solution. To it a 10% solution of sucrose (490 ml) is added, previously neutralized to phenolphthalein solution. The mixture is shaken vigorously for 5 minutes, and then at frequent intervals during four hours. The solution (250 ml) is filtered off and titrated with 1N HCl, using phenolphthalein solution as indicator. Each ml of 1N HCl is equivalent to 0.03705 g of Ca(OH)$_2$.

$$Ca(OH)_2 + 2HCl \rightleftharpoons CaCl_2 + 2H_2O$$

CALCIUM HYDROXIDE SOLUTION

Calcium hydroxide solution (lime water) contains not less than 0.15 per cent w/v of Ca(OH)$_2$, containing in each 100 ml, not less than 140 mg of Ca(OH)$_2$. It is prepared by adding calcium hydroxide (3g) to purified water (1000 ml) in a lead-free bottle, and shaking, occasionally during a period of one hour. The excess of calcium hydroxide is allowed to settle. When used, the required clear colourless supernatant liquid is drawn off by means of a siphon. It has an alkaline taste and is alkaline to litmus.

Uses : Calcium hydroxide is internally used as an antacid; as lime water in infantile diarrhoea and vomiting (astringent). Lime water is added to milk to prevent formation of large clots of curd, to increase digestibility; in some skin lotions and oily preparations to form calcium soaps of fatty acids which produce water-in-oil emulsions.

Calcium hydroxide pastes are used in dentistry. Calcium hydroxide is also used as pesticides; as egg preservative; and in dehairing hides. As an astringent, it is used in betel leaves for chewing. As a mild antacid, it neutralizes gastric acid and acts as a source of calcium.

Calcium is used medicinally as a fluid electrolyte and a topical astringent. Soda lime, prepared by combination of calcium hydroxide and sodium hydroxide, is used for its ability to absorb CO_2 from expired air in metabolic function test.

SODIUM HYDROXIDE
(Caustic Soda)

NaOH; Mol. Weight = 40.0

Sodium hydroxide contains not less than 97.0 per cent of total alkali calculated as NaOH and not more than 2.5 per cent of Na$_2$CO$_3$.

Preparation

1. When Milk of lime is added to hot sodium carbonate

solution (20%), sodium hydroxide and precipitate of calcium carbonate are obtained. The reaction is reversible.

$$Na_2CO_3 + Ca\,(OH)_2 \rightleftharpoons 2NaOH + CaCO_3\downarrow$$

The precipitated calcium carbonate is separated, the clear liquid containing sodium hydroxide is evaporated and the molten product is converted into sticks, pellets, or masses.

2. Sodium hydroxide is manufactured by the electrolysis of sodium chloride. For this purpose a mercury diaphragm cell, known as *Castner - Kellner cell*, is used. It consists of a large rectangular trough with a layer of mercury at the bottom. Sodium is electrolyzed from a concentrated brine solution with a graphite anode and a mercury cathode to produce a dilute sodium amalgam. The amalgam reacts with water to form a dilute hydroxide solution in cathode compartment in pure form.

Hydrogen and chlorine are the useful by-products at the anode

At cathode (-) : $Na^+ \longrightarrow Na$

$$2Na + 2H_2O \longrightarrow 2NaOH + H_2$$

At anode (+) : $Cl^- \longrightarrow Cl$

$$Cl + Cl \longrightarrow Cl_2$$

Sodium hydroxide solution is removed periodically and water added. The concentrated solution is evaporated to get fused sodium hydroxide.

3. Sodium hydroxide is also prepared from sodium metal and water vapour at low temperature.

Physical Characters : Dry sodium hydroxide is very deliquescent, white sticks, pellets, spherical particles, fused masses or scales; m.p. $318°$. It is hard and brittle and shows a crystalline fracture; strongly alkaline and corrosive to animal and vegetable tissues and to aluminium metal in moist condition and rapidly destroys organic tissues. When exposed to air it rapidly absorbs moisture and carbon dioxide. One gram dissolves in 0.9 ml water, 0.3 ml boiling water, 7.2 ml absolute alcohol, also soluble in glycerol. When sodium hydroxide is dissolved in water or mixed with an acid, considerable heat is generated. Solutions should be filtered through glass wool or asbestos and the solution should be stored in hard glass bottles, using rubber stoppers. If glass-stoppered bottles are used, the solution will dissolve the glass and the stopper will stick in the neck of the bottle.

Chemical Properties

1. Sodium hydroxide is a strong alkali. It changes the colour of indicators and neutralizes all acids or acid oxides producing salts.

$$NaOH + HCl \longrightarrow NaCl + H_2O$$

Sodium hydroxide is highly ionized in solution making it one of the strongest bases available.

2. It precipitates hydroxides of metals by reacting with the salts of all metals in solution.

$$Fe_2(SO_4)_3 + 6NaOH \longrightarrow 2Fe\,(OH)_3 \downarrow + Na_2SO_4$$
Ferrous   Red ppt.
sulphate

Hydroxides of zinc and aluminium are soluble in excess of sodium hydroxide

$$Zn(OH)_2 + 2NaOH \longrightarrow Na_2ZnO_2 + 2H_2O$$
Sodium
zincate

$$Al(OH)_3 + NaOH \longrightarrow NaAlO_2 + 2H_2O$$
Sodium meta
aluminate

    Sodium hydroxide catalyzes the hydrolysis of esters. It is used as a saponifying agent. It reacts with fats to produce glycerin and sodium salts of fatty acid (soap).

$$
\begin{array}{l}
CH_2 - OCO\text{-}C_{17}H_{35} \\
CH - OCO\text{-}C_{17}H_{35} \\
CH_2 - OCO - C_{17}H_{35}
\end{array}
+\; 3\ NaOH \rightarrow 3\ C_{17}\,H_{35}\ COO^- \ Na^+ \;+\;
\begin{array}{l}
CH_2OH \\
CH - OH \\
CH_2OH
\end{array}
$$

Stearin   Soap   Glycerin

3. Ammonium salts are decomposed with sodium hydroxide and form ammonia.

$$NH_4Cl + NaOH \longrightarrow NaCl + NH_3 \uparrow + H_2O$$

5. Sodium hydroxide solution reacts with zinc, aluminium, tin and silicon to form hydrogen.

$$Zn + NaOH + H_2O \longrightarrow NaHZnO_2 + H_2$$

$$4S + NaOH \longrightarrow 2Na_2S + Na_2S_2O_3 + 3H_2O$$
$$Si + 2NaOH + H_2O \longrightarrow Na_2SiO_3 + 2H_2$$

Test for Purity : Tests for aluminium, iron, and matter insoluble in hydrochloric acid; arsenic; heavy metals; potassium; chloride; lead; carbonate; sulphate; clarity and colour of solution.

Aluminium, iron and matter insoluble in hydrochloric acid are estimated gravimetrically. The insoluble matter and hydroxides of aluminium and iron are collected together, washed with aluminium nitrate solution, ignited and weighed.

Heavy metals are detected by treating the substance and standard lead solution with hydrogen sulphide solution separately and comparing the colour of both the solutions.

To an acidified solution with acetic acid, sodium cobaltinitrite solution is added. If precipitate is formed, then potassium is present.

The substance dissolved in water with the addition of nitric acid complies with the limit test for chlorides. When the solution is prepared by addition of nitric acid, it complies with the limit test for sulphates.

Test for Identification : A solution (1 in 20) gives the reactions of sodium.

Assay : Sodium hydroxide is a strong base which can be assayed by titrimetry. The procedure involves titrating a solution containing a weighed sample of NaOH with 1N H_2SO_4. Two end points are determined.

A weighed amount of the substance (1.5g) dissolved in carbon dioxide free water (40ml) is titrated with 1N sulphuric acid using phenolphthalein solution as indicator. When the pink colour of the solution is discharged, volume of acid solution required recorded, methyl orange solution added and the titration is continued until a persistent pink colour is produced. Each ml of 1N H_2SO_4 is equivalent to 0.040g of total alkali, calculated as NaOH and each ml of acid consumed in the titration with methyl orange is equivalent to 0.106 g of Na_2CO_3.

This type of assay is needed because of the ease with which NaOH absorbs CO_2 from the air to form sodium carbonate.

Uses : A 2.5% solution in glycerol is used as a cuticle solvent and to remove warts. An escharotic preparation of sodium hydroxide and calcium oxide, known as London paste, is used for adjusting the pH of solutions. NaOH solutions are used to neutralize acids and make sodium salts; to treat cellulose in making viscose rayon and cellophane. NaOH solutions hydrolyze fats and form soaps; they precipitate alkaloids and most metals (as hydroxides). It is an ingredient of Soda Lime and Sodium Hypochlorite solution.

Ingestion of sodium hydroxide causes vomiting, prostration and collapse. It is corrosive to all tissues.

BUFFERS

Buffers are the solutions of electrolytes which do not change their pH values on :

(i) Standing for a long time.

(ii) Exposure to atmospheric conditions.

(iii) Slight dilution, and

(iv) Addition of small amounts of acids or bases.

Thus buffer systems are pairs of related chemical compounds capable of resisting large changes in the pH of a solution caused by the addition of small amounts of acids or bases.

Buffer Action

In a buffer containing acetic acid and sodium acetate, the acid is a weak electrolyte and sodium acetate is a strong electrolyte. The dissociation of acetic acid is suppressed due to common acetate ion (CH_3COO^-) and the solution contains less proton (H^+) concentration and more Na^+ and CH_3COO^- ions. When a small amount of an acid is added, its protons combine with CH_3COO^- to yield undissociated CH_3COOH and the pH of the solution does not change. When a small amount of base is added, the OH^- ions are neutralized by acetic acid and pH is not effected.

$$CH_3COO^- + H^+ \rightleftharpoons CH_3COOH$$

$$CH_3COOH + OH^- \rightleftharpoons CH_3COO^- + H_2O$$

In the same way, addition of small amount of base OH^- to a basic buffer containing NH_4OH and NH_4Cl combines with NH_4^+ ion and the pH does not change. When a small quantity of an acid is added, NH_4OH neutralizes it and pH is not changed.

$$NH_4^+ + OH^- \rightleftharpoons NH_4OH$$

$$NH_4OH + OH^- \rightleftharpoons NH_4^+ + H_2O$$

The pH of acidic buffer can be determined by the equation:

$$pH = pKa + \log [salt]/[acid].$$

The maximum buffer action is obtained when the concentration of the acid and the base are equal, i.e.,

$$pH = pKa + \log 1 = pKa + OH = pKa$$

The pH of an alkaline buffer solution containing a weak base and its salt with a strong acid can be calculated as :

$$pH = 14\text{-}pOH = 14 - (pKa + \log [\text{conjugate acid}]/[\text{base}]$$

Buffer Capacity : Buffer solutions do not change pH upon addition of strong acid or strong base. The buffering action is determined in terms of buffer capacity which is defined as the moles of strong acid or strong base required to change the pH of one litre of buffer solution by one unit. The greater the buffer capacity, the better is the buffer as it can tolerate more acid or base without significant changes in pH.

Physiological Buffers : The pH of blood in human body is about 7.3-7.4 which is controlled by buffering mechanism. In the body acidic metabolites, e.g. CO_2, proteins and amino acids, are produced in greater amounts than the basic metabolites like, bicarbonate ions. The resulted pH produced due to neutralization is slightly alkaline. When alkaline pH is increased, metabolic acidosis is developed.

A buffer solution is prepared by dissolving a solution of a weak acid with the solution of one of its salts with a strong base or by mixing the solution of a weak base with the solution of one of its salts with a strong acid. The pH of a mixed solution of an acid and its salt is dependent on the ratio of their concentrations. A change in ionic strength of a solution changes the activity factors and consequently the pH values.

Buffer solutions are required as pH standards or for conducting some biochemical and other experiments, which are sensitive to the pH values of the reaction media and which produce an acid or a base during the course of the reaction. Normal or deci-normal solutions of strong acids and bases would act as buffers of low and high pH value. Buffers of intermediate pH values are prepared by mixing weak acids along with their salts for acid buffers and weak bases along with their salts for alkaline buffers.

The buffer should not react with other chemicals in a pharmaceutical preparation. The buffer pair should not participitate in oxidation-reduction reactions; alter the solubility of other components; form complexes with active ingredients; or participitate in acid-base reactions other than those required as part of the buffer function. The buffer should not change pharmacological properties of the active ingredients. The buffers composed of common biochemical acids and conjugate bases serve as nutrient media for microorganisms and support microbial growth.

Maintenance of pH is necessary for chemical stability and solubility of the drug. The pH is altered due to alkali in the glass of some containers, and gases in the air such as CO_2 and NH_3, which can dissolve in the solution giving acidic or basic reactions.

The alkaline buffers should be protected from the absorption of atmospheric CO_2, which would finally produce a drop in the pH.

Certain buffer systems, e.g. borates, are toxic when taken internally. However, borate buffers can be used for topical, (ophthalmic) preparations. Weak acids and congugate bases lacking toxicity are found as common biochemicals in the body.

Standard Buffer Solutions

Standard buffer solutions are solutions of standard pH. They are used for reference purposes in pH measurements and for carrying out many pharmacopoeial tests which require adjustments to or maintenance of a specified pH. For the preparation of standard buffer solutions, all the crystalline reagents except boric acid should be dried at $110°$ to $120°$ for one hour before use. Freshly boiled and cooled water should be used. The prepared solutions should be stored in chemically resistant; glass-stoppered bottles of alkali free glass and used within 3 months of preparation. Any solution which has become cloudy or show any other evidence of deterioration should be discarded.

Standard buffer solutions for various ranges of pH values between 1.2 and 10.2 may be prepared by appropriate combinations of 0.2N hydrochloric acid or 0.2N sodium hydroxide and of 0.2M solutions as described below.

1. **Hydrochloric Acid, 0.2N :** Hydrochloric acid is diluted with freshly boiled and cooled under water to contain in 1000 ml 7.292g of HCl. It is standardized by volumetric titration.

2. **Sodium Hydroxide, 0.2N :** Sodium hydroxide is dissolved in water to produce a 40 to 60 per cent w/v solution and allowed to stand. Taking precautions to avoid absorption of carbon dioxide, the clear supernatant liquid is siphoned off and diluted with carbon dioxide free water to a suitable volume of the liquid to contain

in 1000 ml 8.0g of NaOH. It is standardized by volumetric reagents and solutions.

0.2N sodium hydroxide must not be used later than one month after preparation.

3. **Potassium Hydrogen Phthalate, 0.2M :** 40.846g of potassium hydrogen phthalate is dissolved in water, and diluted with water to 1000 ml.

4. **Potassium Dihydrogen Phosphate, 0.2 M :** 27.218 g of potassium dihydrogen phosphate is dissolved in water, and diluted with water to 1000 ml.

5. **Boric Acid and Potassium Chloride 0.2 M :** 12.366 g of boric acid and 14.911 g of potassium chloride are dissolved in water, and diluted with water to 1000 ml.

6. **Potassium Chloride, 0.2 M :** 14.911 g of potassium chloride is dissolved in water and diluted with water to 1000 ml.

Composition of Standard Buffer Solutions

Hydrochloric Acid Buffer : Potassium chloride solution (50ml) is placed in a 200 ml volumetric flask, specified volume (85.0 to 7.8 ml) of hydrochloric acid solution is added to adjust pH from 1.2 to 2.2 and then water is added to volume.

Acid Phthalate Buffer : Potassium hydrogen phthalate solution (50 ml) is placed in a 200 ml volumetric flask, the specific volume (49.5 to 0.1 ml) of the hydrochloric acid solution is added to adjust pH (2.2 to 4.0), and than water is added to volume.

Neutralized Phthalate Buffer : Potassium hydrogen phthalate solution (50 ml) is placed in a 200 ml volumetric flask, the specified volume of the sodium hydroxide solution (3.0 to 42.3 ml) is added to adjust pH (4.2 to 5.8), then water is added to volume.

Phosphate Buffer : Potassium dihydrogen phosphate solution (50 ml) is placed in a 200 ml volumetric flask, the specified volume (3.6 to 46.1 ml) of the sodium hydroxide solution is added to adjust the pH (5.8 to 8.0), then water is added to volume.

Alkaline Borate Buffer : The boric acid and potassium chloride solution (50 ml) is placed in a 200 ml volumetric flask, the specified volume (3.9 to 43.7 ml) of the sodium hydroxide solution is added to adjust pH (8.0 to 10.0), than water is added to volume.

Other Buffer Solutions

Acetate Buffer pH 2.8 : Anhydrous sodium acetate (4 g) is dissolved in about 840 ml of water, sufficient glacial acetic acid (about 155 ml) is added to adjust the pH to 2.8 and diluted with water to 1000 ml.

Other acetate buffer of pH 3.5 to 5.0 are similarly prepared by dissolving calculated amount of sodium acetate or ammonium acetate as mentioned in the Indian Pharmacopoeia.

Acetic Ammonia Buffer pH 3.7, Ethanolic : To 5 N acetic acid (15 ml), alcohol (60 ml) and water (24 ml) are added, the pH of the solution adjusted to 3.7 with 10 N ammonia and diluted with water to 100 ml.

Acetone Solution, Buffered : Sodium acetate (15 g) and sodium chloride (42 g) are dissolved in water, 0.1 N hydrochloric acid (68 ml) and acetone (150 ml) added, and diluted with water to 500 ml.

Ammonia Buffer pH 10.0 : Ammonium chloride (5.4 g) is dissolved in 5 N ammonia (70 ml) and diluted with water to 100 ml.

Barbitone Buffer pH 8.6 : To 0.1 N hydrochloric acid (129 ml), sufficient 0.1 M barbitone solution is added to produce 1000 ml.

Copper Sulphate Solution pH 3.2, Buffered : Anhydrous disodium hydrogen phosphate (7.0 g) is dissolved in sufficient water to produce 247 ml and a 2.1% w/v solution (about 753 ml) of citric acid added until the pH of the solution is between 3.15 and 3.25. The resulting solution (999 ml) is mixed with 1 ml of a 0.51 per cent w/v solution of copper sulphate.

Copper Sulphate Solution pH 4.0, Buffered : Copper sulphate (0.25 g) and ammonium acetate (4.5 g) are dissolved in sufficient 2 N acetic acid to produce 100 ml.

Glycerin Solution pH 7.2, Buffered : The pH of a 50% w/v solution of glycerin in carbon dioxide free water is determined. If pH of the solution is above 5.5, the buffered glycerin is prepared by method (A), and if pH is below 5.5, prepared by method (B).

A. To glycerin (500 ml), a mixture (500 ml) of M disodium hydrogen phosphate (17.5 ml), M potassium dihydrogen phosphate (7.5) and carbon dioxide free water (475 ml) are added.

B. To glycerin (500 ml), a mixture (500 ml) of M disodium hydrogen phosphate (42 ml), M potassium dihydrogen phosphate (8 ml) and carbon dioxide free water (450 ml) are added.

If necessary, the pH is adjusted to 7.2 with M disodium hydrogen phosphate or M potassium dihydrogen phosphate, as required. Suitable quantities of the buffered glycerin are distributed in screw-capped bottles and sterilized by heating in an autoclave at 121° for one hour.

Glycine Buffer Solution (Aminoacetate Buffer Solution) : Sodium bicarbonate (42 g) and potassium bicarbonate (50 g) are mixed with water (180 ml) and a solution containing glycine (37.8 g) and strong ammonia solution (15 ml) in water (180 ml) is added. It is diluted with water to 500 ml and stirred until solution is complete.

Imidazole Buffer pH 7.4 : Imidazole (3.40 g) and sodium chloride (5.84 g) are dissolved in water, N hydrochloric acid (18.6 ml) is added and diluted with water to 1000 ml.

Palladium Chloride Solution, Buffered : To palladium chloride (0.5 g), hydrochloric acid (5 ml) is added and warmed on a water bath. Hot water 9200 ml) is added in small portions with continued heating until solution is complete. It is cooled and diluted with sufficient water to produce 250 ml. To 50 ml of the resulting solution, M sodium acetate (10 ml) and N hydrochloric acid (9.6 ml) are added and sufficient water mixed to produce 100 ml.

Phosphate Buffer pH 4.0, Mixed : Disodium hydrogen phosphate (5.04 g) and potassium dihydrogen phosphate (3.01 g) are dissolved in sufficient water to produce 1000 ml and the pH adjusted to 4.0 with glacial acetic acid.

Phosphate Buffer pH 6.8, Mixed : Disodium hydrogen phosphate (28.8 g) and potassium dihydrogen phosphate (11.45 g) are added in sufficient water to produce 1000 ml.

Phosphate-Buffered Saline pH 7.4 : Disodium hydrogen phosphate (1.38 g), potassium dihydrogen phosphate (0.19 g) and sodium chloride (8 g) are added in sufficient water to produce 1000 ml. Immediately before use, the pH is adjusted, if necessary.

Buffer Solution pH 2.5 : To 0.2 M potassium hydrogen phthalate (25 ml), 0.1 N hydrochloric acid (37 ml) is added, and diluted with sufficient water to produce 1000 ml.

3

ANTIOXIDANTS

Antioxidants are chemically reducing agents. They are used in pharmaceutical preparations containing easily oxidized substances for maintaining these substances in their reduced form. The antioxidant is oxidized in place of the active constituent. If the active component is oxidized, the antioxidant reduces it back to its normal oxidation state.

The mechanism of antioxidants is based on oxidation - reduction (redox) reactions. The transfer of electrons from one compound to the other and the loss of electrons are used to balance the oxidation states on both sides of the half-reaction similarly to Brönsted acid-base reactions. The reaction of oxidized compound (OX_1) and reduced compound (Red_1) can be represented as :

$$Ox_1 + e^- \rightleftharpoons Red_1$$

Redox reactions take place in electrochemical cells where the electron transfer takes place through a system of electrodes. The electrical potential is measured with a potentiometer or a voltmeter.

An antioxidant in a pharmaceutical preparation should be physiologically inert; usually the concentrations employed are sufficiently low. The possible toxicity of both the reducing agents and its oxidized product must be assessed. Antioxidant selection should consider possible solubility problems between the reducing agent and the drug. Preparations containing calcium should be adjusted to an acidic pH if an antioxidant containing the sulphite ion (SO_3^{-2}) is used. Sulphite compounds will cause the precipitation of calcium from solutions at neutral to alkaline pH. When bisulphites are added as antioxidant, it will form addition compounds with many unsaturated organic functional groups e.g., ethylene bonds and carbonyl groups. Very strong reducing agents (e.g. hypophophorus acid and hypophosphites) will form explosive mixtures when combined in dry form or in concentrated solutions with strong oxidizing agents.

HYPOPHOSPHORUS ACID

H_3PO_2; Mol. Weight = 66.0

Hypophosphorus acid is a monobasic and reducing agent. It is a colourless or slightly yellow odourless liquid, containing 30 to 32 per cent of H_3PO_2. It is conveniently prepared by treating NaH_2PO_2 with an ion-exchange resin. The water-free acid forms deliquesc crystals; m.p. 26.5°; supercools to a colourless, odourless, oily liquid. It is decomposed by heat into H_3PO_4 and spontaneously flammable PH_3. It is miscible with water, alcohol and ether. It is stored in airtight containers.

Hypophosphorus acid contains only one ionizable hydrogen. Therefore, it reacts as a monoprotic acid and is assayed by titrating against 1N sodium hydroxide to a methyl orange end point.

The oxidation state of the central phosphorus atom is +1. It is a very powerful reducing agent. It can easily reduce many compounds to form phosphorus acid (H$_3$PO$_3$) and an oxidation state of +3, and finally phosphoric acid (H$_3$PO$_4$) with oxidation state of +5. It on reduction forms phosphine which interacts with mercuric halide papers. Therefore, it is oxidized to phosphoric acid by reacting with potassium chlorate and hydrochloric acid. Excess of chlorine formed by interaction of chlorate and HCl is removed by boiling and then by treatment with stannous chloride.

Hypophosphorous acid is oxidized by sulphuric acid to form sulphur dioxide and sulphur. The mixture of hypophosphorus acid with any oxidizing agent can produce an incompatibility and can be exploded. In diluted form it is very effective reducing agent or antioxidant.

It reacts with molecular iodine to form iodide ions and decolourizes acidic solutions of potassium permanganate immediately.

$$H_3PO_2 + 2I_2 + 2H_2O \longrightarrow 4HI + H_3PO_4$$
$$5H_3PO_2 + 4KMnO_4 + 6H_2SO_4 \longrightarrow 2K_2SO_4 + 4MnSO_4$$
$$+ 5H_3PO_4 + 6H_2O$$

Test for Purity : Tests for barium; calcium; iron; chloride; sulphate; phosphoric acid; oxalic acid; weight per ml.

Barium and calcium are determined by adding dilute sulphuric acid to dilute hypophosphorus acid and allowing to stand for one hour. No turbidity is produced.

For detecting phosphoric and oxalic acids, calcium chloride solution and dilute ammonia solution are added to the dilute hypophosphorus acid. Not more than a slight turbidity is produced.

Incompatibility : Combination of hypophosphorous acid with oxidizing agents such as nitrates, chlorates or permanganates forms explosive mixtures in concentrated amounts. In dilute solution it is a very effective antioxidant.

Assay : The acid (10 g) is diluted with water (50 ml) and titrated with 0.5 N sodium hydroxide, using methyl orange solution as indicator. Each ml of 0.5 N sodium hydroxide is equivalent to 0.03300 g of H_3PO_2.

Uses : Hypophosphorus acid is used as an antioxidant. Earlier hypophosphates were used in tonics. It prevents the formation of free iodine in diluted hydriodic acid and hydriodic acid syrup. It also prevents the formation of both ferric ions and molecular iodine in ferrous iodine syrup. Salts of hypophosphorus acid, e.g. sodium and ammonium hypophosphite, are present as a preservative in certain food and preparations.

SULPHUR DIOXIDE

SO_2; Mol. Weight = 64.06

Sulphur dioxide contains not less than 97.0 per cent, by volume of SO_2. It occurs in volcanic gases and in atmosphere formed due to burning of sulphur compounds in coal.

Preparation

1. Sulphur dioxide is manufactured by burning sulphur in air or by roasting metallic sulphides like copper, iron or zinc.

$$S + O_2 \longrightarrow SO_2\uparrow$$
$$4FeS_2 + 11O_2 \longrightarrow 8SO_2\uparrow + 2Fe_2O_3$$
$$2ZnS + 3O_2 \longrightarrow 2ZnO + 2SO_2\uparrow$$

2. Sulphuric acid is reduced to sulphur dioxide when heated with sulphur, copper or mercury.

$$SO_2 + Cl_2 \longrightarrow SO_2Cl_2$$
$$2H_2SO_4 + S \longrightarrow 3SO_2\uparrow + 2H_2O$$
$$2H_2SO_4 + Cu \longrightarrow CuSO_4 + SO_2\uparrow + 2H_2O$$

Treatment of sulphuric acid with sulphites or bisulphites also produces sulphur dioxide.

$$H_2SO_4 + Na_2SO_4 \longrightarrow Na_2SO_4 + SO_2\uparrow + H_2O$$

Physical Characters : Sulphur dioxide is a colourless gas with a typical pungent small of burning sulphur. It condenses readily under pressure to a colourless liquid which boils at about -10°. It is soluble in water (36 in 1) and alcohol (114 in 1) at 20° and normal pressure; soluble in chloroform and ether. When passed into water it yields a clear colourless solution which is strongly acidic to litmus paper. It is stored in cylinders and usually packaged under pressure in liquid form.

Sulphur dioxide forms sulphurous acid in aqueous solution.

$$SO_2 + H_2O \longrightarrow \underset{\substack{\text{Sulphurous}\\\text{acid}}}{H_2SO_3} \rightleftharpoons 2H^+ + SO_3^{2-}$$

Chemical Properties

1. Sulphur dioxide is decomposed into sulphur and sulphur trioxide when heated strongly.

$$3SO_2 \longrightarrow S + 2SO_3$$

2. Sulphur dioxide is incombustible. However, strongly burning potassium or magnesium continues to burn in SO_2 and decomposes it into sulphur and oxygen.

$$3Mg + SO_2 \longrightarrow 2MgO + MgS$$
$$4K + 3SO_2 \longrightarrow K_2SO_3 + K_2S_2O_3$$

3. Sulphur dioxide forms addition compounds with barium peroxide, lead oxide, chlorine and oxygen due to remaining two valencies of sulphur.

$$2SO_2 + O_2 \rightleftharpoons 2SO_3$$
$$SO_2 + Cl_2 \xrightarrow{\text{Light}} \underset{\text{Sulphuryl chloride}}{SO_2Cl_2}$$
$$PbO_2 + SO_2 \xrightarrow{\text{Heat}} PbSO_4$$

4. Sulphur dioxide acts as a strong reducing agent in the presence of moisture or an oxidising agent. Acidified potassium permanganate is decolourized and potassium dichromate is turned green. Halogens are reduced to halogen acids and ferric salts are converted to ferrous salts.

$$2KMnO_4 + 5SO_2 + 2H_2O \longrightarrow K_2SO_4 + 2MnSO_4 + 2H_2SO_4$$

$$K_2Cr_2O_7 + H_2SO_4 + 3SO_2 \longrightarrow K_2SO_4 + Cr_2(SO_4)_3 + H_2O.$$

$$Cl_2 + SO_2 + 2H_2O \longrightarrow 2HCl + H_2SO_4$$

$$I_2 + SO_2 + 2H_2O \longrightarrow 2HI + H_2SO_4$$

$$Fe_2(SO_4)_3 + SO_2 + 2H_2O \longrightarrow 2FeSO_4 + 2H_2SO_4$$

5. In the presence of moisture sulphur dioxide acts as a bleaching agent.

6. Sulphur dioxide acts as an oxidizing agent.

$$2H_2S + SO_2 \longrightarrow 3S + 2H_2O$$

$$4K + 3SO_2 \longrightarrow K_2SO_3 + K_2S_2O_3$$

$$3Fe + SO_2 \longrightarrow 2FeO + FeS$$

Test for Purity : Test for water; sulphuric acid and non-valatile residue. To determine non-volatile residue, a weighed sample is evaporated and the ramaining matter is weighed. If the non-volatile matter is mixed with water and the mixture titrated with N/100 alkali, the amount of sulphuric acid is obtained.

Water of crystallization, or moisture content in volatile compounds is determined by the Karl Fischer method which is a volumetric procedure. Karl Fischer reagent is a solution of iodine and sulphur dioxide in pyridine with added methanol. When used for the titration of water, two reactions occur.

$$I_2 + SO_2 + 3C_5H_5N + H_2O \longrightarrow 2C_5H_5NHI$$

$$+ C_5H_5N \diagdown \begin{matrix} SO_2 \\ | \\ O \end{matrix}$$

$$\downarrow CH_3OH$$

$$C_5H_5NHSO_4CH_3$$

Each molecule of iodine is equivalent to one molecule of water. The end point is determined visually or electrometrically.

Incompatibility : Under alkaline conditions, sulphur dioxide is converted to bisulphite and sulphite. In buffer solutions, the SO_2 reduces hydroxide ion concentrations due to formation of HSO_3^- and the solution becomes more acidic.

$$SO_2 + OH^- \longrightarrow HSO_3^-$$

Assay (U.S.P.) : Sulphur dioxide is stable at moderate to strong acidic pH. As the pH becomes neutral to alkaline values, sulphur dioxide is converted into bisulphite and sulphite. This fact is used in the assay of SO_2. It is absorbed into 0.1 N sodium hydroxide to form sodium bisulphite which is then titrated against 0.1 N iodine solution to a pale blue end point with starch. In unbuffered medium, sulphur dioxide will reduce hydroxide ion concentrations and cause a shift to more acidic pH.

$$SO_2 + OH \longrightarrow HSO_3^-$$

Gaseous sulphur dioxide (100 ml) is collected over mercury and temperature and pressure upon it are noted. 0.1 N sodium hydroxide (50 ml) is introduced slowly into the air space over the mercury and the sample is absorbed in the solution by shaking. When absorption is complete, the solution is transferred to a conical flask, starch (3 ml) added and titrated with 0.1 N iodine until the solution is pale blue in colour. Each ml of 0.1 N iodine is equivalent to 1.094 ml of SO_2 at a temperature of $0°$ and a pressure of 760 mm of mercury.

Uses : Sulphur dioxide has antioxidant and antimicrobial properties and is used as a preservative for food. It is also used as a fumigant and to disinfect equipment in the wine and food industries and houses. In industry it is used for bleaching wood pulp, fumigating grains and arresting fermentation. Fruits are generally exposed to SO_2 atmosphere to prevent darkening and growth of micro-organisms. A lotion prepared from SO_2 and glycerin is used to cure sore throat in cold, tonsillitis and skin infections.

Sulphur dioxide is highly irritant to the eyes, skin and mucous membrances. Inhalation results in irritation of the respiratory tract which may lead bronchoconstriction and pulmonary oedema.

SODIUM BISULPHITE

$NaHSO_3$; Mol. Weight = 104

Sodium bisulphite consists chiefly of sodium bisulphite ($NaHSO_3$) and sodium metabisulphite ($Na_2S_2O_5$) in varying proportions. It possesses the same properties as the true bisulphite. It yields 58.5 to 67.4% of SO_2.

$$Na_2S_2O_5 + H_2O \longrightarrow 2NaHSO_3$$

Preparation

Sulphur bisulphite is prepared by passing sulphur dioxide into a solution of sodium carbonate until the solution is saturated. Evaporation of the solution gives a mixture of sodium bisulphite and metabisulphite.

$$Na_2CO_3 + 2SO_2 + H_2O \longrightarrow 2NaHSO_3 + CO_2\uparrow$$

$$2NaHSO_3 + SO_2 \longrightarrow Na_2S_2O_5 + H_2SO_3$$

Characters : Sodium bisulphite is a white or yellowish white crystalline powder having pungent odour of burning sulphur and disagreeable taste. On exposure to air it is unstable, loses some SO_2 and is gradually oxidized to sulphate. It is soluble in cold water (2 in 3.5) and alcohol (1 in 70). Its aqueous solution is acidic. It is kept in well-closed containers and in a cool place.

Sodium bisulphite forms water-soluble, stable compounds with aldehydes and ketones and hence it is used to prepare their derivatives and in formulations containing carbonyl compounds.

Test for Purity : Tests for arsenic; heavy metals; and iron.

Assay : The Assay is dependent on iodimetric titration. The substance is allowed to react with iodine. This is acidified with hydrochloric acid and titrated with sodium thiosulphate using starch solutions as indicator. End point is the disappearance of blue colour.

$$2Na_2S_2O_3 + I_2 \longrightarrow Na_2S_4O_2 + 2NaI$$
Sodium
tetrathionate

A weighed amount (0.2g) is transferred to a glass-stoppered flask, 0.1 N iodine added and the stopper of the flask inserted. It is allowed to stand for five minutes, hydrochloric acid (1 ml) added, and the excess of iodine titrated with 0.1N sodium thiosulphate, using starch solution as indicator added towards the end of the titration. Each ml of 0.1 N iodine is equivalent to 0.003203 g of SO_2.

Uses : Sodium bisulphite acts as a disinfectant, antioxidant and bleaching agent, particularly for wool; as antiseptic in fermentation industries; as preservative and bleach in food. It converts water-insoluble menadione (vitamin K analogue) to a highly water soluble form menadione sodium bisulphite without significant loss of activity. It is used as an antiseptic in gastric fermentation, in parasitic skin diseases, to stabilize kidney stones, in injections of epinephrine hydrochloride, phenylnephrine hydrochloride and ascorbic acid, to remove permanganate stains and to stabilize certain dyes and other chemicals.

Concentrated solutions are irritating to skin and mucous membranes.

SODIUM METABISULPHITE

$Na_2S_2O_5$; Mol. Weight = 190.10

Sodium metabisulphite contains not less than 95.0 per cent of $Na_2S_2O_5$ equivelent to not less than 66.0% of SO_2.

It is prepared by saturating hot, concentrated sodium hydroxide solution with sulphur dioxide. Cooling of the solution yields the salt.

$$NaOH + SO_2 \longrightarrow NaHSO_3$$
$$\text{Sodium bisulphite}$$

$$2NaHSO_3 \longrightarrow Na_2S_2O_5 + H_2O$$

Physical Characters : It occurs as colourless or white prismatic crystals or a white or yellowish crystalline powder. It has sulphurous odour. On exposure to air and moisture, it is slowly oxidized to sulphate with disintegration of the crystals.

$$Na_2S_2O_5 + H_2O \longrightarrow 2NaHSO_3$$

It is soluble in water (1 in 2); slightly soluble in alcohol; freely soluble in glycerol. A solution in water is acidic to phenol red. It is stored at a temperature not exceeding 40° in well-filled airtight containers.

Chemical Properties

1. When an acid is added to a solution of sodium metabisulphite, SO_2 gas is formed which is dissolved in solution as sulphurous acid (a solution of SO_2 in water).

$$Na_2S_2O_5 \xrightarrow{H^+} SO_2 \xrightarrow{H_2O} H_2SO_3$$

2. Sodium metabisulphite is a powerful reducing agent. When dissolved in water, it is immediately converted to bisulphite.

$$Na_2S_2O_5 + H_2O \longrightarrow 2NaHSO_3$$

Like sulphur dioxide, it contains sulphur in the +4 oxidation state.

Test for Purity : Tests for acids; arsenic; lead; heavy metals; and thiosulphate.

When the substance is heated with hydrochloric acid, then an opalescence or turbidity of sulphur is formed if thiosulphate is present.

$$Na_2S_2O_3 + 2HCl \longrightarrow 2NaCl + SO_2\uparrow + S + H_2O$$
Thiosulphate

$$Na_2S_2O_5 + 2HCl \longrightarrow 2NaCl + 2SO_2\uparrow + H_2O$$
Metasulphite

For detecting the presence of iron, an acidified solution is treated with bromine and then boiled. Ammonium persulphate and ammonium thiocyanate solutions are added to the reaction mixture. Any colour produced is not darker than that obtained by adding ammonium thiocyanate solution to a mixture of standard iron solution, hydrochloric acid, ammonium persulphate and water.

Tests for Identification

1. A solution (1 in 20) decolourizes iodine solution, and the resulting solution gives the reactions of sulphates.
2. The solution gives the reaction of sodium.

Incompatibility : The bisulphites of alkaline earth metals are less soluble and their sulphites are insoluble. Only alkali metal salts are soluble.

Assay : Like sulphur dioxide, sodium bisulphite and sodium metabisulphite are assayed on the basis of reducing a 0.1 N iodine solution which is added to the solutions in excess. The residual iodine is titrated against sodium thiosulphate to determine the amount reduced by the metabisulphite.

A weighed amount (0.2 g) of the substance is dissolved in 0.1 N iodine (50 ml), hydrochloric acid (1 ml) is added and the excess of iodine titrated with 0.1 N sodium thiosulphate using starch solution, added towards the end of the titration, as indicator. Each ml of 0.1 N iodine is equivalent to 0.004753 g of $Na_2S_2O_5$.

$$NaHSO_3 + I_2 + H_2O \longrightarrow NaHSO_4 + 2HI$$
$$2Na_2S_2O_3 + I_2 \longrightarrow 2NaI + Na_2S_4O_6$$

Uses : Sodium metabisulphite is a strong reducing agent and is used as an antioxidant in pharmaceutical preparations to stabilize injections containing salts of adrenaline, apomorphine and sodium salicylate possessing phenol or catechol nucleus. It also has an antimicrobial action. It is used as a preservative in acidic solutions and syrups. It prevents oxidation of quinone like compounds. It is added to ascorbic acid injection as a reducing agent.

It is used in the food industry as an antioxidant, antimicrobial preservative and anti-browning agent. It is also used in wine-making as an antimicrobial preservative, antioxidant, clarifier; and equipment cleanser. Sodium bisulphite has been used topically to treat dermatological disorders caused by certain parasites.

Ingestion of the metasulphide causes gastric irritation. Large doses of sulphites may cause gastro-intestinal upsets, respiratory or circulatory failure and central nervous system disturbances.

SODIUM THIOSULPHATE

$Na_2S_2O_3$; $5H_2O$; Mol. Weight = 248.17

Sodium thiosulphate contains not less than 99.0 per cent of $Na_2S_2O_3$, $5H_2O$.

Preparation

1. It is prepared by boiling sodium sulphite solution with powdered sulphur. Sodium sulphite is obtained when an aqueous solution of sodium carbonate is reacted with sulphur dioxide and the sodium bisulphite is further reacted with sodium carbonate.

$$Na_2CO_3 + H_2O + 2SO_2 \longrightarrow 2NaHSO_3 + CO_2\uparrow$$
$$2NaHSO_3 + Na_2CO_3 \longrightarrow 2Na_2SO_3 + H_2O + CO_2\uparrow$$
$$Na_2SO_3 + S \longrightarrow Na_2S_2O_3$$

The excess of sulphur is separated by filtration, the filtrate is concentrated and crystallized.

2. Sodium thiosulphate is also prepared by reacting sodium hydroxide with sulphur.

$$6NaOH + 4S \longrightarrow Na_2S_2O_3 + 2Na_2S + 3H_2O$$

Physical Characters

Sodium thiosulphate occurs as colourless, odourless, transparent crystals or a coarse crystalline powder; cooling bitter taste; efflorescent in dry air above $33°$; deliquescent in moist air. It dissolves in its own water of crystallization at about $49°$. It loses all its water at $100°$; decomposes at higher temperature. It is soluble in water (1 in 0.5); pH 6.0 to 8.4; practically insoluble in alcohol. Its solutions are neutral or faintly alkaline to litmus. It is stored in airtight containers, and protected from light and moisture.

Chemical Properties

In sodium thiosulphate sulphur occurs in two different oxidation states. The oxidized sulphur atom is in a +6 state resisting further oxidation. The remaining sulphur atom is in a zero oxidation state. Due to this property the compound acts as a reducing agent or as an antioxidant.

1. Sodium thiosulphate decomposes on heating yielding sulphur dioxide, hydrogen sulphide and sulphur.

2. Aqueous solutions decompose slowly as

$$4Na_2S_2O_3 \longrightarrow 3Na_2SO_4 + Na_2S_5 \longrightarrow Na_2S + 4S$$

3. Dilute acids convert it into thiosulphuric acid which decomposes yielding sulphur dioxide and sulphur.

$$Na_2S_2O_3 + 2HCl \longrightarrow H_2S_2O_3 + 2NaCl$$
$$H_2S_2O_3 \longrightarrow S + SO_2 + H_2O$$

4. Silver halides are dissolved by sodium thiosulphate solution. Therefore, it is used in photography and known as 'hypo'.

$$2Na_2S_2O_3 + AgBr \longrightarrow Na_3[Ag(S_2O_3)_2] + NaBr$$

| Silver | Sodium argento- |
| bromide | thiosulphate |

It must be buffered near pH 8.5 and covered with nitrogen during autoclaving to prevent degradation by oxidation.

$$Na_2S_2O_3 \xrightarrow{O_2} Na_2SO_4 + S \text{ or } Na_2S_4O_6$$

$$Na_2S_2O_3 \xrightarrow{H^+} H_2SO_3 + NaHSO_3 + S\downarrow$$

5. With dilute solution of sodium thiosulphate, silver nitrate gives a white precipitate, changing to yellow, brown and finally black, due to the formation of silver sulphide.

$$Na_2S_2O_3 + 2AgNO_3 \longrightarrow Ag_2S_2O_3 + 2NaNO_3$$

$$Ag_2S_2O_3 + H_2O \longrightarrow Ag_2S + H_2SO_4$$

With a concentrated sodium thiosulphate solution, precipitate is not formed due high solubility of the silver thiosulphate.

$$Ag_2S_2O_3 + 3Na_2S_2O_3 \longrightarrow 2Na\,[Ag\,(S_2O_3)_2]$$

6. Chlorine oxidizes sodium thiosulphate to sodium sulphate. Iodine is decolourized due to formation of tetrathionate.

$$Na_2S_2O_3 + Cl_2 + H_2O \longrightarrow Na_2SO_4 + 2HCl + S$$
$$2Na_2S_2O_3 + I_2 \longrightarrow Na_2S_4O_6 + 2NaI$$

The reaction of the compound with iodine is used to remove iodine stains and chlorine from industrial bleaching operations.

7. Reaction of barium chloride with sodium thiosulphate solution gives white precipitate of barium thiosulphate. Calcium thiosulphate formed from calcium chloride is soluble in water.

$$Na_2S_2O_3 + BaCl_2 \longrightarrow BaS_2O_3 + 2NaCl$$

8. It acts as a reducing agent and reduces ferric chloride solution to form dark violet colour which quickly disappears.

$$3Na_2S_2O_3 + 2FeCl_3 \rightleftharpoons Fe_2(S_2O_3)_3 + 6NaCl$$

$$\underset{\substack{\text{Neutral} \\ \text{solution}}}{2FeCl_3 + 2Na_2S_2O_3} \longrightarrow 2FeCl_3 + 2NaCl + Na_2S_4O_6$$

$$2FeCl_3 + Na_2S_2O_3 + H_2O \xrightarrow{H^+} 2FeCl_2 + 2NaCl + H_2S\uparrow + S$$

This reaction is used to estimate iodine quantitatively.

Test for Purity : Test for arsenic; calcium; heavy metals; chloride; sulphate; sulphite; and sulphide.

Heavy metals are detected by comparing colours formed by addition of hydrogen sulphide solution separately to an acidified solution of the substance and standard lead solution.

When ammonium oxalate solution is added to an aqueous solution, no turbidity is produced indicating the absence of calcium.

The substance dissolved in water with the addition of nitric acid complies with the limit test for chlorides.

For detecting sulphate and sulphite, iodine solution is added to the aqueous solution until a very faint persistent yellow colour is produced. The resulting solution complies with the limit test for sulphates.

Sulphide is detected by treating aqueous solution with sodium nitroprusside to produce a violet colour.

Tests for Identification

1. To a 10 per cent w/v solution, few drops of iodine solution are added. The colour is discharged.
2. A solution (1 in 20) gives the reactions of sodium and of thiosulphates.

Incompatibility : It is incompatible with metal cations due to the precipitation of the metal thiosulphate. In acid solution, these precipitates may darken due to the formation of the related sulphides.

Assay : The assay is based on iodimetric titration. A weighed amount (0.8) dissolved in water (30 ml) is titrated with 0.1 N iodine, using 3 ml of starch solution as indicator as the end point is obtained. Each ml of 0.1N iodine is equivalent to 0.02482 g of $Na_2S_2O_3 . 5H_2O$.

$$2Na_2S_2O_3 + I_2 \longrightarrow Na_2S_4O_6 + 2NaI$$

Uses : Sodium thiosulphate is used as an antidote in the treatment of cyanide poisoning in combination with sodium nitrite. It has antifungal properties and is used to treat pityriasis versicolour; externally in combination with acids to treat various dermatological disease, e.g. ringworm, mange, etc. It is also used as a fixer in photographic work as 'Hypo' solution, as a standard titrant in iodimetric titrations and as an antichlor in bleaching operations.

NITROGEN

N_2; Mol. Weight = 28.

Nitrogen is present more than 75 per cent of atmospheric air. In combined state nitrogen occurs in nitrates, nitrites, ammonium salts, oxides of nitrogen, in proteins, alkaloids and coal. Fertile soils contain nitrogen as ammonium salts and nitrates. Fixed or combined nitrogen is present in many mineral deposits.

Preparation

1. Nitrogen is manufactured by fractional distillation of liquid air. Oxygen is removed from air by burning phosphorus. Phosphorus pentoxide is formed which is dissolved in water leaving behind nitrogen.

$$P_4 + 5O_2 \longrightarrow P_4O_{10} \xrightarrow{6H_2O} 4H_3PO_4$$

Oxygen present in air can be removed by passing over red hot copper gauze which forms copper oxide.

Carbon dioxide of the air is separated by passing it through potassium hydroxide.

2. When a solution of sodium nitrite and ammonium chloride or sulphate is reacted, nitrogen is formed.

$$NaNO_2 + NH_4Cl \underset{-NaCl}{\longrightarrow} NH_4NO_2 \longrightarrow N_2 + H_2O$$

3. Nitrogen is also formed when ammonium dichromate is heated.

$$(NH_4)_2 Cr_2O_7 \longrightarrow N_2 + Cr_2O_3 + 4H_2O$$

4. Oxidation of ammonia with red hot copper oxide or chlorine also produces nitrogen.

$$8NH_3 + 3Cl_2 \longrightarrow N_2 + 6NH_4Cl$$

Physical Characters

Nitrogen is a colourless, odourless and tasteless gas which is non-inflammable and does not support in combustion. It condenses to a liquid, b.p. -195.8°; solidifies to a snow-white mass, mp-210°. It is soluble in water (1 in 65) and alcohol (1 in 9) at normal temperature and pressure. It is stored under compression in metal cylinders.

Chemical Properties

1. Nitrogen neither burns nor support in burning. However, burning of magnesium and aluminium continues in an atmosphere of nitrogen forming nitrides.

$$3\ Mg + N_2 \longrightarrow Mg_3N_2$$
$$2Al + N_2 \longrightarrow 2AlN$$

2. Nitrogen is an inactive gas and combines with other elements with difficulty. With oxygen it combines only in the presence of lightning discharge. With hydrogen it reacts under

pressure and in the presence of a catalyst. With calcium carbide it reacts at high temperature to form calcium cyanamide (a fertilizer).

$$N_2 + O_2 \rightleftharpoons 2NO$$

$$N_2 + 3N_2 \xrightarrow[\text{Fe + Mo}]{\text{200-900 atm}} 2\,NH_3$$

$$\underset{\substack{\text{Calcium} \\ \text{carbide}}}{CaC_2 + N_2} \longrightarrow \underset{\substack{\text{Calcium} \\ \text{cyanamide}}}{CaCN_2 + C}$$

Test for Purity : Test for CO_2.

Uses : Nitrogen is used as a diluent for pure oxygen or other active gases and as an inert gas to replace air in containers holding oxidisable substances, e.g. cod liver oil, olive oil, and multivitamin preparations. Liquid nitrogen is used as a cryotherapeutic agent for the removal of warts and malignant growths, the treatment of cysts in acne vulgaris and for preservation of tissues and organisms. It is also used to retard oxidation in the qualitative test for carbon monoxide. The determination of a patient's nitrogen balance is an important diagnostic parameter.

Nitrogen narcosis has been reported from nitrogen breathed at high pressure.

SODIUM NITRITE

$NaNO_2$; Mol. Weight = 69.0

It contains 97 to 101 per cent of $NaNO_2$, calculated with reference to the substance dried over silica gel for four hours.

Preparation

1. Sodium nitrite is prepared by strongly heating sodium nitrate;

$$2NaNO_3 \longrightarrow 2NaNO_2 + O_2$$

2. It is also prepared by heating sodium nitrate with metallic lead or carbon which reduces it at lower temperature.

$$NaNO_3 + Pb \longrightarrow NaNO_2 + PbO$$

$$2NaNO_3 + C \longrightarrow 2NaNO_2 + CO_2$$

The reaction mixture is cooled and the product is extracted with water. The insoluble lead oxide is filtered off, the filtrate is concentrated and crystallized.

3. The gases formed during the catalytic oxidation of ammonia in sodium carbonate solution on absorption give sodium nitrite.

$$2Na_2CO_3 + 4NO + O_2 \longrightarrow 4NaNO_2 + 2CO_2$$

4. It is also prepared by heating a mixture of sodium nitrate solution and quicklime and then passing air free SO_2 through the solution.

$$NaNO_3 + CaO + SO_2 \longrightarrow CaSO_4 + NaNO_2$$

Physical Characters : Sodium nitrite occurs as white or slightly yellow granular powder or fused masses or sticks; odourless; taste is saline; deliquescent; hygroscopic; very slowly oxidizes to nitrate in air; m.p. 271°. It is soluble in water (1 in 1.5); sparingly soluble in alcohol. Solutions in water are alkaline to litmus.

Chemical Properties

1. Sulphuric acid reacts with sodium nitrite solution forming nitrous acid.

$$2NaNO_2 + H_2SO_4 \longrightarrow Na_2SO_4 + 2HNO_2$$
$$\downarrow$$
$$H_2O + NO + HNO_3$$

2. Sodium nitrite acts as a reducing as well as oxidizing agent. It is readily oxidized by $KMnO_4$ or $KClO_3$.

$$KClO_3 + 3HNO_2 \longrightarrow 3HNO_3 + KCl$$

When nitrites react as oxidizing agents, the reduced product will be nitric oxide (NO) in acidic solution.

3. With aniline hydrochloride at 4°C, nitrous acid forms diazonium chloride;

$$\underset{\text{Aniline}}{C_6H_5NH_2, HCl} + HNO_2 \longrightarrow \underset{\text{Diazonium chloride}}{C_6H_5N_2Cl} + 2H_2O$$

4. Sodium nitrite forms complex ions with metallic salts, eg. $Co^{3+}, Fe^{2+}, Cr^{3+}, Pt^{2+}$. The cobaltic nitrite complex $[Co(NO_2)_6]^{3-}$ is used in analytical chemistry.

5. Sodium nitrite oxidizes Fe^{++} in dilute acetic acid solution forming a typical brown colour of $Fe(NO)^{++}$ whereas sodium nitrate does not.

Tests for Purity : Tests for heavy metals; chloride; sulphate; loss on drying.

Tests for Identification : A solution of it responds to the tests for sodium and for nitrite.

Incompatibility : It is incompatible with acetanilide, antipyrine, phenazone, caffeine citrate, chlorates, hypophosphites, iodides, mercury salts, permanganate, sulphites, tannic acid, vegetable astringent decoctions, infusions or tinctures.

Assay : The assay is based on oxidation reduction titration as discussed for hydrogen peroxide and ferrous sulphate. A weighed amount (1 g) is dissolved in water to make 100 ml. The solution (10 ml) is added by a pipette to a mixture of 0.1 N potassium permanganate (50 ml), water (100 ml) and sulphuric acid (5 ml) immersing the tip of the pipette beneath the surface of the mixture during the addition. The liquid is warmed to 40°, allowed it to stand for five minutes, and 0.1 N oxalic acid (25 ml) added, the mixture heated to about 80° and titrated with 0.1 N potassium permanganate. Each ml of 0.1 N potassium permanganate is equivalent to 0.00345 g of $NaNO_2$.

Uses : Sodium nitrite is used in the treatment of cyanide poisoning in conjugation with sodium thiosulphate. The sodium nitrite produces methaemoglobinaemia and the cyanide ions combine with the methaemoglobin (modified haemoglobin incapable of transporting oxygen) to produce cyanmeth-aemoglobin, thus protecting cytochrome oxidase from the cyanide ions. As the cyanmethaemoglobin slowly dissociates, the cyanide is converted to relatively nontoxic thiocyanate by the sodium thiosulphate and is excreted in the urine. Sodium nitrite is also used as a rust inhibitor, preservative in foods such as cured meats; for manufacturing dyes, photographs and as vasodilator. Nitrites are used in urine solutions for the curing of meals and fish.

Sodium nitrite may cause nausea and vomiting, abdominal pain, dizziness, headache, cyanosis and dyspnoea (difficulty in breathing).

4

GASTROINTESTINAL AGENTS

For the treatment of gastrointestinal disorders of more serious conditions the inorganic drugs used are acidifying agent changing gastric pH, protectives for intestinal inflammation, adsorbents for intestinal toxins and laxatives (cathartic) for constipation.

(A) ACIDIFYING AGENT

The condition of the absence of hydrochloric acid in the gastric secretions (achlorhydria) may be due to free of gastric hydrochloric acid after stimulation with histamine phosphate or due to a lack of gastric hydrochloric acid though there may be stimulation by histamine. The first condition is found in persons with a gastectomy, atrophic gastritis, carcinoma of the stomach, or gastric polyps. The second condition is caused by chronic nephritis and alcoholism, tuberculosis, hyperthyroidism, pellagra (nutritional disorder), spru (frothy diarrhoea) and parasitic infections.

The gastric hydrochloric acid promotes formation of pepsin, a proteolytic enzyme; softens fibrous foods and destroys the bacteria in ingested food materials. When the pH of the gastric contents drops below 6, pepsin in formed from pepsinogen and its activity is greatest below pH 3.5. Thus, a scarcity of hydrochloric acid is responsible for gastrointestinal disorders. The symptoms of achlorhydria include mild diarrhoea, loose motions, epigastric pain, and sensitivity to spicy foods.

Acidifying agents are given orally. After absorption hydrogen ion is formed. Ammonium chloride, ammonium nitrate and calcium chloride are used as acidifying agents. Liver converts ammonium ions to urea which is then excreted as diuretic. The chloride ions form hydrochloric acid, which by reacting with HCO_3^- of blood, depletes the alkali reserve of the body. The excess of acid is eliminated in urine to make the urine acidic.

DILUTE HYDROCHLORIC ACID

Dilute hydrochloric acid is 9.5 to 10.5% w/v of HCl prepared by mixing hydrochloric acid (274 g) with water (726 g). It is stored below 30° in airtight containers of glass or other internal material.

When diluted hydrochloric acid is further diluted with 25 to 50 volumes of water, it may be used as a gastric acidifier to treat achlorhydria caused due to low level of hydrochloric acid on gastric juice.

Tests for Identification : As for concentrated HCl (page 19).

Assay : Accurately weighed sample (10 g) is titrated with 1 N NaOH solution as described under concentrated HCl.

Diluted hydrochloric acid can be used as an acidifying agent. It forms water soluble hydrochloride salts with organic bases; is used to extract basic drugs and to test for alkaline properties.

(B) ANTACIDS

Antacids are substances which reduce gastric acidity, resulting in an increase in the pH of the stomach and duodenum. In addition to increase of pH above 4, they inhibit the proteolytic activity of pepsin. They produce symptomatic relief of the uncomfortable feeling from overeating, heart burn and a growing hungry feeling between meals. The main functions of an antacid are to neutralize excess gastric hydrochloric acid which may cause pain and ulceration and to inactivate the proteolytic enzyme, pepsin. Certain antacids like sodium bicarbonate may raise it above pH 7. Reduction in acidity may inhibit pepsin release and interfere with digestic process. Antacids do not coat the mucosal lining, but may have a local astringent effect. The continual hyperacidity may lead to peptic or duodenal ulcer.

The stomach pH may be from 1 due to high concentration of endogenous hydrochloric acid when empty to 7 when food is taken. In case of hyperacidity, gastritis (a general inflammation of the gastric mucosa) and peptic ulcer may develop. A peptic ulcer may be present in the lower esophagus (esophageal ulcer); stomach (gastric ulcer), duodenum (duodenal ulcer) or on the jejunal side of gastrojejunostomy. The esophageal ulcer occurs when the esophageal sphincter is defective, suffer from heartburn. These people get relief by sleeping in a bed elevated at the head to reduce the flow of gastric fluid from the stomach into the esophagus.

Gastric ulcer occurs in the lesser curvature of the stomach. Patients with this ulcer have a lower secreation of acid. Haemorrhage is more common with gastric than the duodenal ulcers.

An ideal antacid (i) should be quick acting, (ii) should not liberate CO_2, and cause rebound hyperacidity, (iii) should not produce systemic alkalosis, (iv) should not interfere with absorption of food, and (v) should be palatable and inexpensive. The neutralizing capacity of the antacid substance is expressed in milli equivalents (mEq) of hydrochloric acid. Every antacid product must have a total neutralizing capicity of at least 5 mEq of hydrochloric acid per dosage unit. This is enough to raise the pH in an essentially empty stomach to 3.5. The more potent a product is, the more acid it can neutralize. A product that neutralize 2.5 mEq acid per dose is half as potent as one that neutralizes 5 mEq, one that neutralizes 10 mEq is twice as potent.

The choice of preparation usually depends on patient's acceptability. Mixing salts can prevent constipation or diarrhoea. Liquids and powders have a more rapid action, but are bulky to carry. Tablets should be chewed or sucked. Antacids should be given after a meal as their action is then prolonged. Antacids reduce the absorption of tetracycline antibiotics and should not be administered along with these antibiotics. Most of the antacid preparations are available in combination formulations.

Antacids, which locally neutralize the hyperacidity, are broadly grouped into;

(i) *Systemic (absorbable) antacids*, e.g. sodium bicarbonate, which is soluble, readily absorable and capable of producing systemic electrolytic alterations and alkalosis.

(ii) *Non-systemic (non-absorable) antacids*, e.g. aluminium salts, magnesium salts, calcium carbonate and sodium carboxymethylcellulose, which are not absorbed to a significant extent and thus do not exert a systemic effect.

Antiflatuents are generally included in antacid formulations. They act by reducing the surface tension of bubbles in the stomach making them coalesce and more easily expelled by eructation.

Antacids are normally given between meals and at bedtimes when symptoms occur. Gastro-intestinal absorption can be reduced by adsorption on insoluble antacids or changes in gastric emptying time. The effect of a drug may be diminished or enhanced by alterations in the intestinal pH or by the formation of complexes.

ALUMINIUM HYDROXIDE GEL

$Al(OH)_3$; Mol. Weight = 78.0

Aluminium hydroxide gel is an aqueous suspension of hydrated aluminium oxide with different amounts of basic aluminium carbonate and bicarbonate. It contains about 3.5-4.4 per cent of Al_2O_3. It may contain glycerin, sorbitol, sucrose or saccharin as sweetening agent, peppermint oil or other suitable flavours. It may also contain suitable antimicrobial agent.

Preparation

When an aluminium salt (such as aluminium chloride or sulphate) is treated with ammonia or sodium carbonate, a white gelatinous precipitate of aluminium hydroxide is obtained. The intermediate product, aluminium carbonate, is so unstable that it immediately hydrolyzes to yield aluminium hydroxide and carbon dioxide.

$$AlCl_3 + 3NH_4OH \longrightarrow Al(OH)_3 + 3NH_4Cl$$

$$Al(OH)_3 + 3NaOH \longrightarrow Na_3AlO_3 + 3H_2O$$

DRIED ALUMINIUM HYDROXIDE GEL

It consists mainly of hydrated aluminium oxide and varying small quantities of basic aluminium carbonate and bicarbonate. It contains not less than 47.0 per cent of Al_2O_3 in the form of the hydrated oxide.

Physical Characters : Aluminium hydroxide is a white, light, odourless, tasteless amorphous powder containing some aggregates. It is practically insoluble in water and alcohol; soluble in dilute mineral acids and in solutions of alkali hydroxides. It forms gels on prolonged contact with water; pH 5.5-8.0. It absorbs acids and CO_2. It is stored in airtight containers at a temperature not exceeding 30°.

In the presence of an alkali, it behaves as an acid :

$$Al(OH)_3 \rightleftharpoons 3H^+ + AlO_3^{3-}$$

In acidic medium, it acts as a weak base :

$$Al(OH)_3 \rightleftharpoons Al^{3+} + 3OH^-$$

The aluminium hydroxide gels are ideal buffers in the pH 3-5 region due to their amphoteric character.

Test for Purity : Tests for arsenic; ammonium salts; chloride; lead; sulphate; alkalinity; neutralizing capacity; microbial limits; appearance; viscosity; X-ray diffraction pattern; differential thermal analysis.

The presance of ammonium salts is determined by heating the substance with sodium hydroxide to yield ammonia which is collected in standard acid and back-titrated by the usual procedure. The limit of ammonia in aluminium hydroxide is determined to be 0.034 per cent.

Neutralizing capacity is found by measuring pH of suspension of the substance in a medium which is approximately N/20 in respect of hydrochloric acid.

An aqueous solution after addition of hydrochloric acid complies with the limit test for chlorides.

An acidified solution with hydrochloric acid complies with the limit test for sulphates.

The total microbial count does not exceed 100 per ml. It shows the tests for the absence of *E. Coli:* and pseudomonas.

Test for Identification : A solution in dilute hydrochloric acid gives the reactions of aluminium.

Assay : Both the forms are assayed in terms of their aluminium oxide (Al_2O_3) content and their acid consuming capacity.

Accurately weighed substance (5 g) is dissolved in hydrochloric acid (3 ml) and diluted with water (100 ml). To the solution (20 ml), 0.05 M disodium ethylenediaminetetraacetate (40 ml), water (80 ml) and methyl red solution (indicator) are added and the mixture is neutralized with 1 N NaOH. It is warmed for 30 minutes, hexamine (3 g) is added and titrated with 0.05 M lead nitrate, using xylenol orange solution as indicator. Each ml of 0.05 M disodium ethylenediaminetetra acetate is equivalent to 0.002549 g of Al_2O_3.

Uses : Aluminium hydroxide is a gastric antacid. It buffers the gastric acid and so raises the pH and reduces acid induced damage. It is used as a phosphate binder in patients with chronic renal failure and as an adjuvant in the manufacture of adsorbed vaccines. It is not absorbed in the gastro-intestinal tract and does not generate carbon dioxide as in case of metallic carbonates. It is also used in antiperspirants and dentifrices. It does not significantly affect the pepsin activity. It has astringent and demulcent properties by which it forms a protective coating over the ulcer crater. It may also absorb toxins.

Aluminium hydroxide is astringent and may cause nausea, vomiting and constipation; large doses can cause intestinal obstructions.

Aluminium salts are available as liquid, powder or tablets. The choice of preparation depends on patient acceptability. Liquids and powders have a more rapid action but are bulky to carry. Aluminium hydroxide has no effect on the volume of gastric juice nor on the total output of hydrogen ions.

The antacid properties are lost on ageing. The rate of loss is dependent upon the pH used to precipitate the gel.

ALUMINIUM PHOSPHATE

$AlPO_4$; Mol. Weight = 122.0

Aluminium phosphate consists mainly of hydrated aluminium orthophosphate containing not less than 80.0% of $AlPO_4$. It occurs in nature as the minerals *angelite; coeruleolactite; evansite; lucinite; sterretite; variscite; wavellite;* etc. It is prepared by treating aluminium sodium oxide ($NaAlO_2$) with phosphoric acid (H_3PO_4). It may be prepared by drying under suitable conditions the product of interaction in aqueous solution of an aluminium salt with an alkali phosphate such as sodium phosphate.

Characters : It is a white infusible powder containing some friable aggregates; m.p. above 1460°. It is practically insoluble in water, alcohol (95%), solutions of alkali hydroxides or acetic acid; very slightly soluble in concentrated hydrochloric acid and nitric acid. A 4% suspension in water has a pH of 5.5 to 6.5. It is stored in well-closed containers at a temperature not exceeding 30°.

Aluminium phosphate gel is a white, viscous suspension from which small amounts of water may separate on standing. It may contain suitable preservatives. The gel has a pH in the range 6.0 to 7.2.

Tests for Purity : Tests for arsenic; heavy metals; chlorides; sulphate; soluble phosphate; alkalinity; and neutralizing capacity.

For determining neutralizing capacity the substance is passed through a sieve and treated with hydrochloric acid at 37°. The pH of the mixture at 37° is 2.0 to 2.5.

Soluble phosphate is determined by adding sulphuric acid, ammonium molybdate and methylaminophenol - sulphite reagent to an aqueous solution of the substance. The absorbance is measured of the resulting solution. The content of soluble phosphate is calculated from a calibration curve prepared by treatings suitable aliquots of a 0.00286% solution of potassium dihydrogen orthophosphate in the same manner.

Tests for Identification

1. A solution in 2N hydrochloric acid gives the reactions characteristic of aluminium salts.
2. A solution in 2N nitric acid gives the reactions characteristic of phosphate.

Assay : The assay is based on complexometric titration as disassed for magnesium sulphate and calcium gluconate. It is assayed in terms of aluminium phosphate ($AlPO_4$) content. To an acidified solution of weighed amount of the substance (0.8 g), disodium acetate is added and made alkaline with ammonia. Ammonium acetate (7.7 g) is added, pH adjusted to 4.5 with glacial acetic acid and a dithizone in ethanol added. Sufficient ethanol is added and titrated with 0.05 N zine chloride until the colour changes to red. A blank experiment is performed. The difference between the titrations represents the amount of disodium edetate required. Each ml of 0.05 M disodium edetate is equivalent to 6.098 mg of $AlPO_4$.

Uses : Aluminium phosphate is an antacid and used as an adjuvant in the manufacture of adsorbed vaccines. It is used in place of aluminium hydroxide gel where loss of phosphate may be a problem to the patient. The acid consuming ability of the phosphate is dependent on the release of phosphate anions.

$$AlPO_4 \rightleftharpoons Al^{+3} + PO_4^{-3}$$

$$PO_4^{-3} + H_3O^+ \xrightarrow{-H_2O} HPO_3^{-2} \xrightarrow{-H_3O^+} H_2PO_4^- + H_2O$$

Aluminium phosphate is highly water soluble and is absorbed as phosphate anion by gastric acid.

CALCIUM CARBONATE

(Precipitated Chalk)

$CaCO_3$; Mol. Weight = 100.0

Calcium carbonate is found in nature as limestone, marble, aragonite, calcite, vaterite, iceland spar, dolomite and shells of sea animals.

The official drug is the precipitated calcium carbonate containing 98 to 100.5 per cent of $CaCO_3$.

Preparation

Calcium carbonate is precipitated when carbon dioxide is passed through lime-water or a solution of sodium carbonate is added to calcium chloride.

$$CaCO_3 + CO_2 + H_2O \longrightarrow Ca(HCO_3)_2$$
Insoluble   Soluble

$$CaCl_2 + Na_2CO_3 \rightleftharpoons CaCO_3 + 2NaCl$$

Physical Characters : Calcium carbonate occurs as a white, odourless, tasteless microcrystalline powder which is stable in air. It is dimorphous and two crystal forms are of commercial importance :

(i) Aragonite, orthorhombic, m,p, 825° (dec), formed above 30°;

(ii) Calcite, hexagonal rhombohedral, m.p. 1339°, formed below 30°. It is practically insoluble in water; its solubility in water is increased by the presence of carbon dioxide or ammonium salts; practically insoluble in alcohol; soluble with effervescence in acetic acid, hydrochloric acid, and nitric acid. The presence of any alkali hydroxide reduces its stability.

Precipitated calcium carbonate is 98-99% $CaCO_3$.

Calcite widely occurs in nature. Iceland spar is a very pure form of calcite and present as transparent, colourless crystals. Marble and limestone are also calcite having interlocking crystals. Chalk, eggshell, corals, shells of mollusca and bones also contain calcium carbonate in the form of calcite.

Precipitated chalk is prepared as a fine precipitate by adding a solution of ammonium carbonate and ammonia or sodium carbonate to a solution of calcium nitrate.

Hardness of water is due to the presence of calcium and magnesium salts. If bicarbonates are present, water is boiled to produce a carbonate and hardness of water is removed.

Calcium carbonate is stored in well-closed containers.

Chemical Properties

Calcium carbonate is decomposed at about 83° into CaO and CO_2

$$CaCO_3 \xrightarrow{\Delta} CaO + CO_2$$

In the presence of CO_2 calcium carbonate dissolves in water due to the formation of calcium bicarbonate.

$$\underset{\text{Insoluble}}{CaCO_3 + CO_2 + H_2O} \longrightarrow \underset{\text{Soluble}}{Ca(HCO_3)_2}$$

Tests for Purity : Test for aluminium; arsenic; iron; lead; barium; magnesium and alkali metals; phosphate; sulphate; chloride; heavy metals; hydrochloric insoluble matter; soluble alkali; and loss on drying.

A solution of calcium carbonate in hydrochloric acid is boiled to liberate CO_2. When the solution is made alkaline with ammonia, aluminium and iron are precipitated as hydroxides. The hydroxides are filtered off and washed with dilute ammonium chloride solution to prevent peptization of aluminium hydroxide. The adsorbed calcium ions are separated by re-precipitation and the precipitate is washed finally with dilute ammonium nitrate to prevent peptization. The residue containing aluminium, iron, phosphate, and the hydrochloric acid insoluble matter is ignited at about 1000°C. The presence of iron can be determined by the ordinary limit test.

Chloride and soluble alkali may be present when calcium carbonate is not properly washed during its preparation.

An acidified solution with nitric acid complies with the limit test for chlorides.

Acid-insoluble substances are determined by treating calcium carbonate with hydrochloric acid at higher temperature. The solution is filtered, the residue washed with water and dried at 105° for one hour.

Magnesium and alkali metals are detected by neutralizing an acidified solution of the substance with dilute ammonia. Acetic acid and ammonium oxalate solution are added, filtered and dilute sulphuric acid added. The solution is dried, the residue ignited and weighed.

Soluble alkali is determine by neutralizing an aqueous solution with 0.1 N sulphuric acid using methyl orange solution as indicator.

An aqueous solution is acidified with acetic acid and calcium sulphate solution added. If the solution remains clear for not less than fifteen minutes, barium is absent.

Tests for Identification : When calcium carbonate (few mg) is added to acetic acid, effervescence is produced and the resulting solution, after boiling, gives the reactions of calcium.

Incompatibility : Acids, alum, ammonium salts.

Assay : The assay is based on the complexometric titration as discussed for calcium gluconate and magnesium sulphate. Accurately weighed calcium carbonate (0.1 g) is dissolved in dilute hydrochloric acid (3 ml) and water (10 ml). The reaction mixture is boiled for 10 minutes, cooled, and diluted to 50 ml with water. It is titrated with 0.05 M disodium ethylenediamine tetraacetate; sodium hydroxide solution and calcon mixture are added to get and point, and the titration is continued until the colour of the solution changes from pink to a full blue colour. Each ml of 0.05 M disodium ethylenediaminetetraacetate is equivalent to 0.0050 of $CaCO_3$.

Uses : Due to its fast action calcium carbonate is used as an antacid; as a calcium supplement in deficiency states; as a food additive and in homoepathic medicine (Calcarea carbonica; Calc. Carb). Other uses of calcium carbonate are in dentifrices, insecticides, cosmetics, antibiotics and antidiarrhoeal agent. As gastric hydrochloric acid consumes the solubilized calcium carbonate, more compound is dissolved into the solution.

$$CaCO_3 \longrightarrow Ca^{+2} + CO_3^{-2}$$

$$H_3O^+ + CO_3^{-2} \longrightarrow H_2CO_3 \longrightarrow H_2O + CO_2$$

The calcium cations can be absorbed or precipitated as the insoluble calcium phosphate salt in the intestine or as insoluble calcium soap from the hydrolyzed glyceride formed due to digesting of food.

Most calcium carbonate preparations are available with magnesium antacid due to calcium's constipative effect.

Calcium carbonate may cause constipation and hypercalcaemia. The liberation of carbon dioxide may cause discomfort in some patients.

MAGNESIUM CARBONATE

$(MgCO_3)_4$; $Mg(OH)_2$; $5H_2O$; Approx. Mol. Weight = 485

Magnesium carbonate is a hydrated basic magnesium carbonate containing the equivalent of 40.0 to 45.0% of MgO. It occurs in nature as the mineral *magnesite* and *lansfordite*.

Preparation

Magnesium carbonate is precipitated by the addition of sodium carbonate to an aqueous solution of a magnesium salt and saturating it with CO_2.

$$MgCl_2 + 2NaHCO_3 + CO_2 + H_2O \longrightarrow MgCO_3\downarrow + 2NaCl + 2H_2CO_3$$

Usually a basic carbonate, $(MgCO_3)_4$. $Mg(OH)_2$. $5H_2O$, is obtained by precipitation of a magnesium salt with any soluble carbonate.

Heavy Magnesium Carbonate is a hydrated basic carbonate, $(MgCO_3)_3$. $Mg(OH)_2$. $4H_2O$ containing 40 to 45 per cent of MgO.

For its preparation the hot solutions of magnesium sulphate (125 parts) and sodium carbonate (150 parts) in water (250 parts each) are mixed, evaporated to dryness and the residue is treated with water. The insoluble carbonate is filtered, washed and dried in an oven.

Light Magnesium Carbonate, $(MgCO_3)_3$ $Mg(OH)_2$. $3H_2O$ is a hydrated basic carbonate, containing about 40 to 45 per cent of CaO. It is prepared by mixing solutions of magnesium sulphate (125 parts) and sodium carbonate (150 parts) in water (1000 parts each). The combined solution is boiled (15 minutes). The precipitate is filtered, washed and dried in oven.

Characters

Both heavy and light magnesium carbonate are hydrated basic magnesium carbonates containing the equivalent of 40 to 45% of MgO. Both are white, odourless powders or light, white, friable masses. They are stable in air; practically insoluble in water and alcohol but dissolve in dilute acids with strong effervescence. At about 700°, they are converted into MgO.

$$MgCO_3 \longrightarrow MgO + CO_2$$
$$4MgCO_3.Mg(OH)_2.5H_2O \longrightarrow 5MgO + 4CO_2 + 6H_2O$$

Test for Purity : Tests for arsenic; calcium; chloride; copper; iron; lead; sulphate; heavy metals; soluble matter; residue to ignition; substances insoluble in acetic acid.

On ignition the substance losses from 55.0 to 58.0 per cent of its weight.

Test for Identification : A solution in dilute nitric acid gives the reactions of magnesium, and of carbonates.

Assay : The assay is based on the complexometric titration as discussed for calcium gluconate and magnesium sulphate. Accurately weighed substance (0.18g) is dissolved in dilute hydrochloric acid (2 ml). Water (50 ml) and strong ammonia-ammonium chloride solution (10 ml) are added and titrated with 0.05 M disodium ethylenediaminetetraacetate, using 0.1g of mordant black 11 mixture as indicator until the pink colour is discharged from the blue. Each ml of 0.05 M disodium ethylene-diaminetetra acetate is equivalent to 0.002015 g of MgO.

Uses : Magnesium carbonate is an antacid, cathartic and laxative; also used as a food additive, in tooth and face powders.

The antacid properties of magnesium carbonate are due to the carbonate and hydroxide anions reacting with the hydrochloric acid of gastric juice. Due to its slight solubility, it dissolves only as carbonate and the hydroxide is being utilized.

Magnesium carbonate in common with other magnesium salts may cause diarrhoea. The release of CO_2 in the stomach may cause discomfort.

MAGNESIUM OXIDE
(Magnesia)

MgO; Mol. Weight = 40.3

Magnesium oxide contains not less than 98.0% of MgO.

It occurs in nature as the mineral *periclase*. Magnesium oxide after ignition contains about 98 per cent of MgO. It is either the heavy or light variety. Heavy magnesium oxide is a relatively dense white powder with 5 g occupying a volume of about 10 to 20 ml. The light variety is a very bulky white powder with 5 g occupying a volume of about 40 to 50 ml.

Preparation

Magnesium oxide is prepared by gently heating the magnesium carbonate.

$$MgCO_3 \longrightarrow MgO + CO_2$$

When light carbonate is heated to redness, MgO is formed;

$$3MgCO_3 \cdot Mg(OH)_2 \cdot 3H_2O \longrightarrow 4MgO + 3CO_2\uparrow + 4H_2O$$

Characters

Light magnesium oxide is a very light, bulky, white powder whereas heavy magnesium oxide is a dense mass. Both the oxides are odourless, taste slightly alkaline; practically insoluble in water yielding a solution which is alkaline to phenolphthalein but dissolve in dilute acid with slight effervescence. They absorb moisture and CO_2 when exposed to air. The aqueous solutions are alkaline to phenolphthalein; pH of saturated aqueous solution is 10.3. In the presence of acid, the oxide forms the magnesium hydroxide. Therefore, the chemistry and pharmacology are the same as those of magnesium hydroxide.

$$MgO + H_3O^+ \longrightarrow Mg(OH)_2 + 2H_2O$$

Magnesium oxide is soluble in carbonic acid solution.

$$MgO + H_2O + 2CO_2 \longrightarrow Mg^{+2} + 2HCO_3^-$$

Magnesium oxide reacts with acids to form salts.

$$MgO + 2HCl \longrightarrow MgCl_2 + H_2O$$

At very high temperatures it reacts with carbon to form magnesium carbide (MaC_2).

$$CaC_2 + MgO \longrightarrow MgC + CaO + C$$

Magnesium oxide takes CO_2 and water from the air, the light form more readily than the heavy.

Magnesium oxide should be kept in a well-closed container.

Tests for Purity : Tests for arsenic; lead; calcium; copper; iron; heavy metals; chloride; sulphate; colour of solution; substances insoluble in acetic acid; soluble matter; and loss on ignition.

Loss on ignition of magnesium oxide is not more than 5.0 per cent of its weight.

For the test of calcium, it is precipitated as calcium sulphate in aqueous ethanolic solution. The solution is kept for several hours; the precipitate is filtered, washed with aqueous-alcoholic sulphuric acid, dried, ignited and weighed.

The following are the tests of copper :

1. Hydrogen sulphide is passed through a solution of copper salt to yield black precipitate of cupric sulphide.

CuS. The precipitate is insoluble in yellow ammonium sulphide, but soluble in boiling dilute nitric acid.

2. When ammonia solution is added to a solution of a copper salt, a pale blue precipitate of cupric hydroxide, $Cu(OH)_2$, is formed. The precipitate is soluble in excess of the ammonia solution giving a deep blue solution due to formation of the cuprammonium cation, $Cu(NH_3)_4{}^{2+}$.

3. Treatment of a solution of a copper salt, acidified with acetic acid, with potassium ferrocyanide, forms brown precipitate of copper ferrocyanide.

4. When copper compounds are burnt in a flame, colour of the flame becomes green.

Test for Identification : A solution in dilute nitric acid gives the reaction of magnesium.

Calcium oxide is tested by calcination. The weight of calcium sulphate is converted into percentage of calcium oxide as :

136.1 g of calcium sulphate are equivalent to CaO.

Assay : The assay is based on the complexometric titration. A weighed amount of the substance (0.1 g) is dissolved in dilute hydrochloric acid (2 ml). Strong ammonia - ammonium chloride (10 ml) is added and the reaction mixture titrated with 0.05 M disodium ethylenediaminetetracetate, using 0.1 g of mordant black 11 mixture as indicator until the pink colour is discharged from the blue. Each ml of 0.05 M disodium ethylenediaminetetra acetate is equivalent to 0.002015 g of MgO.

Uses : Magnesium oxide is an antacid and possesses osmotic laxative properties. It is also used as a food additive, in hypomagnesemia, gastric ulcers, compounding and preserving fluid extracts due to its absorptive properties and in dentrifices.

Adverse effects are the same as for magnesium carbonate, but without release of carbon dioxide.

MAGNESIUM TRISILICATE

$2MgO, 3SiO_2 . 3H_2O$; Mol. Weight (anhydrous) = 260.86.

Magnesium trisilicate is a hydrated magnesium silicate corresponding to the formula $2MgO, 3SiO_2$ with varying proportions of water of crystallization. It contains about 29 to 32 per cent of MgO and 65 to 68.5 per cent of SiO_2.

Its composition varies according to the conditions of preparation and it contains 3 or 4 moles of water of crystallization. I.P. and B.P. require it to contain not less than 30% and not more than 32.0% of MgO and not less than 66.0% and not more than 69.5% of SiO_2 calculated as residue left on ignition at 1000°C.

Preparation

It is prepared by precipitation from solutions of magnesium sulphate and sodium silicate.

$$2MgSO_4 + 2Na_2O.3SiO_2 \longrightarrow H_2O + Na_2SO_4$$

The precipitate is filtered, washed, dried and powdered.

Magnesium trisilicate is also prepared by adding hydrochloric acid to a solution of sodium silicate followed by addition of precipitated magnesium hydroxide.

Characters : It is an odourless, fine, white, tasteless powder free from gritty particles. It is practically insoluble in water and alcohol; readily decomposed by mineral acids. It is stored in well-closed containers.

Magnesium trisilicate is decomposed with hydrochloric acid into a magnesium salt and silicic acid. In the presence of alkali carbonates it is decomposed into magnesium carbonate and soluble silicate.

$$2MgO. 3SiO_2 + 4HCl \longrightarrow MgCl_2 + H_4Si_3O_8\downarrow$$
$$\text{Trisilicic acid}$$

In stomach, the gelatinous trisilicic acid is formed with gastric hydrochloric acid.

Tests for Purity : Tests for arsenic; chloride; iron; lead; sulphate; heavy metals; chloride; acid absorption; free alkali; soluble salts; and loss on ignition.

Acid absorption is determined with a weighed quantity of the substance and N/20 hydrochloric acid kept at body temperature (37°) for three hours. Free alkali soluble salts are determined by boiling the substance in water, cooling and replacing the water loss by evaporation. The solution is allowed to stand for 15 minutes and filtered. Free alkali is determined by neutralizing with hydrochloric acid using phenolphthalein as indicator. Free salts are determined by evaporating the filtrate to dryness and then ignited.

Development of any pink colour on addition of phenol-phthalein to the aqueous solution indicated the presence of free alkali.

For determining water soluble salts, an aqueous solution is evaporated to dryness. The residue is ignited and weighed.

The presence of heavy metals, chloride and sulphate is determined as mentioned in the limit tests.

Test for Identification : The substance (0.5 g) is boiled with sodium hydroxide solution (10 ml), filtered; the filtrate is acidified with dilute hydrochloric acid and boiled. A white gelatinous precipitate is produced slowly. The residue is washed on the filter paper with water, dissolved in dilute hydrochloric acid and filtered. The filtrate gives the reaction of magnesium.

Assay : It is assayed in terms of silicon dioxide and magnesium oxide and must have a definite magnesium oxide and silicon dioxide ratio. As the amount of silicon dioxide increases with respect to magnesium oxide, antacid property is decreased.

For MgO : A weighed quantity of the substance (1 g) is heated with hydrochloric acid (35 ml) and water (50 ml), cooled, filtered, and the residue washed with water. The filtrate and washings are diluted with water (250 ml) and neutralized with 10N sodium hydroxide solution. Ammonia buffer (pH 10) and mordant black 11 mixture are added, heated to 40° and titrated with 0.05 M disodium ethylenediaminetetra acetate until the colour changes from violet to full blue. Each ml of 0.05 M disodium ethylenediaminetetra acetate is equivalent to 0.002015 g of MgO.

For SiO$_2$: A mixture of the substance (0.7 g), 1N sulphuric acid (10 ml) and water (10 ml) is heated for 90 minutes. It is cooled, decanted onto an ashless filter paper, and the precipitate washed with hot water to remove sulphate ions (filtrate is tested with barium chloride solution and hydrochloric acid). The filter paper is ignited and weighed.

Uses : Magnesium trisilicate is an antacid used to neutralize excess amount of hydrochloric acid in the stomach. It relieves pain in gastric and duodenal ulcers and possibly absorbs the pepsin. When magnesium trisilicate is taken by mouth, magnesium chloride and hydrated silica gel are formed during neutralization. The hydrated silica gel passes into the intestine where it acts as an adsorbent. The silica gel protects ulcers and acts as an antacid. Magnesium chloride has laxative action.

Its side effects are similar to that of magnesium carbonate.

SODIUM BICARBONATE
(Sodabicarb)

$NaHCO_3$; Mol. Weight = 84.01

Sodium bicarbonate contains not less than 99.0 per cent and not more than the equivalent of 100.5 per cent of $NaHCO_3$.

Preparation

1. Sodium bicarbonate is prepared from ammonium bicarbonate and sodium chloride.
2. Sodium carbonate is converted into the bicarbonate by passing carbon dioxide through a saturated solution.

$$Na_2CO_3 + H_2O + CO_2 \longrightarrow 2NaHCO_3$$

Physical Characters

Sodium bicarbonate occurs as a white odourless crystalline powder or granules. It begins to lose CO_2 at about 50° and at 100° it is converted into Na_2CO_3. It is soluble in water (1 in 12); practically insoluble in alcohol. The aqueous solution is alkaline to litmus; alkalinity increases on standing, agitation or heating. It is stored in well-closed containers.

Insoluble precipitates are formed when sodium bicarbonate solutions are mixed with calcium or magnesium salts, cisplatin, dobutamine hydrochloride or oxytetracycline. The following drugs are susceptible to inactivation on mixing with sodium bicarbonate solution; adrenaline hydrochloride, benzyl penicillin potassium, carmustine, glycopyrronium bromide; isoprenaline hydrochloride and suxamethonium chloride.

It is stable in dry air, but slowly decomposes in moist air.

Chemical Properties

1. When sodium bicarbonate is heated, it is decomposed into the normal carbonate, CO_2 and water.

$$2NaHCO_3 \longrightarrow Na_2CO_3 + H_2O + CO_2$$

2. A solution of sodium bicarbonate is alkaline due to hydrolysis (pH 8.2);

$$NaHCO_3 + H_2O \rightleftharpoons Na^+ + H_2CO_3 + {}^-OH$$

Sodium bicarbonate is slightly alkaline and fails to turn phenolphthalein red. On the other hand, in sodium carbonate the carbonate ion is so extensively hydrolyzed that the solution is quite alkaline (pH is 11.6).

$$CO_3^{-2} + H_2O \rightleftharpoons HCO_3^- + {}^-OH$$

3. When a mercuric chloride solution is added to a solution of sodium bicarbonate there is no immediate formation of a precipitate. After some time a reddish precipitate of HgO is formed.

$$2NaHCO_3 + HgCl_2 \longrightarrow 2NaCl + Hg(HCO_3)_2$$
$$Hg(HCO_3)_2 \longrightarrow HgO + H_2O + 2CO_2$$

4. When the bicarbonate is treated with an acid, carbon dioxide is liberated;

$$NaHCO_3 + HCl \longrightarrow NaCl + CO_2 + H_2O$$

Test for Purity : Tests for alkalinity; aluminium; calcium; insoluble matter; arsenic; iron; lead; chloride; sulphate; ammonium compounds.

For detecting the presence of aluminium, calcium and insoluble matter an aqueous solution is boiled with ammonia solution and filtered. The residue is ignited and weighed.

An aqueous solution after addition of nitric acid complies with the limit test for chloride.

An aqueous solution after addition of hydrochloric acid complies with the limit test for sulphates.

Evolution of ammonia on heating the substance with sodium hydroxide indicates the presence of ammonium compound.

An aqueous solution after addition of hydrochloric acid complies with the limit test for iron.

Heavy metals are determined by comparing the colour produced with the substance and with standard lead solution after treatment with hydrogen sulphide solution.

Simultaneous administration of sodium bicarbonate with other drugs inhibits the activity of the drug. Such a therapeutic incompatibility is found when sodium bicarbonate and sodium salicylate are used in equivalent amounts.

Test for Identification : It gives the reactions of sodium, and of bicarbonates.

Assay : Titrate with 0.5 N hydrochloric or sulphuric acid, using methyl orange as indicator.

$$HCl + NaHCO_3 \longrightarrow NaCl + H_2O + CO_2$$

$$2NaHCO_3 + H_2SO_4 \longrightarrow Na_2SO_4 + 2H_2O + 2CO_2$$

Each ml of 0.5 N hydrochloric acid is equivalent to 0.042 g of $NaHCO_3$.

It is a direct titration method. The end point in yellow to pink. The equivalence point of this titration is at about pH 3.6 which corresponds to the colour change methyl orange (pH 2.8 - 4.0, red-yellow). The reaction at the equivalence point is acidic because of the presence of carbonic acid.

$$CO_2 + H_2O \longrightarrow H_2CO_3$$

Uses : Sodium bicarbonate is an electrolyte replenisher, and systemic alkalinising agent used in the treatment of metabolic acidosis (increase in acidity), diarrhoea, acute poisoning from acidic drugs (phenobarbitone and salicylates), and as an antacid to relieve dyspepsia. Solutions of sodium bicarbonate are used as eye lotions, to aid the removal of crusts in blepharitis, as ear-drops, to soften and remove ear wax, and as lubricating fluid for contact lenses.

Administration of sodium bicarbonate by mouth can cause stomach cramps and flatulence. Its large quantities may cause systemic alkalosis, vertigo (loss of power of balancing) and jerky muscular movement.

Sodium bicarbonate is available as mint-flavoured soda-mint tablets. It is self-medicated, inexpensive and easily available drug. It is absorbed from the intestines which produces effects all over the body. It produces carbon dioxide gas in stomach and may cause perforation of a deep ulcer. Its onset of action is quick but the duration of action is short. It may cause rebound acidity due to short duration of action and systemic effects. When taken with milk it may cause milk alkali syndrome, characterized by deposition of calcium of milk on the kidney and increased blood urea.

COMBINATION ANTACID PREPARATIONS

No single antacid completes all the criteria for an ideal antacid, several products are available in the market containing mixtures of antacids. Most of these combination products have constipative effect of calcium and aluminium and laxative effect of magnesium. Some of these products are also a mixture of an antacid with rapid onset of action and one with a longer duration of action.

Aluminium hydroxide magnesium carbonate co-dried gel : It is a co-precipitate of aluminium hydroxide and magnesium carbonate carefully dried to contain a critical proportion of water for antacid activity. It acts as an antacid that is given in doses of up to 1 g.

Algicon Tablets : The tablets are chewable, prepared by aluminium hydroxide-magnesium carbonate co-dried gel (360 mg), magnesium alginate (500g), magnesium carbonate (320 mg) and potassium bicarbonate (100 mg).

The suspension is prepared by combining aluminium hydroxide-magnesium carbonate co-dried gel (140 mg), magnesium alginate (250 mg), magnesium carbonate (175 mg) and potassium bicarbonate (50 mg/5ml). Dose. 1 or 2 tablets or 10 to 20 ml of suspension after meals and at bedtime.

Simeco tablets contain aluminium hydroxide-magnesium carbonate co-dried gel (282 mg), magnesium hydroxide (85 mg) and activated dimethicone (25 mg).

Aluminium Hydroxide gel-Magnesium Trisilicate Combinations :

This is one of the more common combinations. It has laxative, constipative and protective effect.

Magaldrate : It is a chemical combination of aluminium hydroxide and magnesium hydroxide. It contains the equivalent of 28 to 39% magnesium oxide and 17 to 25% of aluminium oxide. It occurs as a white, odourless, crystalline powder which is insoluble in water and alcohol, but soluble in dilute solutions of mineral acids.

Calcium Carbonate Containing Antacid Mixtures : Calcium carbonate with aluminium hydroxide gel yields products which have a rapid onset with prolonged action. Three - part combinations of calcium carbonate, aluminium hydroxide gel and a magnesium containing antacid are also available.

Alginic acid Sodium Bicarbonate-Containing Antacid Mixtures : The tablet is chewed when the contents come in contact with water, the alginic acid reacts with sodium bicarbonate, forming sodium alginate and carbon dioxide. In the acid environment of the stomach, alginic acid is precipitated in the form of a light, viscous gel which floats on top of the stomach contents.

(C) PROTECTIVES AND ADSORBENTS

Inorganic agents used as protectives and adsorbents are used for the treatment of diarrhoea which may be mild or chronic. Mild diarrhoea is caused when some factors impair digestion or absorption, thereby increasing the bulk of the intestinal tract. Acute diarrhoea results from bacterial toxins, chemical poisons, drugs, allergy, and disease, carcinomas, gastrointestinal surgery, chronic inflammatory conditions, and various absorptive defects. Diarrhoea is a serious condition in which loss of fluids and electrolytes can readily lead to dehydration and electrolyte imbalance. Some of the bacterial toxins stimulate the flow of electrolytes into the intestines, thereby increasing the intestinal osmotic load. Most products used for the treatment of diarrhoea consist of an adsorbent protective, an antidiarrhoeal and antibacterial agent. The ideal antidiarrhoeal agent acts directly on the smooth muscles of the gut to produce a spasm like effect which reduces peristalsis (worm-like movement of stomach) and increases segmentation. The antibacterials are only effective if there is an actual infection in the intestinal tract. The adsorbent protectives adsorb toxins, bacteria, and viruses along with providing a protective coating of the intestinal mucosa. They include bismuth salts, activated charcoal and special clays.

BISMUTH SUBCARBONATE

$[(BiO_2)_2 \ CO_3]_2^- \ H_2O$

Bismuth subcarbonate contains not less than 82.5% of Bi and 79% of Bi_2O_3. It is a basic salt of variable composition.

Its composition varies with the conditions of preparation. It is prepared by dissolving metallic bismuth in 50 per cent nitric acid and the solution is concentrated by evaporation. The solution is then added to a cold solution of sodium carbonate with constant stirring. The precipitated basic carbonate is filtered, washed with an equal volume of cold water and dried below 60°. Repeated washings of the precipitate decompose the subnitrate into hydroxide.

$$2Bi + 8HNO_3 \longrightarrow 2Bi\,(NO_3)_3 + 2NO + 4H_2O$$

$$\text{Bi (NO}_3)_2 \xrightarrow[\text{Na}_2\text{CO}_3]{\text{H}_2\text{O}} \text{(BiO)}_2 \text{CO}_3$$

It is a white, heavy, odourless, tasteless, microcrystalline slightly hygroscopic powder; practically insoluble in water and in alcohol, readily soluble with effervescence in nitric acid and hydrochloric acids. It is kept in well-closed containers and protected from light.

Bismuth subcarbonate is stable in pure air but is slowly effected by light. It darkens in air containing traces of hydrogen sulphide. It is decomposed to Bi_2O_3 and nitrogen oxides when heated to red heat.

Incompatibility : It is incompatible with bicarbonates, soluble iodides, gallic acid, calomel, salicylic acid, tannin and sulphur.

Tests for Purity : Tests for chloride; nitrate; alkalis and alkaline earth metals; arsenic; copper; lead; silver; sulphate; loss on drying; and clarity and colour of solution.

Sodium carbonate and other basic compounds are determined in a solution from which the bismuth has been separated as sulphide by addition of sulphuric acid, drying, ignition of the residue, and weighing of the residual metallic sulphates.

Sulphate is detected by precipitation as barium sulphate; copper by formation of the blue colour with ammonia; lead by precipitation as the sulphate; and silver by precipitation as silver chloride in the solution from which bismuth has been removed as sparingly soluble basic nitrate, $BiONO_3$.

For determining alkalies and alkaline-earth metals hydrogen sulphide is passed through an acidified solution. The precipitate formed is filtered, the filtrate dried, sulphuric acid added to the filtrates, ignited and the residue weighed.

Copper is detected by addition of ammonia to an aqueous solution. It is filtered and sodium diethyl dithiocarbamate is added. Any colour produced is not more intense than that produced by treating at the same time and in the same manner a solution containing copper standard solution.

Lead is determined by atomic absorption spectrophotometry.

Silver is detected by treating a solution in nitric acid with hydrochloric acid to produce an opalescence.

The presence of nitrate is found out by treating the substance with indigo carmine and sulphuric acid. It is titrated with indigo carmine until a stable blue colour is produced.

Tests for Identification : It gives the reactions characteristic of bismuth compounds and of carbonate.

Assay : The substance (0.5 g) is dissolved in nitric acid, diluted to water (250 ml) and carried out complexometric titration of bismuth. Each ml of 0.1 N disodium edetate is equivalent to 20.90 mg of Bi.

Uses : Bismuth subcarbonate is used as an antacid, mild astringent, dusting powder, antiseptic, protective and adsorbent. It has been used in the form of bismuth subnitrate and iodoform paste as a wound dressing, and as topical protective in lotions and ointments.

There is a risk of the nitrate being reduced to nitrite with the development of methaemoglobinaemia.

KAOLIN

Al_2O_3, $2SiO_2$, $2H_2O$

Kaolin (China clay) is a purified, natural, hydrated aluminium silicate of variable composition. It is derived from the decomposition of feldspar of granitic rocks. Kaolin consists mainly of aluminium silicate with traces of compounds of magnesium, calcium and iron. It is usually found together with the vegetable carbohydrate, pectin.

Preparation

Kaolin is prepared when the rock is mined, excavated and the impurities are washed with water and then powdered. The rock is elutriated with water and large-sized particles are separated. The turbid liquid is allowed to settle, heavy kaolin containing large particles and colloidal kaolin containing particles of small size are separated and dried.

Properties

Kaolin is slightly plastic-like and is normally white. It has an earthy or clay-like taste. Its colour may be tinged grey, yellow brown, blue or red due to impurities. It is unctuous and soapy to touch; its surface takes a high polish on rubbing. Its fusion point is in between 1700-1800°. On heating it losses water. It is not affected by dilute hydrochloric or nitric acid, but is decomposed by prolonged boiling or treatment with concentrated sulphuric acid. It becomes more resistant to acids if it is first heated to white heat. When moistened with water, it assumes a darker colour and develops a marked clay-like odour.

Heavy kaoline is purified natural form of variable composition. Its particles are 20 μm in diameter, flat and irregularly arranged. With water plastic-like form is obtained which is less sticky. It is a fine white or greyish-white earthy mass or powder; unctuous when moist. It is practically insoluble in water and in organic solvents. When the aqueous suspension is kept for some time, the whole kaolin settles below leaving a clear supernatant liquid. Heavy kaolin polarizes light brightly.

Light kaolin is a native form, freed from most of its impurities by elutriation, and dried. It contains a suitable dispersing agent. The particles are small, less than 2 μm in diameter and have various shapes and sizes. They do not polarize light. Light kaolin is a white, light, odourless unctuous powder free from gritty particles. It is practically insoluble in water and mineral acids. A sticky mass is obtained with water. Its aqueous suspension remains turbid permanently and only a small fraction is deposited.

Natural Light Kaolin is light kaolin which does not contain a dispersing agent.

Tests for Purity : Tests for arsenic; carbonate; chloride; sulphate calcium; heavy metals; loss on drying (15%); iron; loss on ignition (1%); soluble matter in mineral acids; organic impurities; absorption power; swelling power; particle sizes; alkalinity or acidity.

Development of pink colour due to addition of phenolphthalein to an aqueous suspension indicates the presence of alkaline nature.

For determining lead, the substance is digested with nitric acid. The reaction mixture is centrifuged and in the supernatant liquid limit test for lead is carried out.

Iron is detected by triturating kaolin with water. Sodium salicylate is added; the mixture does not acquire more than a slight reddish tint.

If no effervescence occurs on addition of sulphuric acid to the aqueous solution, carbonate is absent.

For determining soluble matter an acidified solution is filtered. Dilute sulphuric acid is added to the filtrate, evaporated to dryness, ignited and weighed.

Absorption power is determined by shaking the substance with 0.37% methylene blue solution, centrifuging and diluting the solution. The solution is not more intensely coloured than a solution of methylene blue.

Swelling power is detected by triturating the ubstance with water; the mixture should not flow.

Uses : Kaolins are adsorbent, antidiarrhoeal, and when given by mouth, adsorb toxic and other substances from the alimentary tract and increase the bulk of the faeces. They are employed in the symptomatic treatment of diarrhoea and to coat irritated intestinal mucosa in case of diarrhoea, dysentery and intestinal fermentation. Externally, light kaolin is used as a dusting-powder and food additive.

Heavy kaolin is used in the preparation of kaolin poultice, which is applied with the intention of reducing inflammation and alleviating pain.

(D) SALINE CATHARTICS

Saline cathartics (purgatives) are agents that fasten and increase evacuation from the bowels. Laxatives are mild cathartics that are used for short-term therapy. Cathartics are used to ease defecation in patients with painful haemorrhoids (piles) or other rectal disorders; to avoid excessive staining and concurrent increase in abdominal pressure in patients with hernias; to avoid potentially hazardous rises in blood pressure during defecation in patients with hypertension, cerebral, coronary, or other arterial diseases; to relieve acute constipation; and to remove solid material from the intestinal tract prior to certain roentgenographic (X-rays) studies. Material is propelled through the intestinal tract by peristaltic movements which are wave-like contractions at 2 to 25 cm per second. The contents are carried out through the small intestine in about 3.5 to 4 hours. The last part of a meal leaves the ileum about 8 or 9 hours after ingestion. The products of digestion are held up at the ileocolic sphincter for sufficient period to complete intestinal digestion and absorption.

In the colon a strong peristaltic wave occurs about 3 or 4 times a day. The contents may be expelled into the rectum by one of these massive movements and the individual feels a sensation of fullness in the rectum and an intention to defecate. The frequency of defecation varies from person to person, ranging from once every two or three days to up to three bowel movements per day.

Difficult evacuation of the feces is known as constipation. It may be due to dry and hard fecal material, intestinal atony, intestinal spasm, emotions, drugs, and diet. Laxatives may be used for evacuation which are of four types :

(i) stimulant,

(ii) bulk forming,

(iii) emollient, and

(iv) saline.

The stimulant laxatives, e.g. phenolphthalein, aloin, extracts of cascara, rhubarb and senna, castor oil, etc. act by local irritation on the intestinal tract increasing peristaltic activity. The bulk-forming laxatives, e.g. psyllium seed, methyl cellulose, sodium carboxymethyl cellulose and karaya gum, are made of cellulose and other non-digestible carbohydrates. They swell when moistened increasing bulk stimulate peristalsis. The emollient laxative act either as stool softeners or as lubricants facilitating the expulsion of compacted fecal.

Mineral oil is the main lubricant laxative while an anionic surface active agent, d-octyl sodium sulphosuccinate, acts as stool softener. The saline cathartics of the fourth group are the salts of poorly absorbable anions and cations and act by increasing the osmotic load of the gastrointestinal tract. The body relieves the hypertonicity of the gut by secreting additional fluids into the intestinal tract. Peristalsis is stimulated by the resulting increased bulk. Poorly absorbed anions that are used as saline cathartics are biphosphate ($H_2PO_4^-$), phosphate (HPO_4^-), sulphate, and tartrate. The poorly absorbed cations are the soluble magnesium salts. The saline cathartics are water soluble and are used with excess amounts of water. This prevents excess loss of body fluids and reduces nausea and vomiting.

Certain salts, when given orally, are not completely absorbed and are retained in the gastrointestinal tract. Such preparations exert an osmotic effect and, therefore, hold considerable amounts of water, thus increasing the intestinal bulk. This acts as a mechanical stimulant causing an increase in the intestinal motor activity and evaluation. The efficacy of the saline laxative is related to the osmotic activity exerted by the unabsorbed fraction within the intestinal lumen. Magnesium sulphate, milk of magnesia, magnesium citrate, potassium sodium tartrate, etc. are the common saline cathartics. These compounds act in the intestine and full cathartic doses produce a watery evacuation within 3 to 6 hours. Because of their quick onset of action, they are given early in the morning before breakfast. They do not cause irritation and there is very little griping. Adequate fluid intake is necessary to avoid dehydration.

They are used for bowel evacuation before radiological, endoscopic and surgical procedures, and also to expel parasites and toxic materials.

Small amounts of these drugs may be absorbed in the blood causing occasional toxicity. The absorption of magnesium may cause marked central nervous system depression while that of sodium may worsen the existing congestive cardiac failure.

MAGNESIUM SULPHATE

$MgSO_4 . 7H_2O$; Mol. Weight = 246.47.

Magnesium sulphate contains not less than 99.0 per cent of $MgSO_4$. Monohydrate form of magnesium sulphate occurs in nature as the mineral *kieserite*. The heptahydrate form (*bitter salts; epsom salts*) occurs in nature as the mineral *epsomite*.

Preparation

1. In laboratory magnesium sulphate is prepared by neutralizing hot, dilute sulphuric acid with magnesium, or its oxide or carbonate. The solution is filtered, concentrated and crystallized.

$$MgCO_3 + H_2SO_4 \longrightarrow MgSO_4 + H_2O + CO_2$$
$$MgO + H_2SO_4 \longrightarrow MgSO_4 + H_2O$$

2. On commercial scale it is manufactured by reacting sulphuric acid with magnesite or with powdered and calcined dolomite. Magnesium sulphate so formed dissolves in the solution and the sparingly soluble calcium sulphate is deposited. The liquid is filtered, the filtrate is concentrated and crystallized.

$$MgCO_3 . CaCO_3 + 2H_2SO_4 \longrightarrow MgSO_4 + CaSO_4 + 2CO_2 + 2H_2O$$
Dolomite

3. Magnesium sulphate is also prepared from the native sulphate (*kieserite*), $MgSO_4 . H_2O$ by dissolving in hot water. When the solution is cooled, rhombic crystals of hepta-hydrate deposits.

Dried magnesium sulphate is prepared by heating the heptahydrate at 100° to lose about 25% of its weight.

Physical Characters

Magnesium sulphate occurs as odourless, brilliant, colourless crystals or a white crystalline powder; with bitter, saline and cooling taste. It effloresces in warm dry air. Each g represents about 4.1 mmol of magnesium and of sulphate. It is soluble in water (1 in 1.5) and very soluble in boiling water; practically insoluble in alcohol. A 5% solution in water has a pH of 5.0 to 9.2. On exposure to dry air at ordinary temperature it loses about 1 mole of water; at 70-80° loses 4 moles of water; at 100° loses 5 moles and at 120° loses 6 moles of water; loses the last mole of water at about 250°; rapidly reabsorbs water when exposed to moist air. It is stored in well-closed containers.

Tests for Purity : Tests for arsenic; iron; lead; zinc; chloride; heavy metals; acidity or alkalinity; loss on drying (51.1%); and clarity and colour of solution.

For detecting iron, a solution of magnesium sulphate is heated on a steam both. A gradual development of a brownish turbidity is observed.

Zinc is determined by precipitation as white zinc ferrocyanide.

A 10% solution is neutral to phenol red solution.

Test for Identification : A solution (1 in 20) gives the reactions of magnesium, and of sulphates.

Incompatibility : Alkali carbonates and bicarbonates, tartrates, soluble phosphates and arsenates. Potassium and ammonium bromides in concentrated solutions form a precipitate of double sulphate.

Assay : The assay is based on the complexometric titration carried out with ethylenediamine tetra-acetate (EDTA). It forms complexes with almost all the metal ions which are water soluble, stable and the formation is instantaneous and quantitative. Since EDTA is less water-soluble, disodium salt ($Na_2H_2Y.H_2O$) is used as titrant. The titration is carried out in the presence of a buffer such as strong ammonia-ammonium chloride solution using mordant black 11 mixture as indicator. The end-point is the change of colour from pink to blue.

$$(HOOC.CH_2)_2 \, NCH_2CH_2N \, (CH_2\text{-}COOH)_2$$
$$EDTA$$
$$Mg^{2+} + H_2Y^{2-} \longrightarrow MgY^{2-} + 2H^+$$

To a weighed amount of the substance (0.3 g) dissolved in water (50 ml), strong ammonia ammonium chloride solution (10 ml) is added. The reaction mixture is titrated with 0.05 M disodium ethylenediamininetetraacetate using 0.1 of mordant black 11 mixture as indicator, until the pink colour is discharged from the blue. Each ml of 0.05 M disodium ethylenediamine tetraacetate is equivalent to 0.00602 g of $MgSO_4$.

Uses : Magnesium sulphate is used in the treatment of magnesium deficiency. It acts as a saline laxative and has anticonvulsant properties. It is used to control seizuses associated with acute uraemia (failure of renal function); hypothyroidism and eclampsia (convulsions arising in pregnancy). Externally it is used for local inflammations and infected wounds. It is also used in the treatment of cholecystitis (inflammation of gall bladder), sea-sickness, hypertension, to lower intercranial pressure, tetanus spasm and as wet dressing for carbuncles (infection of hair follicle and subacious gland) and boils.

Excessive use of magnesium sulphate causes hyper-magnesaemia, gastro-intestinal irritation and watery diarrhoea.

SODIUM POTASSIUM TARTRATE

COONa CH (OH). CH (OH). COOK, $4H_2O$;

NaK $C_4H_4O_6$, $4H_2O$; Mol. Weight = 282.17.

It contains 99 to 104% of NaK $C_4H_4O_6$. $4H_2O$

Sodium potassium tartrate is prepared by boiling a solution of sodium carbonate and potassium bitartrate for some time and allowing the reaction mixture to stand at 60°. The solution is filtered, concentrated and crystallized.

$$2KHC_4H_4O_6 + Na_2CO_3 \longrightarrow 2KNaC_4H_4O_6 + CO_2 + H_2O$$

Physical Characters : Sodium potassium tartrate occurs as odourless, colourless, crystals or white crystalline powder, with a cooling saline taste. It effloresces slightly in warm dry air, the crystals often being coated with a white powder, m.p. 70-80°; at 100° loses three moles of water; becomes anhydrous at 130-140°; at 220° begins to decompose and gives off inflammable vapours having the odour of burnt sugar leaving behind residue of potassium and sodium carbonates. It is soluble in water (1 in 1); practically insoluble in alcohol. The aqueous solution is slightly alkaline to litmus, pH 7-8. It is stored in airtight containers.

Chemical Properties

1. It gives characteristic reactions of sodium, potassium and tartrates.

2. When an equal volume of acetic acid is added to 5% solution of the salt, a white crystalline precipitate of potassium bitartrate is obtained after 15 minutes.

3. On ignition it gives the odour of burning sugar and forms an alkaline residue consisting of sodium and potassium carbonates which effervesces with acids.

Assay : A weighed amount (2 g) is heated until carbonized, cooled, and the residue boiled with 50 ml of water and 0.5 N sulphuric acid (50 ml). It is filtered, washed with water and the filtrate and washings are titrated with 0.5 N sodium hydroxide, using methyl orange solution as indicator. Each ml of 0.5 N sulphuric acid is equivalent to 0.07056 g of NaK $C_4H_4O_6$. $4H_2O$.

$$2NaKC_4H_4O_6 + 5O_2 \longrightarrow K_2CO_3 + Na_2CO_3 + 6CO_2 + 4H_2O$$

Tests for Purity : Tests for arsenic; chloride; iron; heavy metals; sulphate; loss on drying; acidity and alkalinity.

Incompatibility : Acids, calcium or lead salts, magnesium sulphate, silver nitrate.

Uses : Sodium potassium tartrate is used as a laxative and food additive in the form of a stabilizer in cheese and meat products. It causes watery evacuation of bowels without causing irritation. It is also used in Seidlitz powder, Fehling's solution, as antimony potassium tartrate, and bismuth potassium tartrate.

5

TOPICAL AGENTS

Topical agents are for external use only on the body surface. Topical application of drugs may be accomplished within body cavities that open to the outside (e.g. the oral, vaginal, and colonic cavities). Topical agents are divided into two main categories based on their action or use as (i) protective, (ii) antimicrobial, and (iii) astringent compounds.

They are not placed in eyes, nose or mouth. Before applying the medicine, hands are washed thoroughly, skin area is cleaned with soap and water each time before application, unless otherwise directed by the physician. After applying the medicine, the hands are washed and dried gently with a clean towel. This avoids accidentally getting any medicine in eyes, nose or mouth. The prescribed amount of the medicine is used. Any other creams, lotions or cosmetics should not be used over the already applied medicine. If the condition persists or becomes worse, or if a constant irritation, such as burning or itching occurs, the physician should be consulted. Only the medicine that is actually touching the skin will work. A thick layer of creams and ointments is not more effective than a thin layer. In case of lotions, the liquid preparation is shaken well before using. A small amount of medicine is applied to the affected part and spreaded lightly. The containers, aerosols and sprays are shaken well each time before using. The containers are held straight up and about 6 to 8 inches away from the affected skin. The affected area is sprayed for 2 to 3 seconds and eyes, nose or mouth to be avoided. It should not be sprayed near food. Some sprays may contain alcohol which may catch on fire. While using the spray, it should not be smoked and fired on open flame or heater. The aerosol should not be punctured, broken or burnt even if empty.

(A) PROTECTIVES

Protectives are agents which are applied to the skin to protect certain areas from irritation. These substances are insoluble and chemically inert. The absorption of the compounds through the skin makes it difficult to wash them off due to their insolubility and diminishes metallic properties on tissue. Unreactive nature of the compounds prevent interactions between the protective substance and the tissue. Ideal protectives are biologically inactive and efficient adsorbents useful for adsorbing moisture from the surface of the skin. Protective and adsorbent action becomes maximum with decreasing particle size. Small particles occupy a larger surface area, allowing them to adhere to each other, stick better to the surface of the skin, and adsorb moisture more efficiently. Fine powder particles also offer a smooth substance which is easy to apply and aids in preventing irritation due to rubbing or friction.

Protectives are usually applied as ointments, dusting powders and suspensions to the areas of the skin which are subjected to constant irritation due to moisture and/or friction, or areas which have already become irritated or inflamed due to friction and allergy. If a fluid is exuding from the area to which the protective is to be applied, adsorbent-type protectives should not be used. These substances will mix with the exudate and form a crust on drying which adheres to the open tissue.

BENTONITE
(Wilkinite)

Bentonite is a natural, colloidal, hydrated aluminium silicate consisting mainly of *montmorillonite*, Al_2O_3. $4SiO_2$. H_2O. It may also contain calcium, magnesium and iron. The silica content may be less than shown, and the water content depends upon the treatment to which the natural substance has been subjected. The most common type is volclay bentonite, composed of about 90% *montmorillonite* $[Al_2Si_4O_{10}(OH)_2. nH_2O]$. Other components are *feldspar* $(K_2O. Al_2O_3. 6SiO_2)$ and aluminosilicate containing SiO_2, Al_2O_3, Fe_2O_3, CaO, MgO and some Na and K.

Characters : It occurs as a very fine odourless, pale buff, or cream-coloured to greyish-white powder with a yellowish tint; free from grit; taste is slightly earthy. It is insoluble in water but swells into a homogeneous mass occupying about 12 times the volume of the dry powder; insoluble in, and does not swell in organic solvents. A 5% suspension of purified bentonite has a pH of 9.0 to 10.0. It is stored in tightly closed containers.

Tests for Purity : Tests for sedimentation volume; swelling powder; alkalinity; arsenic; gel formation; coarse particles; pH; loss on drying; and gritty particles.

Sedimentation volume is determined by mixing the substance (6 g) with light magnesium oxide (0.3 g) and water (200 ml), shaking for 1 hour and placing the suspension in a cylinder. After 24 hours the volume of the clear supernatant liquid is not greater than 2 ml.

Swelling power is detected by adding the substance (2g) in sodium laurylsulphate and allowing to stand for 2 hours. The apparent volume of the sediment at the bottom of the cylinder is not less than 24 ml.

Coarse particles are determined by triturating the substance with sodium hexametaphosphate solution, separating the colloidal suspension by syphon and the coarse particles by a sieve of nominal mesh aperture 125 μm. The weight of the particles on the sieve is not more than 5 mg.

pH is between 9.0 and 10.5, determined in a 2% w/v suspension in water.

Tests for Identification

1. The substance is fused with anhydrous sodium carbonate, water added and filtered. The residue is dissolved in dilute hydrochloric acid; the solution gives the reactions of aluminium.

2. To the filtrate hydrochloric acid is added; a gelatinous precipitate is produced.

Uses : Bentonite is used as pharmaceutical aid (suspending agent). It absorbs water readily to form gels. It is used as suspending and stabilizing agent and as an adsorbent or clarifying agent.

CALAMINE

$ZnCO_3$, Fe_2O_3 or ZnO, Fe_2O_3.

Calamine (I.P.) is zinc oxide with a small proportion of ferric oxide. It contains not less than 98.0 per cent of ZnO.

Calamine (B.P.) is the basic zinc carbonate coloured with ferric oxide, yielding on ignition 68 to 74% of oxides of zinc and iron. It is a fine amorphous, impalpable, odourless, pink or reddish-brown powder, the colour depending on the variety and amount of ferric oxide present and the process by which it is incorporated. It is practically insoluble in water; soluble with effervescence in hydrochloric acid.

Tests for Purity : Tests for barium salts; calcium; lead; chloride; sulphate; alcohol-soluble dyes; alkaline substances; acid-insoluble matter; water-soluble dyes; and residue on ignition (68-74%).

Acid-insoluble substances are determined by dissolving calamine (1 g) in warm dilute hydrochloric acid (25 ml). Any insoluble residue is collected on a tarred filter washed with water, dried to constant weight at 105° cooled and weighed. The weight should not exceed 20 mg.

For detecting alkaline substances, calamine (1g) is digested in warm water (20 ml), and phenolphthalein (2 drops) added. If a red colour is produced, not more than 0.2 ml of 0.1 N sulphuric acid is required to discharge it.

To a solution (A) of calamine in water and glacial acetic acid, 5N ammonia and ammonium oxalate (2.5%, w/v) are added. If the solution remains clear after two minutes, it indicates the absence of calcium. A clear solution obtained on addition of potassium chromate solution to the solution (A) suggests the absence of lead in calamine.

Tests for Identification

1. The substance (1 g) is shaken with dilute hydrochloric acid and filtered; the filtrate gives the reactions of zinc.
2. Calamine (1 g) is boiled with dilute hydrochloric acid (10 ml) and filtered. A few drops of ammonium thiocyanate solution are added to the filtrate; a reddish colour is produced.

Assay : A weighed amount of the substance (1.5 g) is digested with 1N sulphuric acid (50 ml), filtered and the residue washed with hot water. To the filtrate and washings, ammonium chloride (2.5 g) is added and titrated with 1 N sodium hydroxide using methyl orange solution as indicator. Each ml of 1N sulphuric acid is equivalent to 0.04068 g of ZnO.

Uses : Calamine is a topical protectant and has a mild astringent action on the skin. It is used as a dusting-powder, cream, lotion, or ointment in a variety of skin conditions, including urticaria (skin eruption), eczema, and the effects of sunburn. Calamine lotion contains calamine and zinc oxide (1%) suspended with

Bentonite and calcium hydroxide. Phenolated calamine lotion contains phenol (2%) which is used as a local anaesthetic and antipyretic.

SILICONE POLYMERS

$CH_3[Si(CH_3)n.O]_3 Si(CH_3)_3$

Silicone polymers (dimethicone) may be prepared by hydrolyzing a mixture of dichlorodimethylsilane, $(CH_3)_2SiCl_2$, and chlorotrimethylsilane, $(CH_3)_3SiCl$. The hydrolyzed products contain active silanol groups (SiOH) through which condensation polymerization proceeds. By varying the proportion of chlorotrimethylsilane, which acts as a chain terminator, silicones of varying molecular weight may be prepared.

As the molecular weight increases, the products become more viscous. The various grades are distinguished by numbers relating to the viscosity. The physical properties depends on the size and type of the radical and the molecular configuration of the polymer (linear, cyclic, degree of crosslinking). The products have remarkably high thermal and chemical stability and unusual release from sticking and surface properties.

The products occur as clear colourless, odourless liquids; insoluble in water, alcohol, acetone and methyl alcohol and soluble with chlorinated hydrocarbons, ether and xylene; very slightly soluble in absolute alcohol and isopropyl alcohol; also miscible with amyl acetate, cyclohexane, kerosene, toluene and ethyl acetate.

The polymers are stored in airtight containers.

Uses : Silicone polymers are water-repellent and have a low surface tension. They are used in barrier creams for protecting the skin against water-soluble irritants. Creams, lotions and ointments containing the silicone polymers are employed for the prevention of bedsores and napkin rash and to protect the skin against trauma due to colostomy discharge. They are also used as lubricants for hypodermic syringes and in the treatment of flatulence. Dimethicone or Simethicone is a mixture of dimethyl polysiloxanes and silica gel.

Injections of silicone polymers may cause a granulomatour reaction. They adhere very well to the skin and exclude contact with air. Therefore, they should not be applied over broken skin or wounds. Contact with the eyes should be avoided.

TALC

$Mg_6 (Si_2O_5)_4 (OH)_2$ or $3MgO, 4SiO_2, H_2O$

Talc is a finely powdered, purified, natural hydrous magnesium silicate containing a small amount of aluminium silicate and iron. The natural lumps are known as *soapstone, foliated, fibrous* or *steatite*. The most desirable form for cosmetic and pharmaceutical purposes is the foliated talc which has a plate-like structure. The actual composition of talc is variable, containing MgO (28-31.2%), SiO_2 (57-61.7%) and H_2O (3-7%).

Preparation : Talc is prepared by boiling finely powdered talc with dilute hydrochloric acid, allowing the insoluble talc to settle, decanting the supernatant liquid and removing the acid by washing with water. The impurities such as iron, calcium oxide, aluminium oxide and ferric oxide are removed in this process.

Physical Characters : Talc occurs as a very fine, light, homogeneous, white, or greyish-white, odourless, impalpable, and unctuous powder, which adheres readily to the skin. It is practically insoluble in water and in dilute mineral acids and dilute solutions of alkali hydroxides. It is sterilized by exposure to ethylene oxide or by heating so that the whole of the material is maintained at 160° for 1 hour. It is preserved in well-closed containers.

Chemical Reactions : Chemically, talc may be considered to be a hydrated magnesium silicate.

When talc is heated to red heat (850-1000°C), it loses water and the natural mineral *enstatite*, $Mg_4Si_4O_{12}$, is formed.

When a mixture of talc, anhydrous sodium carbonate and anhydrous potassium carbonate is fused in a platinum crucible, magnesium carbonate is formed.

$3MgO. 4SiO_2.H_2O + Na_2CO_3 + 2K_2CO_3$

$\longrightarrow 3MgCO_3 + Na_2SiO_3 + 2K_2SiO_3 + H_2SiO_3.$

The reaction on further treatment with hydrochloric acid yields insoluble silica.

$MgCO_3 + 2HCl \longrightarrow MgCl_2 + H_2O + CO_2$

$Na_2SiO_3 + 2HCl \longrightarrow 2NaCl + SiO_2 + H_2O$

$K_2SiO_3 + 2HCl \longrightarrow 2KCl + SiO_2 + H_2O$

$SiO_2 + H_2O \xrightarrow{100°} SiO_2$

Soluble   Insoluble

Tests for Purity : Tests for iron carbonates; calcium; chloride; organic substances; acidity; alkalinity; acid soluble matter (less than 1%); water soluble matter (0.2%); loss on drying (not more than 4.8%); and loss on ignition (not more than 6%).

Acidity is determined by shaking talc (5g) with carbon dioxide free water (25 ml) for one minute, filtering and adding to the filtrate bromothymol blue solution (0.5 ml). The solution is not acid and requires not more than 0.3 ml of 0.1 N hydrochloric acid.

If talc does not show effervescence by adding in dilute hydrochloric acid, carbonates are absent.

Talc is liable to be heavily contaminated with bacteria, including *Clostridium tetani, Cl.* welchii, and *Bacillus anthracis*. When used in dusting-powders, it should be sterilized.

Tests for Identification

1. A mixture of the substance (0.5 g), anhydrous sodium carbonate (0.2 g) and anhydrous potassium carbonate (2 g) are fused, cooled, and hydrochloric acid is added until it ceases to cause effervescence. More acid is added and the mixture is dried. The residue is boiled with water, filtered, and to the filtrate ammonium chloride (2g) and dilute ammonia solution (5 ml) are added. The solution is filtered, disodium hydrogen phosphate solution added to the filtrate; a white crystalline precipitate of magnesium ammonium phosphate separates.

2. The substance (0.5 g) is fused with anhydrous sodium carbonate (4 g), dissolved the melt in hot water and filtered. To the filtrate hydrochloric acid is added to produce a strong acid reaction and dried. The residue gives the reactions of silicates.

Uses : Purified talc is used in massage and as a dusting powder to allay irritation and prevent chafing. It is usually mixed with starch or boric acid to increase absorption of moisture, and zinc oxide. It is also used as a lubricant in making pills, tablets and for dusting tablet molds; to clarify liquids by filtration. Talc poudrage has been used to treat recurrent spontaneous pneumothorax (collection of air in the pleural cavity) and pleural effusions.

Contamination of wounds or body cavities with talc is liable to cause granulomas. Prolonged or intense aspiration of talc may produce pneumoconiosis. Talc is used in preparations which may be perfumed for cosmetic purposes, or medicated with antimicrobial agents, such as boric acid.

Due to its insoluble and chemically inert and non-adsorptive nature, talc is used as a filtering aid.

TITANIUM DIOXIDE

TiO_2; Mol. Weight = 79.90

Titanium dioxide contains not less than 98.0 per cent of TiO_2, calculated with reference to the dried substance. It is found in nature as the minerals *rutile* (tetragonal), *brookite* (orthorhombic), *anatase* or *octahedrite* (tetragonal), *ilmenite* ($TiFeO_3$) and *perovskite* ($TiCaO_3$). Titanium exhibits three or four valencies. For example, titanous chloride, $TiCl_3$, a reducing agent, is readily oxidized to the tetrachloride, $TiCl_4$ due to loss of the fourth electron.

Preparation

Titanium dioxide is prepared commercially by treating the mineral *ilmenite* with hydrogen chloride and chlorine.

$$2FeTiO_3 + 4HCl + Cl_2 \longrightarrow 2TiO_2 + 2FeCl_3 + 2H_2O$$

It may be prepared by direct combination of titanium and oxygen; by treatment of titanium salts in aqueous solution; by the reaction of volatile, inorganic titanium compounds with oxygen; and by oxidation or hydrolysis of organic compounds of titanium.

Characters : Titanium dioxide is a white, or almost white, infusible, odourless, tasteless powder. It is practically insoluble in water, dilute mineral acids, and organic solvents; slowly soluble in hot concentrated sulphuric acid; soluble in hydrofluoric acid. A 10% suspension in water is neutral to litmus. It is also made soluble by fusion with potassium bisulphate or with alkali hydroxides or carbonates to form alkali titanates. *Titania* is a name applied to large TiO_2 crystals suitable for used in jewellary. These crystals have a refractive index (2.7) higher than diamonds (2.4), but lack the hardness of diamonds. It has high refractive index and, therefore, high opacity.

Titatium dioxide is kept in well-closed containers.

The reactivity of the oxide depends on a previous heat treatment. When hydrogen peroxide is added to dilute sulphuric acid solution of the oxide, an orange-red colour of titanium peroxide, TiO_3, is produced immediately.

Tests for Purity : Tests for arsenic; barium; lead; heavy metals; iron; antimony; heavy metals; loss on drying; loss on ignition; water-soluble matter; acid-soluble matter; clarity and colour of solution; acidity or alkalinity.

For determining barium, the substance is dissolved in hydrochloric acid, filtered and the filtrate washed water. Dilute sulphuric acid is added to the filtrate; the solution remains clear for not less than thirty minutes when barium is absent.

Acidity or alkalinity is determined by neutralizing aqueous solution of the substance with 0.01 N hydrochloric acid or with 0.02N sodium hydroxide using 0.1 ml of bromothymol blue solution as indicator.

A weighed amount of the substance is dissolved in water containing ammonium sulphate and filtered. The filtrate is evaporated to dryness and ignited to get water soluble matter.

For heavy metals the solution prepared in the test for barium is diluted. To the solution, thioacetamide reagent and acetate buffer (pH 3.5) are added. Any brown colour produced is not more intense than that produced by similarly treating a mixture of 1.0 ml of standard lead solution.

For detection of iron, to solution A obtained in identification test (A) bromine water is added. Excess of bromine is removed by passing a current of air and potassium thiocyanate solution added with shaking. After five minutes, any red colour in the solution is not more intense than the colour obtained by treating standard iron solution and sulphuric acid solution (20%) in the same manner.

Tests for Identification

1. A mixture of the substance (0.5 g), anhydrous sodium sulphate (5 g), water (10 ml) and sulphuric acid (10 ml) is boiled until clear, cooled, and 25% sulphuric acid (30 ml) is added. The solution is diluted with water and divided in two parts A and B. To part A (5 ml), strong hydrogen peroxide solution (0.1 ml) is added; an orange-red colour is produced.

2. To part B (5 ml) one piece of granulated zinc is added. After 45 minutes a violet-blue colour is produced.

Assay : Reaction of titanium dioxide with hydrogen peroxide in dilute sulphuric acid produces titanium peroxide (TiO_3) which gives an orange red colour with solution. This reaction is used in the official identification of the compound.

Assay : A weighed amount (0.3 g) is mixed to sulphuric acid (20 ml) and ammonium sulphate (8 g), heated until white fumes appear, cooled and diluted with water. The reaction mixture is re-heated, cooled, filtered and strong ammonia solution is added to the filtrate. The solution is diluted with water, strong hydrogen peroxide solution and 0.05 M disodium ethylenediamine tetra- acetate are added and the pH of the solution adjusted to 5.0 with sodium hydroxide solution. Hexamine (5g) is added and the solution is titrated with 0.05 M zinc chloride using xylenol orange solution as indicator. Each ml of 0.05 M disodium ethylenediamine tetraacetate is equivalent to 0.003995 g of TiO_2.

Uses : Titanium dioxide is applied to the skin as a mild astringent and protective application in eczema; used for the relief of pruritus and in certain exudative dermatoses. It reflects ultraviolet light and is used to prevent sunburn. It is an ingredient of certain face powders and other cosmetics. It is used to pigment and opacity hard gelatin capsules and tablet coatings and as a delustring agent for regenerated cellulose. Purified grades may be used in food colours. It is also used in sun-tan preparation due to its high refractive index (2.7). This high refractivity makes the compound useful for preparation of various sun creams and sun screen products. As a solar ray protective, it is useful in a concentration of 5 to 25% in ointments or lotions. It is also used as a white pigment in cosmetics and paints.

ZINC OXIDE

ZnO; Mol. Weight = 81.34

Zinc oxide contains not less than 99.0 per cent of ZnO.

It occurs as the mineral *zincite.*

Commercially zinc oxide is prepared by heating metallic zinc to bright redness in the presence of preheated air (French Process). The zinc vapours burn to form oxide which is obtained as a fine, white powder.

$$2Zn + O_2 \longrightarrow 2ZnO$$

In an another procedure a mixture of zinc sulphate solution and sodium carbonate solution is boiled to precipitate zinc carbonate which is filtered and washed. When zinc carbonate is ignited, carbon dioxide, and zinc oxide are formed.

$$ZnSO_4 + Na_2CO_3 \longrightarrow ZnCO_3 + Na_2SO_4$$

$$ZnCO_3 \xrightarrow{\text{heat}} ZnO + CO_2$$

Zinc oxide is also prepared from *franklinite* (American process) or from zinc sulphide.

Physical Characters

Zinc Oxide is a white or faintly yellowish-white, odourless, amorphous very fine soft powder, free from grittiness. It gradually absorbs carbon dioxide from air to form basic zinc carbonate, $Zn_2(OH)_2CO_2$; sublimes at normal pressure; practically insoluble in water and in alcohol; soluble in dilute mineral acids, in solutions of alkali hydroxides; ammonia and ammonium carbonate solution to form salts. When treated with dilute hydrochloric acid, the oxide forms the Lewis acid, zinc chloride.

$$ZnO + 2HCl \longrightarrow ZnCl_2 + H_2O$$

$$ZnO + 2NaOH \longrightarrow Na_2ZnO_2 + H_2O$$

When freshly ignited, it contains 99 to 100.5% of ZnO. When heated to 400°C or 500°C, the oxide develops a yellow colour that disappears on cooling.

Ammonia solution and ammonium carbonate form basic ammonia complexes with zinc oxide which are soluble in basic ammonia.

$$ZnO + 4NH_2OH \longrightarrow Zn(NH_3)_4(OH)_2 + 3H_2O$$

$$ZnO + 2(NH_4)CO_3 \longrightarrow Zn(NH_3)_4(OH)_2 + CO_2 \uparrow + H_2O$$

It is stored in well-closed containers.

Tests for Purity : Tests for arsenic; iron; lead; metallic zinc; sulphate; alkalinity; carbonate; substances insoluble in acids; oily impurities; and loss on ignition.

Lead is precipitated as yellow zinc chromate from acetic acid solution. The zinc chromate dissolves in the solution.

Metallic zinc is tested by displacement of lead from a solution of lead acetate.

Alkalinity is determined by treating aqueous solution with phenolphthalein. If red colour is produced, it is titrated with 0.1 N hydrochloric acid to discharge it.

If an aqueous solution on treatment with dilute sulphuric acid produces no effervescence and the resulting solution is clear and colourless, carbonate and substances insoluble in acids are absent.

For detecting iron, the acidified solution of the substance should comply with the limit test for iron.

Tests for Identification

1. It becomes yellow when strongly heated; the yellow colour disappears on cooling.
2. A solution in dilute hydrochloric acid gives the reactions of zinc.

Assay : The assay is based on acidimetry-alkalimetric titration. The end point is yellow to pink. Weighed amounts of the substance (1.5 g) and ammonium chloride (2.5 g) are dissolved in 1 N sulphuric acid (50 ml) and the excess sulphuric acid is titrated with 1 N sodium hydroxide using methyl orange as indicator. Each ml of $1 N H_2SO_4$ is equivalent to 0.04069 g of ZnO.

Uses : Zinc oxide is applied to the skin as a mild astringent, as a soothing and protective application in eczema, and as a protective to slight excoriations often with coal tar. Zinc oxide reflects ultraviolet radiation and is used in sunscreens, and in the treatment of skin ulcerations and other skin problems.

A mixture of zinc oxide and strong solution of zinc chloride is converted into an oxychloride which sets into a hard mass. This mass is used in some dental cements. Mixed with clove oil or eugenol, zinc oxide is used as a temporary dental filling. The antimicrobial-astringent action is due to the release of a small amount of zinc ions due to hydrolysis in the acidic moisture on the skin. It is an ingredient of calamine, zinc gelatin, zinc oxide ointment and zinc oxide paste.

Freshly formed fumes, as from welding, may cause metal fume fever with chills, fever, tightness in chest, cough and leukocytes.

ZINC STEARATE

$[\{CH_3 (CH_2)_{16} CO_2\}_2 Zn]$

$Zn\ C_{36}H_{70}O_4$; Mol. Weight = 632

Zinc stearate is a compound of zinc with a mixture of solid organic acids obtained from fat, and consists mainly of variable proportions of zinc stearate $([CH_3(CH_2)_{16} CO_2]_2 Zn)$ and zinc palmitate ($[CH_3(CH_2)_{14} CO_2]_2Zn$, and usually with some excess of zinc oxide. It contains 10-12% of Zn.

It is prepared from stearic acid and a solution of zinc acetate or some other soluble salt. A calculated amount of commercial stearic acid, which is a mixture of palmitic acid and oleic acid, is added with stirring to a hot solution of sodium hydroxide. The solution of sodium stearate is allowed to cool and a solution of zinc acetate is added. The precipitated zinc stearate is filtered, washed, and dried.

Characters : Zinc stearate occurs as a very fine, light, soft, bulky powder, free from gritty particles; with slight characteristic odour, m.p. 120°. It is unctuous to the touch; readily adheres to the skin; is insoluble in water, alcohol, ether; soluble in benzene. It repels water; and is decomposed by hot mineral acids yielding stearic, and palmitic acids. It is neutral to moistened litmus paper, and stored in well-closed containers.

It is hydrolyzed by heating in dilute mineral acids to form a soluble zinc salt and an insoluble oily layer of stearic and palmitic acids.

Tests for Purity : Tests for arsenic; cadmium; lead; alkalies; alkaline earths; free fatty acids; acid value of the free fatty acid; acidity or alkalinity; colour of solution; chloride; sulphate; clarity and colour of solution of the fatty acids.

For the test of alkali and alkaline earth metals, a sample is dissolved in dilute hydrochloric acid, and a solution of ammonical ammonium sulphide is added to precipitate zinc as zinc sulphide. The sulphide is filtered off to separate liberated fatty acids, the filtrate is acidified with sulphuric acid, dried, ignited and the residue is weighed.

For determining free fatty acids, an ethereal solution is dried to get a residue of the acids. Test for lead is performed in an HNO_3 digested residue of the substance.

Tests for Identification

1. The substance (1 g) is added to a mixture of water (25 ml) and hydrochloric acid (5 ml) and boiled. An oily layer of fatty acids is produced on the surface of the liquid and the lower aqueous layer, after neutralization, gives the tests of zinc.

2. The oily layer is separated on a filter paper wetted with water and washed with water until free from sulphate. The fatty acid is collected, dried and melted (m.p. 54°).

Assay : The assay is based on complexometric titration as in case of magnesium sulphate. A weighed amount of the substance (1 g) is boiled with 0.1 N sulphuric acid (50 ml) until the fatty acid layer is clear. It is cooled, filtered, and washed with water. To the filtrate and washings, strong ammonia-ammonium chloride solution (15 ml) and eriochrome black T solution (0.2 ml) are added. The solution is heated to about 40° and titrated with 0.05 M disodium ethylenediaminetetra acetate until the solution is deep blue in colour. Each ml of 0.05 M disodium ethylenediaminetetra acetate is equivalent to 0.004069 g of ZnO.

Uses : Zinc stearate has mild astringent and antimicrobal properties. It is used in dusting powders and ointments as a soothing and protective agent in the treatment of skin inflammation. It is used either alone or with other powders or in the form of a cream. As it is not wetted by moisture, the product is more desirable in dermatological problems where large amount of fluid exuded.

Zinc stearate is also added as a lubricant to the granules in tablet-making.

Zinc stearate inhalation has caused fatal pneumonitis, (pulmonary inflammation), especially in children.

(B) ANTIMICROBIALS

Antimicrobials include antiseptic, germicide, and disinfectant agents as well as sterilization process. *Antiseptic* is any agent which either kills or inhibits the growth of microorganisms, i.e. growing on man especially or living tissue in general, e.g. bacteria, fungi, protozoans, viruses, etc; thus preventing harmful effects of infection. Germicide agents kill microorganisms. *Disinfectant* agents destroy microorganisms, but not usually bacteria spores. It does not necessarily kill all microorganisms, but reduces them to a level which is harmful neither to health nor the perishable substances. According to their specific properties, disinfectants may be classified as *bacteriocides, sporicides, viricides* and *fungicides. Sterilization* is the total removal or destruction of all living microorganisms which is done by chemicals or by mechanical processes like heat or radiation methods.

The mechanisms of action of inorganic antimicrobial agents may be by oxidation, halogenation and protein precipitation. Primary chemical interactions or reactions that occur between the agent and microbial protein causing death of the microbe or inhibition of its growth. Oxidizing agents are generally nonmetals and some anions, e.g. hydrogen peroxide, metal peroxides, permanganates, halogens and certain oxo-halogen anions. They reduce some groups present in most proteins, e.g. sulphhydryl (-SH) group in cysteine. As the proteins has a specific function in the microorganism, e.g. enzyme, hence the reduction of sulphhydryl group forming the disulphide bridge will alter the conformation of the protein and thereby changes its function; causing destruction of the microorganism.

Halogenation occurs with antiseptic. These compounds serve as a source of chlorination of primary and secondary amides. Similar reaction can take place with the peptide linkage of protein molecules to alter the function of specific proteins. The substitution of the chlorine atom for the hydrogen produces changes in the hydrogen bonding responsible for the proper conformation of the protein molecule.

Metallic ions having large charge or radius ratio or strong electrostatic fields interact proteins. This property is found in transition metal cations, e.g. Cu (II), Ag (I) and Zn (II). Aluminium (III) also precipitates proteins due to its charge and small ionic radius. Except the alkali and alkaline earth metals, most metal cations precipitate proteins. The interaction of metal ions with protein is nonspecific and at sufficient concentration, they will react with the microbial protein and host. Some metals, e.g., mercury, arsenic and antimony, show some enzyme specificity and form strong covalent bonds with specified enzyme systems. The protein precipitant properties of metal cations can be changed according to the concentration at the site of action.

BORAX
(Sodium Borate, Sodium Tetraborate)

$Na_2B_4O_7$; Mol. Weight = 201.2

$Na_2B_4O_7 . 10H_2O$; Mol. Weight = 381.37.

Borax is the sodium salt of pyroboric acid which occurs naturally in lakes of Tibet, Srilanka, India and California. It contains not less than 99.0% of $Na_2B_4O_7 . 10H_2O$.

Preparation

1. The mineral borate is boiled with a concentrated solution of sodium carbonate. The solution is filtered, concentrated and cooled to crystallize borax.

$$Ca_2B_6O_{11} + 2Na_2CO_3 \cdot \longrightarrow 2CaCO_3 + Na_2B_4O_7 + 2NaBO_2$$

Sodium
metaborate

A current of carbon dioxide gas is passed through the mother liquor to convert the metaborate into borax.

$$4NaBO_2 + CO_2 \longrightarrow Na_2CO_3 + Na_2B_4O_7$$

2. Naturally occurring crude borax (Tincal) is dissolved in water, filtered, the filtrate is concentrated and cooled to crystallize borax.

Physical Properties : Borax occurs as odourless transparent colourless crystals, crystalline masses or white crystalline powder. It effloresces in dry air, the crystal often being coated with white powder; m.p. 75°. It loses 5 moles of water at 100° and 9 moles of water at 150°; becomes anhydrous at 320°. It is soluble in water (1 in 20); boiling water (1 in 1) and glycerol (1 in 1); practically insoluble in alcohol. The aqueous solution is alkaline to litmus and phenolphthalein; pH is about 9.5. It is stored in a cooled place in airtight containers.

Chemical Properties

1. The alkalinity of aqueous solutions of borax is due to its hydrolysis :

$$Na_2B_4O_7 + 2H_2O \rightleftharpoons 2NaOH + H_2B_4O_7$$

In concentrated solution, hydrolysis is only partial.

$$Na_2B_4O_7 + 3H_2O \longrightarrow 2NaBO_2 + 2H_3BO_3$$

2. With some metallic salts it gives coloured beads due to formation of metal metaborates.

$$Na_2B_4O_7 + CoO \longrightarrow 2NaBO_2 + Co(BO_2)_2$$

Cobalt oxide	Sod.	Cobalt
	meta	metaborate
	borate	(Blue)

Tests for Purity : Tests for arsenic; iron; lead; calcium; heavy metals; carbonate; free boric acid; chloride; sulphate; alkalinity; clarity and colour of solution, ammonium salt.

A solution prepared in distilled water complies with the limit tests of ammonium, arsenic, calcium, heavy metals and sulphate.

Identification Tests for Borax and Boric Acid

1. *Turmeric paper* is dipped in a solution of borate containing HCl or H_2SO_4. On drying the paper turns brownish red.

When the paper is treated with dilute ammonia solution, or sodium hydroxide or potassium hydroxide solution, the colour changes to blue, green or greenish black.

2. When a mixture of borate, alcohol and concentrated sulphuric acid is ignited in a porcelain dish, the flame turned green due to formation of volatile esters. The esters burn with their characteristic flame.

$$3CH_3OH + H_3BO_3 \longrightarrow (CH_3)_2 BO_3 \uparrow + 3H_2O$$
$$\text{Trimethyl borate}$$

$$3C_2H_5OH + H_3BO_3 \longrightarrow (C_2H_5)_3 BO_3 \uparrow + 3H_2O$$

$$2(CH_3)_3 BO_3 + 9O_2 \xrightarrow{\text{Green flame}} B_2O_3 + 6CO_2 + 9H_2O$$

3. Metal oxides obtained from coloured cations, on fusion with meta- or tetraborates, give typical coloured glasses called borax beads :

$$CuO + Na_2B_4O_7 \longrightarrow Cu (BO_2)_2 + 2NaBO_2$$
$$\text{Blue colour}$$

In case of copper compounds, the reducing flame may give a red opaque beads containing copper.

$$2Cu (BO_2)_2 + 4NaBO_2 + 2C \longrightarrow 2Cu + 2CO_2 \uparrow + 2Na_2B_4O_7.$$

Incompatibilities : Borax is incompatible with gums, alkaloidal salts, zinc sulphate, mineral acids and metallic salts.

Assay : The assay is based on acidimetry and alkalimetry tetration. To an aqueous solution of mannitol (20 in 100), phenolphthalein is added and neutralized with 0.1N sodium hydroxide until the colour of the solution changes to pink. The substance (3g) is dissolved and titrated with 1 N sodium hydroxide until the colour of the solution again becomes pink. Each ml of 1N sodium hydroxide is equivalent to 0.1907 g of $Na_2B_4O_7.10H_2O$.

Uses : Borax is used as pharmaceutical aid (alkalizing agent); as antiseptic, detergent and astringent for mucous membranes. Its activity is the same as that of boric acid due to its hydrolysis to boric acid in aqueous solution. It is used externally in 1 to 2% solutions as an eye wash and as a wet dressing for wounds.

Ingestion of borax can cause severe vomiting, diarrhoea, shock and death.

CHLORINATED LIME

CaOCl (Cl). H_2O

Chlorinated lime (bleachining powder or chlorine of lime) contains not less than 30% w/w of available chlorine. It consists of calcium chloro-hypochlorite, and is a complex chemical compound of indefinite composition, presumably consisting of varying proportions of $Ca(OCl)_2$, $CaCl_2$, chlorine ions, $Ca(OH)_2$ and H_2O in its molecular structure. It is relatively unstable chlorine carrier in solid form. Maximum available chlorine content approaches 39%.

Preparation : Bleaching powder is prepared on commercial scale by the action of chlorine on pure, dry calcium hydroxide (slaked lime). The slaked lime is spread in lead chambers and chlorine is passed into the chambers from 12 to 24 hours to saturate the lime.

$$Ca(OH)_2 + Cl_2 \longrightarrow Ca(OCl)Cl + H_2O$$

Physical Properties : Chlorinated lime is a dull white powder, containing not less than 30% w/w of chlorine. It has strong odour of chlorine. On exposure to air it becomes moist and rapidly decomposes to release hypochlorous acid. Carbon dioxide being absorbed and chlorine evolved. It is partly soluble in water and alcohol. Aqueous solutions are strongly alkaline. It is stored in well-closed containers.

Chemical Reactions

1. When shaken with cold water and filtered, the cold filtrate gives the reactions of chlorides and hypochloride ions while on heating it shows the presence of chloride and chlorate ions.

$$CaOCl_2 \longrightarrow Ca^{++} + Cl^- + ClO^-$$
$$3ClO^- \longrightarrow ClO_3^- + 2Cl^-$$

2. Treatment of chlorinated lime with dilute acids liberates hypochlorous acid which behaves as an oxidizing and bleaching agent.

$$2CaOCl_2 + H_2SO_4 \longrightarrow CaCl_2 + CaSO_4 + 2HClO$$
$$HClO \longrightarrow HCl + O$$

On treatment with excess of dilute acid or CO_2, the whole of chlorine is liberated.

$$CaOCl_2 + H_2SO_4 \longrightarrow CaSO_4 + H_2O + Cl_2$$

$$CaOCl_2 + CO_2 \longrightarrow CaCO_3 + Cl_2$$

This amount of chlorine is called as "available chlorine" which is about 35.38% in a good sample.

3. In the presence of cobalt chloride, chlorinated lime is decomposed to liberate oxygen.

$$2CaOCl_2 \longrightarrow 2CaCl_2 + O_2$$

Auto-oxidation of bleaching powder gives calcium chloride as :

$$6CaOCl_2 \longrightarrow Ca(ClO_3)_2 + 5CaCl_2$$

Tests for Identification

1. It evolves chlorine copiously on addition of 2N sulphuric acid.
2. When shaken with water and filtered, the filtrate yields reactions characteristic of calcium salts and chloride.

Assay : The assay is based on the iodometric and iodimetric tetration. An aqueous suspension of the substance is treated with acetic acid in the presence of excess of potassium iodide.

$$Ca(OCl) Cl + CH_3COOH \longrightarrow Ca(CH_3COO)_2 + HCl + HOCl$$
$$\text{Hypochlorous acid}$$

$$HOCl + HCl \longrightarrow H_2O + Cl$$

$$2KI + Cl_2 \longrightarrow 2KCl + I_2$$

Hypochlorous acid and hydrochloric acid react to form chlorine which displaces an equivalent amount of iodine from potassium iodide. The liberated iodine is titrated with a standard solution of sodium thiosulphate using starch solution as an indicator. The end point is disappearance of blue colour.

$$2Na_2S_2O_3 + I_2 \longrightarrow Na_2S_4O_6 + 2NaI$$
$$\text{Sodium}$$
$$\text{tetrathionate}$$

The substance (4 g) is triturated with successive small quantities of water, diluted with water (1000 ml) and shaken. The resulting suspension (100 ml) is mixed with a solution containing potassium iodide (3 g) in water (100 ml), acidified with 6N acetic acid and the liberated iodine titrated with 0.1 N sodium thiosulphate. Each ml of 0.1N sodium thiosulphate is equivalent to 3.545 mg of available chlorine, Cl.

Uses : Chlorinated lime has a rapid bactericidal action. It is used for the chlorination treatment of water in swimming pools, to disinfect faeces, urine, and other organic material, as a cleansing agent for lavatories, drains, and effluents and in the preparation of surgical chlorinated soda solution (Dakin's solution) employed as a wound disinfectant. A mixture of chlorinated lime and boric acid solution (eusol) is used as a disinfectant lotion and wet dressing. It kills most of bacteria, some fungi, yeasts, algae, viruses, and protozoa.

Ingestion of the chlorinated lime causes irritation and corrosion of mucous membranes with pain and vomiting. A fall in blood pressure, delirium, and coma may occur. Inhalation of fumes may cause laryngeal and pulmonary irritation, pulmonary edema and death.

HYDROGEN PEROXIDE SOLUTION

H_2O_2; Mol. Weight = 34.02

Hydrogen peroxide is an aqueous solution containing 29 to 31% w/w of H_2O_2, corresponding to about 100 times its volume of available oxygen. It may contain suitable stabilizing agent.

Preparation

1. **From Barium Peroxide :** Treatment of a thin aqueous cream of barium peroxide with cold dilute sulphuric acid forms hydrogen peroxide :

$$BaO_2 + H_2SO_4 \longrightarrow BaSO_4 + H_2O_2$$

   When carbon dioxide is passed slowly through ice-cold paste of barium peroxide, hydrogen peroxide is produced. The precipitated barium carbonate is filtered off.

$$BaO_2 + CO_2 + H_2O \longrightarrow BaCO_3 + H_2O_2$$

   Hydrogen peroxide can also be prepared by decomposing barium peroxide with phosphoric acid.

2. **From Sodium Peroxide :** Calculated amount of sodium peroxide is decomposed by addition of ice-cold dilute sulphuric acid. Most of the sodium sulphate is crystallized on cooling as the decahydrate and the hydrogen peroxide is distilled under 10 mm pressure.

$$Na_2O_2 + H_2SO_4 \longrightarrow Na_2SO_4 + H_2O_2$$

3. **By Electrolytic Process :** Commercially hydrogen peroxide is prepared by electrolysis of 50% sulphuric acid followed by vacuum distillation. In the first step persulphuric acid

is formed which on vacuum distillation is converted into hydrogen peroxide.

$$Na_2O_2 + H_2SO_4 \longrightarrow Na_2SO_4 + H_2O_2$$

$$2H_2SO_4 \longrightarrow H_2S_2O_8 + H_2$$

Persulphuric
acid

$$H_2S_2O_8 + 2H_2O \longrightarrow 2H_2SO_4 + H_2O_2$$

4. **From Ammonium Sulphate :** Ammonium sulphate and sulphuric acid are mixed to form ammonium bisulphate and the cold solution is electrolyzed to yield ammonium peroxydisulphate.

$$(NH_4)_2SO_4 + H_2SO_4 \longrightarrow 2NH_4HSO_4$$

Ammonium
bisulphate

$$\downarrow$$

$$(NH_4)_2S_2O_8 + H_2$$

Ammonium
peroxydisulphate

Ammonium peroxydisulphate is distilled directly, or treated with sulphuric acid and distilled at reduced pressure to yield strong hydrogen peroxide solution.

$$(NH_4)_2S_2O_8 + 2H_2O \longrightarrow 2NH_4HSO_4 + H_2O_2$$

$$(NH_4)_2 S_2O_8 + H_2SO_4 \longrightarrow H_2S_2O_8 + (NH_4)_2 SO_4$$

$$H_2S_2O_8 + 2H_2O_2 \longrightarrow 2H_2SO_4 + H_2O_2$$

In an another procedure ammonium peroxydisulphate is converted into intermediate less soluble potassium peroxy-disulphate with potassium bisulphate and then hydrolyzed with steam.

$$(NH_4)_2 S_2O_2 + 2KHSO_4 \longrightarrow K_2S_2O_8 + 2NH_4HSO_4$$

$$K_2S_2O_8 + 2H_2O \longrightarrow 2KHSO_4 + H_2O_2$$

Physical Properties : Hydrogen peroxide is a clear, colourless, odourless or may have an odour resembling that of ozone; unstable liquid; bitter taste; caustic to skin; distilled in high vacuum; acidic to litmus. It is miscible with water; soluble in ether; insoluble in petroleum ether; decomposed by many organic solvents.

Solutions of hydrogen peroxide gradually deteriorate on standing and are usually stabilized by the addition of acetanilide or similar organic compounds. Agitation or contact with rough surfaces, metals or many other substances accelerates decomposition. It decomposes when in contact with many oxidizing or reducing substances. It is rapidly decomposed by alkalies, and finely divided metals. It is unstable on prolonged exposure to light, and may decompose on heating.

Its stability is increased by adding small amount of sulphuric or phosphoric acid; by addition of inorganic or organic preservatives; chelating or complexing agents such as quinine sulphate, 8-hydroxyquinoline, boric acid, urea, acetanilide, or hexamine. These compounds chelate trace amounts of polyvalent metals making them unavailable to catalyze the decomposition. Many adsorbents, e.g. alumina and silica will remove impurities from hydrogen peroxide solution.

Hydrogen peroxide solution is stored in partially-filled containers having a stabilizing agent and a small vent in the closure, at a temperature of 8 to 15°; protected from light.

Chemical Reactions

1. **Decomposition :** Pure hydrogen peroxide when kept in suitable containers decomposes very slowly, even in concentrated solution. It decomposes into water and oxygen rapidly in alkaline solution or in the presence of copper, iron or manganese ions, or when heated to 100°C.

$$2H_2O_2 \longrightarrow 2H_2O + O_2$$

The oxygen acts as an oxidizing agent on bacteria, providing antiseptic action.

2. **Oxidation Reactions :** Hydrogen peroxide is a strong oxidizing agent and reacts many organic materials. It oxidizes lead sulphide to lead sulphate, arsenites to arsenates, sodium sulphite to sodium sulphate, ferrous sulphate to ferric sulphate, potassium ferrocyanide to potassium ferricyanide and liberates iodine from potassium iodide solution.

$$PbS + 4H_2O_2 \longrightarrow PbSO_4 + 4H_2O$$

$$Na_2AsO_3 + H_2O_2 \longrightarrow Na_3AsO_4 + H_2O$$

Sodium	Sodium
arsenite	arsenate

$$Na_2SO_3 + H_2O_2 \longrightarrow Na_2SO_4 + H_2O$$

Sodium	Sodium
sulphite	sulphate

$$KNO_2 + H_2O_2 \longrightarrow KNO_3 + H_2O$$

Potassium   Potassium
nitrite   nitrate

$$2FeSO_4 + H_2SO_4 + H_2O_2 \longrightarrow Fe_2 (SO_4)_3 + 2H_2O$$

Ferrous   Ferric
sulphate   sulphate

$$2K_4Fe (CN)_6 + H_2O_2 \longrightarrow 2K_3Fe (CN)_6 + 2KOH$$

Potassium   Pot ferricyanide
ferrocyanide

$$2KI + H_2O_2 \longrightarrow 2KOH + I_2$$

3. **Reducing Properties :** Hydrogen peroxide behaves as a reducing agent towards other oxidizing agents. It reduces silver oxide to silver, potassium permanganate to potassium sulphate and manganese sulphate, ozone to oxygen, chlorine to hydrochloric acid and potassium ferricyanide to potassium ferrocyanide.

$$H_2O_2 + O \longrightarrow H_2O + O_2$$

$$Ag_2O + H_2O_2 \longrightarrow 2Ag + H_2O + O_2$$

$$2KMnO_4 + 3H_2SO_4 + 5H_2O_2 \longrightarrow K_2SO_4 + 2MnSO_4$$
$$+ 8H_2O + 5O_2$$

$$O_3 + H_2O_2 \longrightarrow 2O_2 + H_2O$$

$$Cl_2 + H_2O_2 \longrightarrow 2HCl + O_2$$

$$2K_3Fe (CN)_6 + 2KOH + H_2O_2 \longrightarrow 2K_4Fe (CN)_6 + 2H_2O + O_2$$

4. **Acidic Nature :** Hydrogen peroxide is slightly acidic in nature though in dilute solution it is neutral towards litmus. It reacts alkalies and carbonates to form their respective peroxides.

$$2NaOH + H_2O_2 \longrightarrow Na_2O_2 + 2H_2O$$

$$Ba(OH)_2 + H_2O_2 \longrightarrow BaO_2 + 2H_2O$$

$$Na_2CO_3 + H_2O_2 \longrightarrow Na_2O_2 + CO_2 + H_2O$$

5. **Colour Reaction :** When hydrogen peroxide is added to an acidified aqueous solution of potassium chromate containing ether, a deep colour is formed between the ether and the aqueous solution due to a perchromic acid (CrO_2-O-O-CrO_2-OH) which is fairly stable in ethereal solution. The test is very sensitive even when the dilution of H_2O_2 is 0.0015%.

Hydrogen peroxide reacts with diphenyl phenol in the presence of an enzyme, *Catalase*, which decomposes H_2O_2 into water and oxygen. The liberating oxygen oxidizes the phenols into blue-coloured quinones.

Tests for Purity : Tests for acidity; barium; slabilizing agent; and non-volatile matter.

For testing the presence of a preservative, H_2O_2 is extracted with chloroform, the chloroform-layer is evaporated under reduced pressure and the residue is weighed.

Acidity is determined by titrating diluted solution with 0.1 N sodium hydroxide using methyl red solution as an indicator.

To 10 ml of H_2O_2, 1 ml of dilute sulphuric acid is added. If no turbidity is produced, barium is absent.

Incompatibilities : Reducing agents, oxidizing agents, alkalies, organic matter, heavy metal ions, heat, agitation, iodides, permanganates, copper, manganese ion and their salts; calcium and strontium salts.

Tests for Identification

1. It decomposes with effervescence when made alkaline and heated, evolving oxygen.
2. To one drop of H_2O_2, dilute sulphuric acid, potassium chromate solution and solvent ether are added and shaked; the ethereal layer is coloured blue.
3. To 1ml, sulphuric acid (1N, 0.2 ml) and potassium permanganate solution (0.02N) are added. The solution becomes colourless with evolution of gas.

Assay : The assay is dependent on the oxidation-reduction (redox) titration. Hydrogen peroxide is titrated with a standard solution of potassium permanganate in the presence of sulphuric acid at room temperature. Potassium sulphate itself acts as an indicator. The end point is appeared as a permanent pink colour.

$$2KMnO_4 + 3H_2SO_4 + 5H_2O \longrightarrow K_2SO_4 + 2MnSO_4 + 8H_2O + 5O_2$$

Hydrogen peroxide (10 ml) is diluted with water (250 ml); 5N sulphuric acid (5ml) is added to the solution (25 ml) and titrated with 0.1N potassium permanganate to a permanent pink end-point. Each ml of 0.1 N $KMnO_4$ is equivalent to 0.00170 g of H_2O_2.

Uses : Hydrogen peroxide is used as a disinfectant, anti-infective and deodorant. Antimicrobial effect of the liberated oxygen is reduced in the presence of organic matter. It is used as mild oxidizing antiseptic to cleanse wounds and ulcers in concentrations up to 6%. It destroys most pathogenic bacteria, e.g., *Escherichia coli*, *Staphylococces aureus*, and *typhoid bacilli*. Hydrogen peroxide solution (1.5%) is used as a mouth-wash in the treatment of acute stomatitis and as a deordant gargle. In dentistry it is used to clean septic sockets and root canals. Hydrogen peroxide ear-drops have been used for the removal of wax. It is also employed as bleaching and oxidizing agent. The effervescent action removes dirt, bacteria and debris from the surface of a wound or difficult-to-reach areas, e.g. the ear canal.

Strong solution of hydrogen peroxide produce irritating burns on the skin and mucous membranes with a white eschar. Continued use of H_2O_2 as a mouth-wash may cause reversible hypertrophy of the papillae of the tongue.

IODINE

I_2; Mol. Weight = 253.8

Iodine contains not less than 99.5 per cent of I. It occurs in the combined state as iodides in California oil-well brines, sea water, sea-weeds, Chile salt-petre mother liquors, and various brines.

Preparation

1. **From Seaweeds :** Dried seaweeds of *Laminaria* species is burnt and the ash, called *kelp*, containing 0.4-1.3% iodates, is extracted with water. The aqueous extract is concentrated and crystallized to separate sulphates and chlorides of sodium and potassium. The small amounts of sulphides and thiosulphates present, are decomposed by adding sulphuric acid and the precipitated sulphur is separated. The acid solution contains soluble iodides and small amounts of bromides and chlorides. The solution is treated with chlorine to precipitate iodine which is collected and purified by sublimation. This iodine contains iodine chloride (ICl) and iodine bromide (IBr). When it is sublimed with a small amount of potassium iodide, potassium chloride and potassium bromide are formed with the production of iodine.

$$KI + ICl \longrightarrow KCl + I_2$$
$$KI + IBr \longrightarrow KBr + I_2$$

2. **From Caliche :** The mother liquor left after the crystallization of sodium nitrate from the solution of *Caliche* (crude Chile salt petre) contains some iodine as sodium iodate. This is treated with a calculated amount of sodium bisulphite to precipitate iodine liberated due to reduction of sodium iodate.

$$2NaIO_3 + 5NaHSO_3 \longrightarrow 3NaHSO_4 + 2Na_2SO_4 + I_2 + H_2O$$

The precipitated iodine is filtered, dried and purified by sublimation.

Physical Characters : Iodine occurs as heavy bluish-black or greyish-violet, brittle plates or small crystals or scales, with a metallic sheen and a distinctive penetrating irritant odour; sharp, acrid taste; violet corrosive vapour, m.p. 113.6°. It is slowly volatile at room temperature; very slightly soluble in water; soluble in alcohol (1 in 8), chloroform (1 in 30); slightly soluble in glycerol and very soluble in concentrated solutions of iodides, carbon disulphide, solvent ether and carbon tetrachloride. Solutions of iodine in aqueous solutions of inorganic iodides are brown. Chloroform, carbon tetrachlorride, carbon disulphide and phosphorus trichloride give violet solutions. The solubility in solutions of iodides (e.g. sodium iodide) is due to the formation of triiodide ion (I_3). Both the iodide and triiodide do not show antibacterial activity. The triiodide ion is converted into I_2 and I, thus retaining antibacterial potency.

Iodine is stored in glass stoppered bottles.

Chemical Properties

1. Iodine is a halogen but it is less active than chlorine and bromine. Iodine combines readily with elements like antimony, phosphorus, potassium, mercury and many other metals yielding the corresponding iodide.

$$2Sb + 3I_2 \longrightarrow 2SbI_3$$
$$P_4 + 6I_2 \longrightarrow 4PI_3$$
$$Hg + I_2 \longrightarrow HgI_2$$

2. In aqueous medium iodine behaves as an oxidizing agent. It oxidizes hydrogen sulphide to sulphur, sulphur dioxide to sulphuric acid, nitrites to nitrates, sulphites to sulphates, arsenites to arsenates and sodium thiosulphate to sodium tetrathionate.

$$I_2 + H_2O \longrightarrow HI + HIO$$

$$H_2S + I_2 \longrightarrow S + 2HI$$
$$SO_2 + 2H_2O + I_2 \longrightarrow H_2SO_4 + 2HI$$
$$KNO_2 + I_2 + H_2O \longrightarrow KNO_3 + 2HI$$
$$Na_2SO_3 + I_2 + H_2O \longrightarrow Na_2SO_4 + 2HI$$
$$Na_2AsO_3 + I_2 + H_2O \longrightarrow Na_3AsO_4 + 2HI$$
$$2Na_2S_2O_3 + I_2 \longrightarrow Na_2S_4O_6 + 2NaI$$

3. With cold sodium hydroxide solution, iodine reacts to form a hypoiodide which hydrolyzes to give hypoiodous acid.

$$2NaOH + I_2 \xrightarrow{\quad -NaI \quad} NaIO + H_2O \longrightarrow HIO + NaOH$$

With hot or even in cold on long contact, iodine reacts with alkali to form iodate.

$$6NaOH + 3I_2 \longrightarrow 5NaI + NaIO_3 + 3H_2O$$
$$\text{Sodium}$$
$$\text{iodate}$$

$$6NH_4OH + 3I_2 \longrightarrow 5NH_4I + NH_4IO_3 + 3H_2O$$

4. Iodine reacts with liquor ammonia to yield a black explosive powder, nitrogen trioxide.

$$2NH_3 + 3I_2 \longrightarrow NI_3 + 3HI$$

5. Iodine dissociates at 700° to form elemental iodine ($I_2 === 2I$).
6. Iodine reacts with concentrated potassium chlorate solution, in the presence of small amount of nitric acid on heating to produce potassium iodate.

$$2KClO_3 + I_2 \longrightarrow 2KIO_3 + Cl_2$$

7. Iodine reacts with organic compounds slowly to form alkyl iodides.

$$CH_4 + I_2 \longrightarrow CH_3I + HI$$
$$CH_2{=}CH_2 + I_2 \longrightarrow CH_2I\text{-}CH_2I$$

8. Iodine acts as a reducing agent and can be oxidized to iodic acid (HIO_3) and iodates by strong oxidizing agents.

$$I_2 + 5Cl_2 \text{ (excess)} + 6H_2O \longrightarrow 2HIO_3 + 10HCl$$
$$3I_2 + 5KClO_3 + 3H_2O \longrightarrow 6HIO_3 + 5KCl$$

9. Iodine reacts with starch mucilage to form a deep blue colour which disappears on heating and reappears on cooling.

Tests for Purity : Tests for chloride and bromide; cyanogen; and non-volatile matter.

Chlorides and bromidess are tested by treating aqueous extract of iodine, previously decolourized with zinc dust, with silver nitrate in the presence of nitric acid. Silver iodide is almost insoluble in dilute ammonia, whereas silver chloride is freely and silver bromide is less soluble. The soluble silver halide is reprecipitated on addition of excess of dilute nitric acid. Cyanogen (ICN) is detected in the solution by the Prussian blue test.

Incompatibilities : It has incompatibility with iodine oxides, hypophosphites, sulphites and many reducing compounds. It reacts with volatile oils, fixed oils, turpentine, ammonia water, ammoniated mercury, alkali hydroxides, and carbonates. It precipitates many alkaloids and gives colour reaction with starch.

Tests for Identification

1. When gently heated, it gives violet coloured vapours which condense, forming a bluish-black crystalline sublimate.
2. With a solution of potassium iodide and starch, a deep blue colour is produced which disappears on boiling but reappears on cooling.

Assay : The assay is based on iodometric titration. The end point is disappearance of blue colour. An aqueous solution of iodine, potassium iodide and dilute acetic acid is titrated with 0.1N sodium thiosulphate, using starch solution as indicator. Each ml of 0.1N sodium thiosulphate is equivalent to 0.01269 g of iodine.

$$2Na_2S_2O_3 + I_2 \longrightarrow Na_2S_4O_6 + 2NaI$$

Sodium
tetraiodate

SOLUTIONS OF IODINE

Strong Iodine Solution or Aqueous Iodine Solution or Lugol's Solution : It is the only official solution of iodine that contains no alcohol and used for internal administration as counter irritant and disinfectant. It is prepared by dissolving iodine (5%, w/v) or potassium or sodium iodide (10%, w/v) in water. Alcoholic solutions (tinctures) are more irritating than strong iodine solution. They dry faster than the aqueous solutions when applied externally due to evaporation of alcohol. Strong aqueous solution and tinctures can be diluted by addition of water without effecting the antiseptic action.

Weak Iodine Solution : It contains iodine (2.5%, w/v) and potassium iodide (2.5%, w/v). For its preparation a weighed amount of iodine is dissolved in aqueous solution of potassium iodide and the required volume is made up by adding sufficient alcohol (90%). Alcoholic content of I.P. grade is from 45 to 48% v/v.

Iodine Tincture : It contains iodine (2%, w/v) and sodium iodide (2.4%, w/v). It is identical to weak iodine solution, but it contains very small amount of alcohol.

Iodine Ampules : They are sealed ampules containing Iodine tincture. The ampules are used for local application in first aid treatment. Generally the ampules are covered with an absorbent material to absorb iodine when the tip is broken. Iodine may be directly applied to a wound from the ampule.

Phenolated Iodine Solution : (Binlton's solution or carbolized iodine solution). It is prepared by mixing strong iodine solution (15 ml), phenol (6 ml), glycerin (165 ml) and sufficient water to make the volume up to 1000 ml. The mixture is heated in a tightly closed glass-stoppered container below 70°C or exposed to sunlight for sometime until the solution becomes colourless or faintly yellow. The solution is used as such externally as an antiseptic mouthwash and as an antibacterial agent.

Uses : Iodine is used as antihyperthyroid, topical anti-infective, germicides, antiseptics and in the manufacture of iodine compounds. Iodine is the essential trace element in the human diet; it is necessary for the formation of thyroid hormones. It is administered as potassium and sodium iodides, as iodised oil injection or as potassium iodate for the treatment of iodide deficiency disorders, such as endemic goitre.

Prolonged use of iodine may produce metallic taste, increased salivation, burning or pain, and coryza. Topical application can give rise allergic reactions.

POVIDONE-IODINE

It is an iodophoric complex of iodine with povidone produced by the interaction between iodine and poly (2-oxopyrrolidin-1-yl ethylene). It contains 9 to 12% of available iodine calculated on the dried basis at 105°C. It occurs as a yellowish-brown amorphous powder with a slight characteristic odour. It loses not more than 8% of its weight on drying. It is soluble in water and alcohol; insoluble in acetone, carbon tetrachloride, chloroform, solvent ether and petroleum ether. Aqueous solutions have a pH of 1.5 to 6.5. The aqueous solution may be made neutral, but less stable, by the addition of sodium bicarbonate.

Solutions do not give the familiar starch test when freshly prepared. It is stored in airtight containers.

Povidone-iodine is an iodophor, i.e. complex of iodine with a carrier organic molecule serving as a solubilizing agent. Such complexes slowly liberate iodine in solution.

Tests for Identification

1. To the aqueous solution starch mucilage is added. A deep blue colour is produced.

2. When a filter paper moistened with starch mucilage is covered on the mouth of the flask containing the aqueous solution, no blue colour is produced on the paper within 60 seconds.

3. To the aqueous solution sodium thiosulphate solution is added dropwise until the colour of the iodine is just discharged. To the solution hydrochloric acid and potassium dichromate are added. A red precipitate is produced.

4. To the solution of test 3 after addition of sodium thiosulphate, ammonium cobaltothiocyanate solution previously acidified with 5N hydrochloric acid is mixed. A blue precipitate is produced.

Assay : The acidified aqueous solution is titrated with 0.02 N sodium thiosulphate determining the end point potentiometrically. Each ml of 0.02 N sodium thiosulphate is equivalent to 2.538 mg of I.

Uses : Povidone-iodine is used as a disinfectant and antiseptic for the treatment of contaminated wounds and pre-operative preparation of the skin and mucous membranes. It is used in gargles and mouthwashes for the treatment of infections in the oral cavity.

Solutions of povidone-iodine release iodine slowly to exert an effect against bacteria, fungi, viruses, protozoa, cysts and spores. The antiseptic activity of povidone-iodine is reduced by alkalies. The main advantages of slow release of iodine are nonirritating effects on tissue, low oral toxicity, its water solubility and its low iodine vapour pressure preventing iodine loss.

Povidone-iodine may produce local reactions.

MERCURY

Hg; Mol. Weight = 200.6.

Mercury contains not less than 99.5% of Hg.

The principal ore of mercury is a red sulphide mineral called *cinnabar*, HgS. The metal is also found in free state in its ore in the form of minute globules.

Preparation : For the extraction of mercury, the ore is crushed, finely powdered and concentrated by *Froth Flotation Process*. The concentrated ore is heated to form mercuric oxide by oxidation of *cinnabar*. The oxide decomposes at 300°C to yield mercury.

$$2HgS + 3O_2 \longrightarrow 2HgO + 2SO_2$$

$$2HgO \longrightarrow 2Hg + O$$

Mercury vaporizes and the vapours are condensed.

Physical Characters : Mercury occurs as a shining, silvery white, very mobile liquid, easily divisible into globules, which readily volatilises on heating; m.p. -38.9°; b.p. 35.6°. Solid mercury is a tin-white, ductile, malleable mass which may be cut with a knife. When pure, it does not tarnish on exposure to air at ordinary temperature, but when heated to near the boiling point, it slowly oxidizes to HgO. It forms alloys with most metals except iron and combines with sulphur at ordinary temperature.

Chemical Reactions

1. Mercury tarnishes slowly in air (auto-oxidation). It forms mercuric oxide on heating at about 300°C which decomposes to give mercury again at higher temperature.

$$2Hg + O_2 \xrightarrow{\text{300°C}} 2HgO.$$

2. Mercury reacts with oxidizing acids like nitric acid to yield mercuric nitrate and nitric oxide. It does not react with dilute HCl, cold H_2SO_4, or alkalies.

$$3Hg + 8HNO_3 \longrightarrow 3Hg(NO_3)_2 + 2NO + 4H_2O.$$

Reaction with concentrated nitric acid forms mercuric nitrate and nitrogen dioxide.

$$Hg + 4HNO_3 \longrightarrow Hg(NO_3)_2 + 2NO_2 + 2H_2O$$

Treating the mercuric nitrate with metallic mercury undergoes auto-oxidation-reduction to produce mercurous nitrate.

$$Hg(NO_3)_2 + Hg \longrightarrow Hg_2(NO_3)_2$$

3. When mercury is treated with concentrated sulphuric acid, sulphur dioxide is formed.

$$2Hg \text{ (excess)} + 2H_2SO_4 \longrightarrow Hg_2SO_4 + SO_2 + 2H_2O$$

$$Hg + 2H_2SO_4 \text{ (excess)} \longrightarrow HgSO_4 + SO_2 + 2H_2O$$

4. Mercury combines directly with halogens and sulphur. Mercuric iodide is formed by simply triturating the metal with solid iodine.

$$Hg + Cl_2 \longrightarrow HgCl_2$$

$$Hg + S \longrightarrow HgS$$

5. Mercury reacts with ammonia solutions in air to form Hg_2NOH (Millon's base).

6. Mercury salts when heated with Na_2CO_3 yield metallic Hg and are reduced to metal by H_2O_2 in the presence of alkali hydroxide.

7. Copper, iron, zinc and many other metals precipitate metallic mercury from neutral or slightly acid solutions of mercury salts. Soluble ionized mercuric salts give a yellow precipitate of HgO with sodium hydroxide and a red precipitate of mercuric iodide with alkali iodide. Mercurous salts give a black precipitate with alkali hydroxides and a white precipitate of calomel with HCl or soluble chlorides. They are slowly decomposed by sunlight.

Tests for Purity : Weight per ml; non-volatile matter.

Tests for Mercury : Most of the mercury compounds sublime unchanged on heating in a dry tube. Characteristic precipitable mercuric compounds are prepared. For example, mercurous salts with dilute HCl give dilute precipitate of mercurous chloride, HgCl, which is insoluble in hot water and turns black on treating with ammonia. With hydrogen sulphide, mercuric salts give a black precipitate of mercuric sulphide, HgS, which is insoluble in nitric acid. The sulphide is soluble in concentrated nitric acid and hydrochloric acid.

Addition of a mercuric compound to a soluble iodide forms red iodide, HgI_2. The yellow mercuric oxide HgO, is formed by addition of sodium hydroxide.

Assay : The assay is based on the modified Volhard's method as discussed for sodium chloride and ammonium chloride. A weighed amount (0.4 g) is dissolved in a mixture (20 ml) of equal parts of water and nitric acid and heated gently until the solution is colourless. Water (150 ml) and sufficient potassium permenganate solution are added to produce a permanent pink colour. The pink colour is decolourized by the addition of a trace of ferrous sulphate and titrated with 0.1 N ammonium thiocyanate at a temperature not exceeding 20°, using ferric ammonium sulphate solution as indication. Each ml of 0.1 N ammonium thiocyanate is equivalent to 0.01003 g of Hg.

Uses : Mercury has cathartic action. The ionizable mercury salts are used as disinfectants, parasiticides and fungicides. The organic mercurials are used as preservatives. A nitrated oxide of mercury is used in homeopathy.

Mercury is readily absorbed via respiratory tract, intact skin, and gastro-intestinal tract. Solutions of salts have violent carrosive effects on skin and mucous membranes; severe nausea, vomiting, abdominal pain, bloody diarrhoea, kidney damage and death.

AMMONIATED MERCURY
(White Precipitate)

NH_2HgCl; Mol. Weight = 252.1

Ammoniated mercury is the mercuric chloride in which one chlorine atom has been replaced by the univalent amino group. It contains not less than 98.0 per cent of NH_2HgCl.

Preparation : Ammoniated mercury is prepared by adding an aqueous solution of mercuric chloride to dilute ammonia solution with constant stirring.

$$HgCl_2 + 2NH_3 \longrightarrow NH_2 + HgCl + NH_4Cl$$

The precipitate is filtered, washed with cold water to remove ammonium chloride and dried at a temperature not exceeding 30°.

Characters : Ammoniated mercury is a white heavy, odourless amorphous powder which is stable in air; but darkens on exposure to light. It is practically insoluble in water and alcohol, soluble in warm hydrochloric, nitric and acetic acids. It is stored in well-closed containers and protected from light.

It is slowly decomposed when dissolved in cold water. In boiling water it is hydrolyzed to a yellow basic compound, NH_2-$HgCl\ H_2O$. When boiled with sodium hydroxide solution, it is decomposed into ammonia, mercuric oxide and sodium chloride.

$$NH_2 . HgCl + NaOH \longrightarrow NH_3 + HgO + NaCl$$

Tests for Purity : Tests for mercurous chloride; carbonates; and sulphated residue.

Mercurous chloride is not soluble in acetic acid and carbonate; gives effervescence in the same test. Ammonium chloride is generally present in the commercial sample of ammoniated mercury in small amount.

Mercurous compounds are detected by dissolving the salt in hydrochloric acid. It is filtered, dried and weighed.

Tests for Identification

1. It is soluble in aqueous solution of sodium thiosulphate with the evolution of ammonia. When this solution is heated gently, a rust-coloured mixture is formed, from which a red precipitate is obtained on centrifugation. If the solution is strongly heated, a black mixture forms.

2. When heated with 1 N sodium hydroxide, it becomes yellow and ammonia is evolved.

3. A solution in warm acetic acid yields with potassium iodide a red precipitate, which is soluble in an excess of the reagent. The solution yields a white precipitate with silver nitrate.

Assay : The assay is based on the neutralization titration (acidimetry-alkalimetry). It is an indirect method where the substance is treated to liberate alkali quantitatively. The compound is treated with water and excess of potassium iodide.

$$NH_2HgCl + 2KI + H_2O \longrightarrow \underset{\text{Insoluble}}{HgI_2} + KCl + KOH + NH_3$$

$$HgI_2 + 2KI \longrightarrow \underset{\text{Soluble}}{K_2HgI_4}$$

$$NH_3 + H_2O \longrightarrow NH_4OH$$

$$KOH + NH_4OH + 2HCl \longrightarrow KCl + NH_4Cl + H_2O$$

The liberated alkalies, i.e. ammonium hydroxide and potassium hydroxide, are titrated with a standard solution of hydrochloric acid using methyl orange as indicator.

Ammoniated mercury (0.25 g) is mixed with water (10 ml), potassium iodide (3 g) added and dissolved and water (40 ml) added again. The mixture is titrated with 0.1 N hydrochloric acid using methyl red as indicator. A blank determination is performed and any necessary correction made. Each ml of 0.1 N hydrochloric acid is equivalent to 12.60 mg of NH_2HgCl.

Uses : Ammoniated mercury was formerly used topically as an anti-infective agent in the treatment of impetigo (infectious skin disease) and other staphylococcal skin infections, in dermatomycoses; in psoriasis; and in crab infestations.

Adverse effects of Ammoniated mercury therapy include allergic reactions, acrodynia and mercury poisoning.

YELLOW MERCURIC OXIDE

HgO; Mol. Weight = 216.6

It contains not less than 99% of HgO, calculated with reference to the substance dried at 105° for one hour.

Preparation

Yellow mercuric oxide is prepared by precipitation of mercuric nitrate or mercuric chloride solution with sodium hydroxide solution. The yellow precipitate is allowed to settle, washed by decantation, filtered, re-washed to separate chloride and dried in air.

$$Hg\,(NO_3)_2 + 2NaOH \longrightarrow \underset{\text{Yellow}}{HgO} + 2NaNO_2 + H_2O$$

$$HgCl_2 + 2NaOH \longrightarrow HgO + 2NaCl + H_2O$$

It is also prepared by decomposing the nitrate by heat or by heating mercury for a long time in air at 300°C.

$$2Hg\,(NO_3)_2 \longrightarrow 2HgO + 4NO_3 + O_2$$

$$2Hg + O_2 \longrightarrow 2HgO$$

Characters : Yellow mercuric oxide is yellow or orange-yellow, heavy, impalpable, amorphous, odourless powder having orthorhombic structure. It is stable in air but becomes discoloured on exposure to light; practically insoluble in water; soluble in dilute HCl or HNO_3 or in solutions of alkali cyanides or iodides forming colourless solutions; slowly soluble in solution of alkali bromides; insoluble in alcohol. It is protected from light; incompatibility with reducing agents.

On heating, the yellow mercuric oxide is converted into red variety but on strong heating it decomposes to give oxygen.

$$2HgO \longrightarrow 2Hg + O_2$$

The red oxide occurs as heavy, orange red, crystalline scales or as a crystalline powder. When it is divided finely, it acquires a yellow colour.

It is preserved in a well-closed container, protected from light.

Tests for Purity : Tests for mercurous salts; chloride; loss on drying; sulphated ash; acidity or alkalinity.

For detecting mercurous salts a solution in dilute hydrochloric acid is not more than slightly turbid.

Assay : The assay is dependent on the volumetric Volhard's method. The substance is dissolved in dilute nitric acid to form mercuric nitrate. This is titrated with a standard solution of ammonium thiocyanate using ferric alum (ferric ammonium sulphate). The end point is the appearance of brick-red colour.

$$HgO + 2HNO_3 \longrightarrow Hg(NO_3)_2 + H_2O$$

$$2NH_4SCN + Hg(NO_3)_2 \longrightarrow Hg(SCN)_2 + 2NH_4NO_3$$

$$3NH_4SCN + Fe^{3+} \longrightarrow Fe(SCN)_3 + NH_4^+$$
$$\text{Ferric}$$
$$\text{thiocyanate}$$

A weighed amount (0.4 g) is dissolved in nitric acid (5 ml) and diluted with water. It is titrated at a temperature not above 20° with 0.1 N ammonium thiocyanate using ferric ammonium sulphate solution as indicator. Each ml of 0.1N ammonium thiocyanate is equivalent to 0.01083 g of HgO.

Uses : Yellow mercuric oxide is used in eye ointments for the local treatment of minor infections including the eradication of crab lice from the eye lashes and inflammation of the eye including conjunctivitis. It has been used as a topical antiseptic, fungicide, in chronic skin conditions, conjunctivitis, corneal ulcers and as oxidizing agent.

During its manufacture and storage, yellow mercuric oxide ophthalmic ointment must not come into contact with metallic utensils or containers except those made of stainless steel, tin, or tin-coated materials.

POTASSIUM PERMANGANATE

$KMnO_4$; Mol. Weight = 158.03

Potassium permanganate contains not less than 99.0 per cent of $KMnO_4$.

Preparation

1. Potassium permanganate is prepared by heating potassium hydroxide with manganese dioxide in the presence of air or an oxidizing agent, such as potassium nitrate or potassium chlorate.

$$2KOH + MnO_2 \xrightarrow{\quad O \quad} K_2MnO_4 + H_2O$$

The greenish product, potassium manganate, is extracted with water and treated with carbon dioxide, or ozonized air to precipitate about one-third of the manganese as the hydrated dioxide. The remaining manganese is converted into $KMnO_4$.

$$3K_2MnO_4 + 2CO_2 \longrightarrow 2KMnO_4 + MnO_2 + 2K_2CO_3$$

If chlorine is passed through the solution in place of carbon dioxide, the whole of the manganese of the manganate is converted into permanganate.

$$2K_2MnO_4 + Cl_2 \longrightarrow 2KMnO_4 + 2KCl$$

Manganate can also be converted into the permanganate by electrolyzing a warm solution :

$$2K_2MnO_4 + 2H_2O \longrightarrow 2KMnO_4 + 2KOH + H_2$$

Any of the above solution is filtered to separate the precipitated potassium manganate. The filtrate is concentrated and cooled to crystallize potassium permanganate.

Physical Properties : Potassium permanganate occurs as odourless dark purple or almost black prismatic crystals or granular powder; almost opaque by transmitted light and of a blue metallic luster by reflected light. It decomposes, with a risk of explosion, in contact with certain organic substances. It is sweet with astringent after taste; stable in air, decomposes at about $240°$ with evolution of oxygen. It is soluble in water (1 in 16), and in boiling water (1 in 3.5); is decomposed by alcohol and many other organic solvents, also by concentrated acids with liberation of oxygen.

Chemical Reactions

1. Potassium permanganate is a strong oxidizing agent. Iodides are oxidized to iodates by alkaline or neutral solution of $KMnO_4$, whereas in acidic solution iodine is liberated from alkali iodides.

$$KMnO_4 + H_2O + KI \longrightarrow 2MnO_2 + KIO_3 + KOH$$

2. With hydrochloric acid, chlorine is liberated.
3. An acidified solution in water is readily reduced by hydrogen peroxide and by organic matter.

   In acidic solution, iodides are oxidized to molecular iodine.

$$2KMnO_4 + 10KI + 8H_2SO_4 \longrightarrow 6K_2SO_4 + 2MnSO_4$$
$$+ 5I_2 + 8H_2O$$

It oxidizes sulphides to free sulphur, ferrous salts to ferric salts and nitrites to nitrates.

Tests for Purity : Tests for chloride and sulphate; colour of solution; water-insoluble matter.

Potassium permanganate is boiled with 95% aqueous alcohol to destroy the purple colour so that the colour should not interfere with the limit tests. The precipitated manganese dioxide is removed by filtration;

$$2KMnO_4 + 3CH_3CH_2OH \longrightarrow 2KOH + 2MnO_2$$
$$+ 3CH_3CHO + 2H_2O$$

A 20 ml portion of the filtrate complies with the limit test for chloride. Another 20 ml portion of the filtrate complies with the limit test for sulphates.

Incompatibilities : It is incompatible with iodides, bromides, alcohol, arsenites, hydrochloric acid, charcoal; organic substances generally; ferrous or mercurous salts, hypophosphites, hyposulphites, sulphites, peroxides and oxalates.

Tests for Identification

1. A solution in water, acidified with sulphuric acid and heated to 70°, is decolorised by hydrogen peroxide solution.
2. Heated to redness, it decrepitates, evolves oxygen, and leaves a black residue which with water forms potassium hydroxide solution. The resulting solution when neutralized with dilute hydrochloric acid, gives the reactions of potassium.

Assay : The assay is based on the oxidation reduction (redox) titration, which is carried out with a standard solution of oxalic acid in the presence of sulphuric acid at 70°C throughout the entire titration. Potassium permanganate itself serves as an indicator. End point is obtained as a permanent pink colour.

An aqueous solution is titrated with 0.1 N oxalic acid solution containing sulphuric acid (5 ml). The temperature is kept at about 70° throughout the entire titration. Each ml of 0.1 N oxalic acid is equivalent to 0.00316 g of $KMnO_4$.

Uses : Potassium permanganate possesses oxidizing properties and oxidizes proteins and other bioorganic substance. Therefore, it acts as a disinfectant and deodorant. It is also astringent, anti-infective and bactericidal. Solutions are used to clean ulcers or abscesses, as wet dressings and in baths in eczematous conditions and acute dermatoses. Solutions have also been used in bromhidrosis (evil smelling perspiration), in mycotic infections such as athlete's foot, in poison ivy dermatitis and as a stomach wash-out in the treatment of poisoning by morphine, opium and strychnine.

The crystals and concentrated solutions of potassium permanganate are caustic and irritant to tissues. Repeated use of dilute solutions may cause corrosive burns.

SILVER NITRATE

$AgNO_3$; Mol. Weight = 169.9

Silver nitrate contains not less than 99.5 per cent of $AgNO_3$.

Preparation : Silver nitrate is prepared by dissolving the metallic silver in hot concentrated nitric acid.

$$Ag + 2HNO_3 \longrightarrow AgNO_3 + NO_2 + H_2O$$

The solution is dried completely and the product crystallized from water.

Properties : Silver nitrate occurs as colourless or white transparent crystals or crystalline odourless powder; taste is bitter and metallic. It is not photosensitive when pure; presence of trace amounts of organic material promotes photoreduction, and it becomes grey or greyish-black; m.p. 212°, forming a yellowish liquid. It is soluble in water (1 in 0.5) and in alcohol (1 in 27). Its solubility is increased in boiling water or alcohol.

The aqueous and alcoholic solutions are neutral to litmus. It is stored in airtight non-metallic containers and protected from light.

Silver nitrate is reduced by hydrogen sulphide in the dark. It is decomposed at 440° into metallic silver, nitrogen, oxygen and nitrogen oxides.

$$2 \text{ AgNO}_3 \longrightarrow 2\text{Ag} + 2\text{NO}_2 + \text{O}_2$$

It gives a black stain when comes in contact with skin or cloth due to reduction to metallic silver;

$$2\text{AgNO}_2 + \text{H}_2\text{O} \longrightarrow 2\text{Ag} + 2\text{HNO}_3 + \text{O}$$

Silver ion precipitates both bacterial and human protein. Antibacterial, astringent, irritant and corrosive nature depend upon the concentration applied. The ions precipitate protein molecule containing $-\text{SH}$, $-\text{NH}_2$, $-\text{COOH}$ and heterocyclic residues, e.g., histidine. Silver preparations darkens the skin due to the deposition of free silver below the epidermis.

Tests for Purity : Tests for aluminium, bismuth, copper and lead; foreign salts; acidity or alkalinity; clarity and colour of solution.

A dark precipitate of silver oxide, Ag_2O, is produced when ammonia is added to a solution of silver nitrate. The precipitate is soluble in excess of ammonia to give clear solution. Bismuth and lead give a white turbidity on addition of ammonia to their solutions which is not soluble in excess of ammonia. Copper forms a blue solution due to formation of cuprammonium ion, $\text{Cu (NH}_3)_4{}^{2+}$.

For determining foreign substances, the acidified solution with 2N hydrochloric acid is filtered, the filtrate dried and the residue weighed.

Incompatibility : Silver nitrate is incompatible with a range of substances like alkalies, antimony salts, arsenites, bromides, carbonates, chlorides, iodides, thiocyanates, ferrous salts, hypophosphites, morphine salts, oils, phosphates, tannic acid, tartrates, vegetable decoctions and extracts.

Test for Identification : A solution (1 in 50) gives the reactions of silver, and of nitrates.

Assay : The assay is based on the modified Volhard's method. An aqueous solution of the substance (0.5 g in 50 ml), acidified with nitric acid (2 ml), is titrated with 0.1 N ammonium thiocyanate, using ferric ammonium sulphate solution as indicator. Each ml of 0.1 N ammonium thiocyanate is equivalent to 0.01699 g of AgNO_3.

Uses : Silver nitrate possesses disinfectant, astringent and irritant properties and is used for prophylaxis of ophthalmia, in stick form as a caustic to destroy warts and other skin growths, in cosmetics to dye eyebrows, eye lashes and in homoeopathic medicine; and as hair dye.

The bactericidal action is due to precipitation of tissue proteins and chloride ions in the tissue fluids caused by slow release of silver ions from the silver proteinase and silver chloride. Silver nitrate solutions (0.01 - 10%) prevent micro-organism activity. A 10% solution is used in the treatment of infected ulcers in mouth. A 1% silver nitrate ophthalmic solution is employed locally in the eyes of infants for the prophylaxis.

Adverse effects include pain in the mouth, sialorrhoea, diarrhoea, vomiting, coma and convulsions.

MILD SILVER PROTEIN

It is prepared by addition of silver oxide to gelatin solution in the presence of alkali, or from silver oxide and serum albumin, or by suspending moist silver oxide in a solution of casein. The mixture is heated until no precipitate is obtained on the addition of a solution of sodium chloride. The mixture is then evaporated to dryness. It contains not less than 19 per cent and not more than 23 per cent of silver.

It occurs as brown, dark-brown, or almost black, odourless, lustrous scales or granules; somewhat hygroscopic. It is freely soluble in water; forming a colloidal solution; almost insoluble in alcohol, chloroform and ether. It is kept well closed and protected from light. Solutions should be freshly made and protected from light.

Mild silver protein is differentiated from strong silver protein by the fact that no or very little precipitate of silver chloride is formed by addition of sodium chloride solution to a filtrate obtained by treating an aqueous solution of the silver protein with solid ammonium sulphate and filtering. Under the same conditions strong silver protein gives a heavy precipitate of silver chloride. It is incompatible with acids and most neutral and acid salts in concentrated solutions.

Colloidal solutions of mild silver protein have no astringent or irritant effect, therefore, they are applied to sensitive areas and mucous membranes. Solutions of mild silver proteins should be freshly prepared or contain a suitable stabilizer.

STRONG SILVER PROTEIN

It is a compound of silver and protein, containing 7.5 to 8.5% of silver in the form of colloidal solutions with sucrose as the stabilizing agent. It is prepared by adding a silver nitrate solution to a solution of peptone. The precipitate is digested with protalbumose until a solution is obtained which is evaporated in a moderate vacuum. Instead of the silver nitrate solution silver oxide may be suspended in the peptone solution. The suspension is shaken until the silver peptone has formed. The digested and dried product is identical with that obtained from silver nitrate.

Strong silver protein is differentiated from mild silver protein in that its silver, most of which is present in ionic form, is found in the filtrate obtained as described under mild silver protein, and gives a heavy precipitate with sodium chloride solution. Although strong silver protein contains about one-third as much silver as mild silver protein, it is more irritating and stands midway between silver nitrate and mild silver protein in both germicidal and irritant action.

It occurs as pale yellowish orange to brownish black, odourless powder; somewhat hygroscopic. It is freely soluble in water, almost insoluble in alcohol, ether and chloroform. It is kept well closed and protected from light. Solutions should be freshly prepared with cold water and be dispensed in amber-coloured bottles.

Uses : Silver protein solutions have antibacterial properties; due to the presence of low concentrations of ionized silver, are used on mucous membranes in the nose, throat, and conjunctiva of the eye. The mild form is less irritating but less active; it is used in nasal solutions. The solutions are employed to irritate the urethra and bladder; to treat gonococcal infections, i.e. gonococcal conjunctivitis; infections of the respiratory tract and as a prophylactic medication against respiratory infections.

(C) ASTRINGENTS

Dilute solution of a metal cation has a local or surface protein precipitant activity on a tissue. This activity is called as astringent. The substance is applied to skin or mucous membranes and does not destruct the host tissue. Astringents will cause the constriction of capillaries and small blood vessels. They are used to stop bleeding from small cuts, to harden the skin to reduce the volume of exudate from wounds and skin eruptions and as antiperspirants in deodorants due to their ability to constrict pores, for mouth ulcers, hyperhidrosis and haemorrhoids, and destroy microorganisms. Some have been taken internally for diarrhoea.

Astringents may stimulate the growth of new tissues when applied topically to wounds. However, the concentrated solutions will produce an irritant or corrosive effect. Corrosive effect is used to remove undesirable tissue, e.g. warts.

The concentrations of water-soluble compounds can be altered to control the antimicrobial and astringent action. Higher concentrations may be used on the skin and not in the eye. Soluble compounds may be administered in a vehicle like glycerin or polyethylene glycol, which would slow their release to the site of action. Ointments also release the antimicrobial agents in a controlled manner. Complex formaton with a ligand, e.g. povidone-iodine, also provides a controlled release of some of these agents, reducing toxicity and activity at host cell. The compounds may be used in the form of suspensions, ointments, or creams to slow release their antimicrobial action. The insolubility property of the compound is helpful in controlling activity.

ALUM

K_2SO_4. $Al_2(SO_4)_3$. $24H_2O$ (Potash alum)

$(NH_4)_2 SO_4$. $Al_2(SO_4)_3$. $24H_2O$ (Ammonia alum)

$AlK(SO_4)_2$ $12H_2O$; Mol. Weight = 474.4

Alum contains 99 to 100.5% of $AlK(SO_4)_2$ $12H_2O$.

When a mixture of potassium sulphate and aluminium sulphate is dissolved in water and concentrated, a double salt is separated in the form of crystals. All double salts with similar composition and properties are called *alums*. Alums are sulphates of a univalent metal (or ammonium) and a trivalent metal.

Preparation : The official alums are prepared by adding a hot, concentrated solution of potassium or ammonium sulphate to a hot solution of aluminium sulphate in equivalent amount. The alum is crystallized on cooling the solution. Large octahedral crystals are formed on slow crystallization.

Physical Characters

Alums occur as odourless, transparent, colourless crystals, white granules or powder; taste is styptic. Alum crystals are sometimes opaque on the surface due to formation of traces of basic salt. On heating potash alum melts at water bath. It loses whole of the water of crystallization below 200°, forming a white residue of anhydrous aluminium and potassium sulphates.

Ammonia alum melts at 95°; becomes anhydrous at 250° and decomposes above 280° leaving a residue of aluminium oxide. It is soluble in water (1 in 7), freely soluble in glycerol; practically insoluble in alcohol. The aqueous solution is acidic to litmus; pH 4.6. Alum should be kept in a well-closed container.

The chemistry of alum is that of aluminium ion, potassium and ammonium ions, and sulphate.

Tests for Purity : Tests for arsenic; heavy metals; iron; zinc; clarity and colour of solutions; ammonium ions.

The solution of alum complies with the limit tests for ammonium, heavy metals and iron.

The presence of alkali salts in ammonia alum is detected by dissolving a weighed quantity of the substance in water, adding excess of ammonia to precipitate aluminium as hydroxide, filtering, drying, and weighing the residue after ignition to remove ammonium salt.

Zinc is detected by the opalescence caused by its ferrocyanide. Heavy metals are detected by passing hydrogen sulphide through a slightly acid solution of the salt and comparing the colour with that given by a very dilute standard solution of lead nitrate.

Tests for Identification

1. Its aqueous solution gives the reactions typical of sulphate and of aluminium.
2. The aqueous solution (10 ml) is shaken with sodium hydrogen carbonate (0.5g) and filtered. The filtrate gives the reactions of sulphate and of potassium salts.

Incompatibility : It is incompatible with alkali hydroxides, borax and carbonates, phosphates, salts of calcium, lead and mercury tannins, phenols and salicylates.

Assay : Complexometric titration of aluminium is carried out, using 0.9 g dissolved in 20 ml of water. Each ml of 0.1 N disodium edetate is equivalent to 47.44 mg of AlK. $(SO_4)_2.12H_2O$.

Uses : Alum precipitates proteins and is a powerful topical astringent. Alum is used as a haemostatic agent; as mouthwashes or gargles; as bladder irrigations; for hyperhydrosis; to harden the epidermis and as a mordant in the dyeing industry.

Large doses of alum are irritant and may be corrosive; gum necrosis and gastro-intestinal haemorrhage have occurred. Adverse effects on muscle and kidneys have been reported.

ZINC SULPHATE

$ZnSO_4.7H_2O$; Mol. Weight = 287.54

Zinc sulphate containts about 99.0 per cent of $ZnSO_4.7H_2O$. It is prepared by boiling slight excess amount of metallic zinc with dilute sulphuric acid until liberation of hydrogen is ceased.

$$Zn + H_2SO_4 \longrightarrow ZnSO_4 + H_2$$

The solution is filtered to separate unreacted zinc, concentrated and crystallized.

Characters : Zinc sulphate occurs as colourless, transparent crystals or crystalline powder; odourless; taste is astringent and metallic. It is efflorescent in dry air. It is very soluble in water; freely soluble in glycerin and insoluble in alcohol. Aqueous solutions are acid to litmus due to hydrolysis of the salt, pH is about 5.

Zinc sulphate is stored in tightly closed containers.

Incompatibility : It is incompatible with alkali carbonates and hydroxides, astringent decoctions and infusions.

Tests for Purity : Tests for acidity; alkali and alkaline earths; aluminium; copper, magnesium, manganese and nickel; arsenic; iron; chloride; clarity and colour of solution.

Alkali and alkaline earths are detected by precipitation of zinc in an aqueous solution of the substance by means of ammonium sulphide solution. The precipitate is filtered, sulphuric acid is added to the filtrate, evaporated to dryness, ignited and the residue is weighed.

Dilute ammonia solution is added in excess to an aqueous solution of zinc sulphate and allowed to stand. The solution remains colourless, and no precipitate is produced within thirty minutes indicating the absence of aluminium, copper, magnesium, manganese and nickel.

For determining heavy metals, potassium cyanide solution is added to an aqueous solution of the substance in a Nessler cylinder (A). Into a similar matched Nessler cylinder (B) standard lead solution and potassium cyanide solution are added. Then sodium sulphide solution is added to each cylinder, mixed and allowed to stand for five minutes. The solution in cylinder A is not darker than that in cylinder B.

Assay : The assay is based on the complexometric titration forming a well-defined simple complex between zinc and disodium ethylenediamine tetra-acetate. The titration is carried out in the presence of a buffer, e.g. strong ammonia-ammonium chloride solution using erichrome black T solution as the indicator. The end point in appeared as a deep blue colour.

$$Zn^{2+} + H_2Y^{2-} \longrightarrow ZnY^{2-} + 2H^+$$

To a solution of the substance (0.3 g) in water (100 ml) strong ammonia-ammonium chloride solution (5 ml) and eriochrome black T solution (0.1 ml) were added and the reaction mixture titrated with 0.05 M disodium ethylenediaminetetra-acetate until the solution was deep blue in colour. Each ml of 0.05 M disodium ethylenediaminetetra acetate is equivalent to 0.01438 g of zinc sulphate.

Uses : Zinc sulphate is given to treat conditions associated with zinc deficiency such as acrodermatitis enteropathica. Externally, zinc sulphate is used as an astringent in lotions and eye-drops. Zinc sulphate has also been used internally as an emetic. It is an ingradient of an ophthalmic astringent known as zinc sulphate ophthalmic solution.

(D) SULPHUR AND SULPHUR COMPOUNDS

Sulphur occurs both in free state and in combination, mainly as sulphides and sulphates. Free elementary form is found in a variety of allotropic forms (rhombic, monoclinic, liquid, plastic and amorphous) in volcanic regions of Sicily, Italy, Japan, South America, Russia and Iceland. In combined state sulphur occurs as sulphates of calcium (gypsum, $CaSO_4$), barium (barytes, $BaSO_4$) and magnesium (epsom salt, $MgSO_4. 7H_2O$); sulphides of zinc (zinc blends, ZnS), lead (galena, PbS), copper (copper pyrites, CuFeS) and mercury (ethiops mineral, HgS). Traces of sulphur occurs in volcanic gases, eggs, proteins, garlic, onions, mustard, hair and wool.

Preparation

1. **Sicilian Process :** Sulphur containing clay, limestone and other rocky impurities is heated in sloppy kilns. The melted sulphur flows down the slope where it solidifies. About 33 per cent of sulphur is lost during burning in this process. Crude sulphur is further purified by distillation in large iron retorts. In the beginning when the walls are cold, sulphur vapours condenses on the walls to form a yellow powder (flowers of sulphur). When the inside temperature

is raised up to 120°, the condensate remains liquid which may be run into cylindrical moulds.

2. **Louisiana or Frasch Process :** In Louisiana sulphur occurs at a depth of 160 to 1500 meters. Holes are bored and a pipe is driven through the quicksand down to sulphur beds. Superheated water and hot air are sent through the pipes surrounding the central pipe. Sulphur-water emulsion is driven which is purified.

Physical Characters : Sulphur occurs as a pale yellow, odourless, amorphous or microcrystalline powder. It is insoluble in water; sparingly soluble in alcohol and ether; soluble in carbon disulphide, benzene and toluene. It is incompatible with topical mercurial compounds; and stored in well-closed containers.

Chemical Properties

1. Sulphur burns in air at 250°C with a pale blue flame yielding sulphur dioxide and sulphur trioxide.

$$S + O_2 \longrightarrow SO_2 + SO_3$$

2. Sulphur combines with elements like carbon, hydrogen, chlorine, fluorine, lithium, sodium, potassium, copper, mercury, silver and all other metals.

$$C + 2S \xrightarrow{\text{Red heat}} CS_2$$
$$H_2 + S \longrightarrow H_2S$$
$$Cl_2 + 2S \longrightarrow S_2Cl_2$$
$$Fe + S \longrightarrow FeS$$

3. Sulphur reduces hot concentrated sulphuric and nitric acids.

$$2H_2SO_4 + S \longrightarrow 3SO_2 + 2H_2O$$
$$6HNO_3 + S \longrightarrow H_2SO_4 + 6NO_2 + 2H_2O$$

4. Sulphur reacts with alkalies on heating to yield sulphides and thiosulphates.

$$12S + 3Ca(OH)_2 \longrightarrow 2CaS_5 + CaS_2O_3 + 3H_2O$$
$$4S + 6NaOH \longrightarrow 2Na_2S + Na_2S_2O_3 + 3H_2O + Na_2S_5$$

5. With oxidizing agents (e.g. potassium nitrate) sulphur forms explosive mixtures.

Tests for Purity : Tests for arsenic; acidity; matter insoluble in carbon disulphide; ash; and water.

Water is more conveniently determined by a volumetric procedure using a solution of iodine and sulphur dioxide in pyridine and methanol (Karl Fischer reagent).

PRECIPITATED SULPHUR

Preparation

1. When a solution of a thiosulphate is acidified with a dilute hydrochloric acid, an unstable thiosulphuric acid is formed which readily decomposes to yield precipitated sulphur.

$$Na_2S_2O_3 + 2HCl \longrightarrow H_2S_2O_3 + 2NaCl$$
$$H_2S_2O_3 \longrightarrow S + SO_2 + H_2O$$

2. For commercial preparation, quicklime is slaked and the product mixed with water. Sublimed or powdered roll sulphur and water are added, and the mixture is boiled for an hour. The liquid is filtered and the filtrate containing a mixture of calcium thiosulphate and calcium polysulphides is treated with hydrochloric acid so that the supernatant liquid should be slightly alkaline. The precipitated sulphur is collected, washed on filter to remove calcium ions and dried.

$$3Ca(OH)_2 + 6S \longrightarrow 2CaS_2 + CaS_2O_3 + 3H_2O$$
$$2CaS_2 + CaS_2O_3 + 6HCl \longrightarrow 3CaCl_2 + 6S + 3H_2O$$

Characters

Precipitated sulphur occurs as a greyish yellow or pale greenish-yellow, soft powder, which is completely amorphous and not gritty; odourless; tasteless.

It burns with a blue flame with the production of SO_2. It is almost insoluble in water and alcohol; completely soluble in carbon disulphide. Under a microscope it consists of grouped amorphous subglobular particle free from crystals.

It is preserved in well-closed containers.

Tests for Purity : Tests for acidity; matter insoluble in carbon disulphide; residue on ignition; water.

Test for Identification : It burns in air to sulphur dioxide, which can be recognized by its characteristic odour.

Assay : Precipitated sulphur is burnt and the gas formed is absorbed in water containing hydrogen peroxide. Water is added and the solution boiled for 2 minutes. It is cooled, phenolphthalein added and titrated with 0.1 N sodium hydroxide. A blank determination is performed and the necessary correction made. Each ml of 0.1 N sodium hydroxide is equivalent to 1.60 of S.

SUBLIMED SULPHUR (Flowers of Sulphur)

When sulphur condenses and falls in the form of a yellow powder in the iron retorts during purification by distillation, it is called *flowers of sulphur* or *sublimed sulphur*. It consists of masses of minute rhombic crystals, mixed with a smaller proportion of amorphous particles, having a faint odour and taste. It is practically insoluble in water and alcohol, and sparingly soluble in olive oil.

Its tests for purity, identification, storage conditions and assay are similar as described under precipitated sulphur.

Uses : Sulphur is a keratolytic, a mild antiseptic and a parasiticide. It is widely used as a dermatological agent in the form of lotions or ointments, in the treatment of of acne, psoriasis, ringworm, lupus erythematosus, dandruff, seborrhoeic conditions and scabies. The scabicidal effect is probably due to its conversion into H_2S and parathionic acid. Lotions of precipitated sulphur with lead acetate have been used to darken grey hair. Sulphur is also used in homoeopathic medicine. When taken by mouth, sulphur is converted in the small intestine into alkali sulphides, which by their irritant action produce a mild laxative effect. It stains the clothes.

SELENIUM SULPHIDE

SeS_2; Mol. Weight = 143.1

Selenium sulphide contains 52 to 55% of Se.

Selenium sulphide (selsun) is prepared by adding selenious acid solution to a solution of aluminium chloride saturated with hydrogen sulphide. The passage of the gas is continued throughout the reaction period. The aluminium chloride acts as a coagulant. The precipitated selenium sulphide is filtered off, washed, and dried.

$$H_3SeO_3 + 2H_2S \longrightarrow SeS_2 + 3H_2O$$

Characters : It occurs as a bright orange to reddish-brown powder with a faint odour of hydrogen sulphide. It is practically insoluble in water and most of organic solvents; very slightly soluble in chloroform and ether. It may discolour metals. It is stored in well-closed containers.

Test for Identification

1. Selenium sulphide is soluble in nitric acid yielding selenious and sulphuric acids.

$$SeS_2 + 16HNO_3 \longrightarrow H_2SeO_3 + 2H_2SO_4 + 16NO_2 + 5H_2O$$

Urea is added to inactivate excess of nitric acid by forming urea nitrate, and destroys any nitrous acid.

$$2HNO_2 + H_2NCONH_2 \longrightarrow CO_2 + 2N_2 + 3H_2O$$

Potassium iodide is then added which yields iodine and selenium forming orange colour which rapidly darkens.

$$H_2SeO_3 + 4HI \longrightarrow 2I_2 + Se + 3H_2O$$

2. The filtrate responds positively to tests of sulphate.

Tests for Purity : Tests for residue on ignition; soluble selenium compounds.

Soluble selenium compounds are detected by adjusting pH of the water soluble extract to 2 to 3 with formic acid, adding aqueous solution of 3,3'-diaminobenzidine tetrahydrochloride and adjusting pH 6 to 7 with ammonia. The solution is shaked with toluene and the absorbance of the toluene solution recorded and compared with the standard solution of selenium.

Assay : The assay is based on the iodometric titration as discussed for chlorinated lime. To the substance (0.1 g) fuming nitric acid is added, heated for 1 hour and diluted with water. To the solution (25 ml) dilute potassium iodide solution and chloroform are added and titrated with 0.02 N sodium thiosulphate until aqueous layer is a pale straw colour. Starch mucilage is added and the titration continued to the complete absence of blue colour in the aqueous layer. Each ml of 0.02 N sodium thiosulphate is equivalent to 0.3948 mg of Se.

Uses : Selenium sulphide has antifungal and antiseborrhoeic activities. It is used as a shampoo in the treatment of dandruff, seborrhoeic dermatitis of the scalp and as a lotion to cure pityriasis versicolour.

Topical application of selenium sulphide can produce irritation of the conjunctiva, scalp, and skin. Scalp oiliness, hair discolouration and hair loss have been reported. In large doses, selenium salts will cause irritation of the gastrointestinal mucosa and damage the renal tubules. Due to danger of introduction into the eyes or mouth, the hands should be thoroughly washed and finger nails cleaned after using selenium sulphide.

6

DENTAL PRODUCTS

Dental caries (tooth decay) is a chronic infectious disease, called dental plague, in which the active agents are members of the indigenous oral flora. It is a colourless sticky mixture of bacterial products, mucin, saliva and foodstuff attached to enamel covering the dentine on the crown. Dental plague is resulted by the combined action of bacteria, *Streptococcus mutans*, on teeth and a periodental disease in which inflammation and swelling of gingiva occurs. The bacteria survive on carbohydrates including the sugar taken in tea and produce acids, especially lactic acids, and proteolytic enzymes. Calcium salts are dissolved in acidic medium, the remaining organic matrix is readily digested by the proteolytic enzymes and cavities are formed. When a cavity deepens, inflammation cf the pulp results. A regular dental care eliminates dental plague.

The drugs containing fluoride ions are used to control dental plague. The best way to prevent caries is maintaining optimal oral hygiene. The teeth should be brushed with a tooth paste and flossed thoroughly twice a day. Fluoride added water supply is the most effective procedure for reducing the dental caries. Sealing the cavities and fissures with inert polymer to prevent the further teeth decay is also valuable. Topical fluoride solutions, mouthwashes and gels are less effective than systemic fluorides.

Modification of food habits such as less frequent eating, particularly less in between meals, and avoidance of use of sugar containing food materials that are retained on tooth surface, are the precautionary measures. Replacing such snacks with fruits or vegetables, cheese or nuts is considered better.

DICALCIUM PHOSPHATE
(Dibasic Calcium Phosphate, Calcium Hydrogen Phosphate)

$CaHPO_4$; Mol. Weight = 136.06

$CaHPO_4 \cdot 2H_2O$; Mol. Weight = 172.1

Dicalcium phosphate is anhydrous or contains two molecules of water of hydration. It contains not less than 30.9 per cent and not more than 31.7 per cent of calcium, calculated with reference to the ignited substance.

Preparation

1. Dicalcium phosphate contains an amount of calcium pyrophosphate $(Ca_2P_2O_7)$ equivalent to not less that 98 per cent of $CaHPO_4$. It occurs in nature as the mineral *monetite*. It is prepared by reacting a neutral solution of calcium chloride and disodium hydrogen phosphate. The white flocculent precipitate of dibasic calcium phosphate is filtered off, washed and dried.

$$CaCl_2 + Na_2HPO_4 \longrightarrow CaHPO_4 + 2NaCl$$

   In the presence of an alkali tribasic calcium phosphate, $Ca_3(PO_4)_2$, is formed.

2. Treatment of powdered mineral, *apatite*, with sulphuric acid forms insoluble calcium sulphate and phosphoric acid. Calcium sulphate is filtered off and to the filtrate calculated amount of calcium hydroxide is added to form the dibasic salt.

$$Ca_3(PO_4)_2 + 3H_2SO_4 \longrightarrow 2H_3PO_4 + 3CaSO_4$$
Apatite   Phosphoric
                                           acid

$$H_3PO_4 + Ca(OH)_2 \longrightarrow CaHPO_4 + 2H_2O$$

Physical Characters : It occurs as a white, odourless, tasteless crystalline powder. It is stable in air; practically insoluble in cold water and alcohol; soluble in dilute hydrochloric and nitric acids. It loses water of crystallization slowly below 100°; is dehydrated at red heat to calcium pyrophosphate. Each g represents nearly 5.8 mmol of calcium and of phosphate. It is stored in well-closed containers.

In the acid of stomach it is converted to the soluble monobasic calcium phosphate and calcium chloride.

$$2CaHPO_4 + 2HCl \longrightarrow Ca(H_2PO_4)_2 + CaCl_2$$

Tests for Purity : Tests for carbonate; chloride; fluoride; sulphate; arsenic; barium; iron; monocalcium and tricalcium phosphates; heavy metals; loss an ignition; loss on drying; acid-insoluble substances; and pH (6 to 7 in 20% suspension in water).

To an aqueous solution dilute sulphuric acid is added. After 15 minutes the solution is not more opalescent than mixture of the solution and water indicating the absence of barium.

When hydrochloric acid is added to an aqueous solution, no effervescence is produced suggesting the absence of carbonate. For determining monocalcium and tricalcium phosphates, methyl orange solution is added to an aqueous solution acidified with hydrochloric acid. Excess of the acid is titrated with sodium hydroxide.

Aqueous solution of the salt complies with the limit tests for arsenic, heavy metals, iron, chloride, fluoride and sulphate.

Tests for Identification

1. The substance is dissolved in dilute hydrochloric acid; the solution gives the reactions of calcium.
2. A solution in dilute nitric acid gives the reactions of phosphates.

Assay : The assay is based on complexometric titration as discussed for calcium gluconate and magnesium sulphate. To the solution of the substance (0.2 g) dissolved in hydrochloric acid, triethanolamine and hydroxynaphthol blue indicator are added and titrated with 0.05 M disodium ethylenediaminetetraacetate until blue end-point is obtained. Each ml of 0.05 M disodium ethylenediaminetetraacetate is equivalent to 0.002004 g of calcium.

Uses : Dicalcium phosphate is used as a calcium replenisher, dietary supplement and as an antacid. Calcium salts are used mainly in the treatment of calcium deficiency. Dicalcium phosphate is also used to reduce dental caries.

Administration of some calcium salts by mouth can cause gastro-intestinal irritation and constipation.

SODIUM FLUORIDE

NaF; Mol. Weight = 42.0

Sodium fluoride contains 98.5 to 100.5% of NaF.

Preparation

1. Sodium fluoride is prepared by neutralizing sodium

hydroxide or sodium carbonate with equivalent amount of 40 per cent hydrofluoric acid or by passing hydrogen fluoride into a solution of sodium carbonate.

$$Na_2CO_3 + 2HF \longrightarrow 2NaF + H_2O + CO_2$$

Sodium fluoride is precipitated in the reaction mixture. The precipitate is contaminated with the acid salt and with fluorosilicate. The fluorosilicate is decomposed when the reaction mixture is treated with sodium carbonate.

$$Na_2SiF_6 + 2H_2O \longrightarrow 2NaF + 4HF + SiO_2$$

The crystal size depends on pH, but too much HF yields sodium bifluoride, $NaHF_2$.

2. Sodium fluoride is also formed when the mineral cryolite $(AlF_3, 3NaF)$ is treated with excess of sodium hydroxide. Aluminium fluoride is soluble in the alkali solution whereas undissolved sodium fluoride is extracted with hot water.

Physical Characters : Sodium fluoride occurs as a white, odourless powder or colourless crystals; m.p. 99.3°. It is soluble in water (1 in 25); practically insoluble in alcohol. Sodium fluoride and its preparations should be stored in air-tight containers; plastic containers should be used for the oral solution.

Chemical Reactions

1. Treatment of sodium fluoride with concentrated sulphuric acid liberates hydrogen fluoride. The gas attacks silica and silicates and hence the glass.

$$Na_2SiO_3 + 6HF \longrightarrow Na_2SiF_6 + 3H_2O$$

2. Sodium fluoride is an ionic salt. It gives reactions for fluoride ion and sodium ion. When it is reacted with red coloured zirconium-alizarin, the yellow colour of alizarin-sulphonic acid is produced. The zirconi-fluoride ion formed in the reaction is colourless.

Tests for Purity : Tests for lead; fluorosilicate; sulphate; clarity and colour of solution; acidity or alkalinity; loss on drying.

Acidity or alkalinity is determined by dissolving potassium nitrate in water. The solution is neutralized with either sodium hydroxide or with hydrochloric acid.

The above neutralized solution is titrated while hot with sodium hydroxide until a red colour is produced. From the amount consumed of the alkali, the amount of flurosilicate is found out.

The solution of sodium fluoride complies with the limit tests for chloride and sulphate.

Tests for Identification

1. The substance is dissolved in water and then calcium chloride solution added. A gelatinous white precipitate is produced which dissolves on adding 5 ml of ferric chloride solution.

2. Alizarin solution (0.1 ml) and zirconyl nitrate solution (0.1 ml) are added to the substance (4 mg). The red colour changes to yellow.

3. The aqueous solution yields reactions characteristic of sodium salt.

Assay : To the substance (80 mg) a mixture of acetic anhydride and anhydrous acetic acid is mixed and heated to dissolve. To it 1, 4-dioxane is added and non-aqueous titration carried out using crystal violet solution as indicator, until a green colour is produced. A blank experiment is operated without the substance being examined. Each ml of 0.1 N perchloric acid is equivalent to 4.199 mg of NaF.

Uses : Sodium fluoride is used as an adjunct to diet and oral hygiene for the prevention of dental caries. It may render the enamel of teeth more resistant to acid; promote remineralization, or reduce microbial acid production. It is also used as insecticide, particularly for roaches and ants; in other pesticide formulations and in the fluoridation of drinking water.

Adverse effects include nausea, vomiting, abdominal distress, diarrhoea, stupor, weakness, tremors, convulsions, collapse, dyspnea, respiratory and cardiac failure and death.

SODIUM METAPHOSPHATE
(Sodium Hexametaphosphate, Maddrell's Salt)

$(NaPO_3)_n$

Sodium metaphosphate is prepared by dehydration of sodium phosphates (e.g. $Na_2H_2P_2O_7$, NaH_2PO_4, Na_2HPO_4).

$$NaH_2PO_4 \rightleftharpoons NaPO_3 + H_2O$$

It occurs as a white powder; practically insoluble in water but soluble in mineral acids.

Sodium metaphosphate is used as a 5% dusting powder in hyperhidrosis and bromidrosis, as a prophylactic against athlete's foot, a water softner and in food industry as emulsifying and chelating agent. It is an ingredient in dentifrices as cleaning and polishing agent and abrasive detergent.

STANNOUS FLUORIDE

SnF_2; Mol. Weight = 156.70

Stannous fluoride contains not more than 71.2 per cent of stannous ions (Sn^{++}) and not less than 22.3 per cent of fluoride (F).

Stannous fluoride is prepared by evaporating a solution of stannous oxide in hydrofluoric acid in the absence of oxygen or by reacting tin with hydrogen fluoride.

$$SnO + 2HF \longrightarrow SnF_2 + H_2O$$
$$Sn + 2HF \longrightarrow SnF_2 + H_2$$

Stannous fluoride occurs as a white crystalline powder with a bitter saline unpleasant taste; m.p. 213°. It is freely soluble in water; practically insoluble in alcohol, chloroform and ether; pH of 0.4% freshly prepared aqueous solution is in between 2.8 to 3.5. Aqueous solutions decompose within a few hours with the formation of a white precipitate; they slowly attack glass.

Preparations are stored in well-closed containers.

Tests for Purity : Tests for antimony; water-insoluble substances; loss on drying; pH.

Tests for Identification

1. When calcium chloride solution is added to a solution of the substance, white precipitate of calcium fluoride is formed.
2. An aqueous solution is mixed with silver nitrate on a spot plate, a brown-black precipitate is formed.
3. The solution is added to mercuric chloride solution; a white, silky precipitate is formed. On further addition of the solution, a brown-black precipitate is formed.

Assay (U.S.P.)

For Stannous Ion : A mixture of stannous fluoride dissolved in 3N hydrochloric acid and potassium iodide is titrated with 0.1 N potassium iodide-iodate, adding starch as the end-point is approached. Each ml of 0.1 N potassium iodide-iodate is equivalent to 5.935 mg of Sn^{++}.

Assay for Fluoride : The standard preparations of 4,5-dihydroxy-3-(p-sulphophenylazo)-2, 7-naphthalene-disulphonic acid trisodium, zirconium oxychloride, hydrochloric acid, and sodium fluoride after addition as indicated in the USP monograph are sereened at a wavelength of maximum absorbance at about 590 nm and the quantily of F is determined.

Uses : Stannous fluoride has similar actions to sodium fluoride and is used as ingredient of caries-preventing tooth pastes, in dentifrices and mouth rinses. It increases teeth discolouration.

STRONTIUM CHLORIDE

$SrCl_2$; Mol. Weight = 158.52

$SrCl_2$. $6H_2O$; Mol. Weight = 266.6

Strontium chloride hexahydrate occurs as colourless, odourless crystals or white granules. It effloresces in air; deliquesces in moist air; at 100° loses 5 moles of water; at 150° all its water is eliminated; m.p. 61° when rapidly heated; the anhydrous salt melts at 868°. It is soluble in water and alcohol. The aqueous solution is neutral. It is kept well-closed.

Uses : Strontium chloride is used as a 10 per cent tooth paste for the relief of dental hypersensitivity or in dentifrice as a tooth temperature desensitizing agent.

Strontium can replace in bone formation and has been used to hasten bone remineralization in diseases, e.g. osteoporosis.

ZINC CHLORIDE

$ZnCl_2$; Mol. Weight = 136.3

Zinc chloride contains 95 to 100.5 per cent of $ZnCl_2$.

Zinc chloride is prepared by heating excess of metallic zinc with mildly concentrated hydrochloric acid. When evolution of hydrogen ceases, the solution is filtered and dried.

$$Zn + 2HCl \longrightarrow ZnCl_2 + H_2$$

Zinc oxide and zinc carbonate may be reacted with the acid in place of zinc metal.

Anhydrous zinc chloride is obtained by passing chlorine or hydrogen chloride over heated zinc or distilling zinc with mercuric chloride.

$$Zn + HgCl_2 \longrightarrow ZnCl_2 + Hg$$

Characters : Zinc chloride occurs as a white, odourless, deliquescent crystalline powder or granules or opaque white masses or sticks; m.p. 290°. It is soluble in water, alcohol and glycerol; freely soluble in acetone. With much water some zinc oxychloride is formed. The aqueous solution is acidic to litmus, pH of 10% solution is of 4.6 to 5.5. It is kept in airtight non-metallic containers.

Zinc chloride always contains some oxychloride, $Zn(OH)Cl$, formed due to hydrolysis, which produces a slightly turbid aqueous solution. Turbid solutions may be cleared by adding gradually a small amount of dilute hydrochloric acid. Solutions of zinc chloride should be filtered through asbestos or sintered glass, since they dissolve paper and cotton wool. Though acidic to litmus, zinc chloride solution may be alkaline to methyl orange.

$$ZnCl_2 + H_2O \longrightarrow Zn(OH)Cl + H^+ + Cl^-$$

Tests for Purity : Tests for oxychloride, sulphate; ammonium salts; calcium; iron; magnesium; alkali and alkaline earths; heavy metals; acidity.

Alkali and alkaline earth metals are detected by dissolving a sample in dilute hydrochloric acid, and the zinc is precipitated as zinc sulphide by addition of ammonical ammonium sulphide solution. The zinc sulphide is filtered off, filtrate is acidified with sulphuric acid, dried, ignited and the residue weighed.

Ammonium salts are detected by heating a solution with sodium hydroxide to evolve ammonia.

For detecting lead, potassium cyanide solution is added to an aqueous solution of zinc chloride in a Nessler cylinder (A). Similarly a mixture of standard lead solution and potassium cyanide solution is placed in Nessler cylinder (B). Sodium sulphide solution is added to each cylinder, the contents mixed and allowed to stand for five minutes. The solution in cylinder A is not more intensely coloured than the solution in cylinder B.

If an aqueous solution becomes cloudy on addition of alcohol and becomes clear again on the addition of 2N hydrochloric acid, oxychloride is absent.

Tests for Identification

1. An aqueous solution is acidified with 2 N hydrochloric acid, until the solution is complete. The resulting solution is complies the tests of zinc.

2. A 5% solution in 2 N nitric acid gives the reactions of chloride.

Assay : The assay is based on the complexometric titration as discussed for zinc sulphate and calcium gluconate. To an aqueous solution of the substance, ammonium chloride, strong ammonia-ammonium chloride solution and eriochrome black T solution are added and titrated with 0.05 M disodium ethylenediaminetetraacetate to a deep-blue end point. Each ml of 0.05 M disodium ethylenediaminetetraacetate is equivalent to 0.006815 g of $ZnCl_2$.

Uses : Zinc chloride is a powerful caustic and astringent (protein precipitant). Weak solutions are used as astringent preparations and as injection for zinc replacement. It is also used as an obtundent in dentistry; as deodorant, disinfecting, embalming material, as a desensitizer of dentin, as mouthwashes, in ulcers, fistulas and pododermatitis.

7

INHALANTS

Drugs used as inhalants may be administered as solid particles, as nebulized particles from solutions or in the form of vapours. They may be sprayed as fine droplets which deposite over the mucous membrane producing local effects, e.g. salbutamol spray is used in bronchial asthma. They can also be administered as gases, e.g. volatile general anaesthetics.

Drugs for inhalation are rapidly absorbed and produce rapid local and systemic effects. Blood levels of volatile substances such as anaesthetics can be controlled as their absorption and excretion through the lungs are governed by the laws of gases. These drugs arrive directly to the left side of the heart through the pulmonary veins and may produce cardiac toxcity. Further, local irritation may result in an increase in the respiratory tract secretions.

OXYGEN

O_2; Mol. Weight = 31.99

Oxygen contains not less than 99.0 per cent of v/v of O_2. The remaining portion consists of argon, nitrogen and hydrogen. It is available in metal cylinders. Argon is present in air as 1%. Oxygen obtained by electrolysis of water contains traces of hydrogen.

Oxygen is the most abundant element on the earth; makes up 46.6% of earth's crust; 20.95% by volume of dry air. In combined state it is present in water (89% by weight) and in plants and animal tissues (50-70%).

Preparation

1. Oxygen is prepared by subjecting liquefied air to fractional evaporation. Nitrogen is more volatile and evaporates first leaving behind oxygen. Argon, present 1 per cent in air, is difficult to separate since its boiling point is only 3° higher than that of oxygen.

2. Oxygen is also prepared by electrolysis of water. Water is made conductor by addition of 20% of an alkali and the electric current is passed. Oxygen evolved is collected at anode. It contains traces of hydrogen and ozone.

3. Oxygen is also prepared by heating some oxygen containing salts, metallic oxides, hypochlorites and by action of concentrated sulphuric acid on manganese dioxide, potassium permanganate or potassium dichromate.

$$2KClO_3 \xrightarrow{\Delta} 2KCl + 3O_2$$
$$2MnO_2 + 2H_2SO_4 \longrightarrow 2MnSO_4 + 2H_2O$$

Physical Characters : Oxygen occurs as a colourless, odourless, tasteless, neutral gas. It is soluble in water (1 in 32) and alcohol (1 in 7) at normal temperature and pressure.

It is stored under compression in metal cylinders usually marketed under pressure in metal cylinders which are usually green-coloured or carry a green label. The cylinder should be stored in a special storage room which should be cooled and free from inflammable materials. The shoulder of the cylinder is painted white and the remainder as black. The cylinder carries a label stating the name of the gas or the symbol 'O_2'

Chemical Reactions : Oxygen combines with a large number of elements and this process is called *oxidation*. It oxidizes phosphorus, nitric oxide, iron, sulphur, carbon, sulphur dioxide, ammonia, etc.

$$P_4 + 5O_2 \longrightarrow P_4O_{10}$$
$$4Fe + 3O_2 \longrightarrow 2Fe_2O_3$$
$$S + O_2 \longrightarrow SO_2 \xrightarrow{O_2} SO_3$$
$$4NH_3 + 5O_2 \longrightarrow 4NO + 6H_2O$$

Oxygen is essential for the production of useful energy in the cell to synthesize adenosine triphosphate (ATP). When ATP is hydrolyzed, energy is released to complete the process. Oxygen requirements in the body can be classified into four major divisions :

1. Anoxic,

2. Anemic,
3. Stagnant, and
4. Histotoxic.

In the anoxic type the oxygen supply to the tissue is inadequate due to lowered tension of oxygen in the blood. Inhalation of oxygen enriched atmospheres containing 40 to 60% oxygen raises the oxygen saturation of arterial blood to normal value in patients with pneumonia and cardiac insufficiency. Oxygen therapy is used in asthma, massive collapse of the lungs, incomplete of lungs at birth, bronchopneumonia, congestive heart failure, coronary thrombosis (formation of a blood clot), cerebral thrombosis, etc. The oxygen is administered by nasal tubes, mask, or in tents at atmospheric pressure in concentrations from 30 to 80%. Sometimes 100% oxygen is given for a short period.

In the anemic type the oxygen tension is normal, but the amount of haemoglobin is inadequate to supply enough oxygen to the tissues. This condition may be due to haemorrhage, defective red blood cell formation, or carbon monoxide poisoning. Oxygen supply for many of these anemic anoxias is not effective. However, in carbon monoxide poisoning, a carbon dioxide-oxygen mixture administration is useful.

The stagnant type of anoxia is found when the general circulation is not sufficient or when circulation is locally retarded. In this case oxygen therapy is not useful. It is treated with cardiotonic drugs to facilitate circulation.

In the histotoxic type, tissue cell oxidation may interfere. Transfer of electrons results reduction of atomic oxygen to the oxide anion and formation of water, the released energy cannot be used by the cell to form ATP. In the end the cell will not be able to obtain useful energy to carry on essential metabolic processes. The toxic substances, e.g. cyanide, block electron transport and stop the cell's capacity to carry out metabolism requiring oxidation and reduction. In such cases oxygen administration will not be effective; the toxic materials are neutralized.

Oxygen may be administered by hyperbaric oxygen therapy in which 100% oxygen is given at 1.5 to 3 atmospheric pressure for air embolism (air bubbles in the blood), carbon monoxide poisoning, gas gangrene, crush injury, myocardial infarction and peripheral and cerebral vascular disease. A pressure chamber is needed.

Tests for Purity : Tests for acidity or alkalinity; carbon monoxide; carbon dioxide; halogens; and oxidizing substances.

For determining carbon monoxide, oxygen and carbon monoxide free air is passed through iodine pentoxide granules. The liberated iodine is titrated with 0.002N sodium thiosulphate. A blank determination is carried out under the same conditions using carbon dioxide-free air. The difference between the volumes of the sodium thiosulphate gives the amount of carbon monoxide in the oxygen sample.

If halogens are absent, no opalescence is produced by passing oxygen in silver nitrate solution.

The colour of the aqueous solution containing soluble starch, potassium iodide and glacial acetic acid, is not changed on passing oxygen. This indicates the absence of oxidising substances.

For detecting carbon dioxide, oxygen is passed through a 0.3 N barium hydroxide solution. Any turbidity produced is not more intense than that produced by adding of a 0.11 per cent w/v solution of sodium bicarbonate in water to 0.3 N barium hydroxide.

Tests for Identification

1. It causes a glowing splinter to burn with a flame.
2. It is absorbed when shaken with alkaline pyrogallol solution, the solution becoming dark brown.
3. When mixed with an equal volume of nitric oxide, red fumes are produced (distinction from nitrous oxide).

Uses : Oxygen is given by inhalation to correct hypoxia, in asthma, in extensive fibrosing alveolitis, after general anaesthesia, in inadequate oxygen supply, in circulatory failure, in treatment of carbon monoxide poisoning, respiratory depression or respiratory failure, in the management of abdominal distension, intestinal gas-filled cysts, and to persons working in pressurized spaces. It is used as a diluent of volatile and gaseous anaesthetics.

At lower pressures pulmonary toxicity occurs causing decrease in vital capacity, cough, and distress. At higher pressures CNS toxicity occurs involving nausea, mood changes, vertigo, convulsions and loss of consciousness.

NITROUS OXIDE
(Laughing Gas)

N_2O; Mol. Weight = 44.01

Nitrous oxide contains not less than 95.0 per cent of N_2O in the gaseous phase. It is manufactured by thermal decomposition of ammonium nitrate at slightly above its melting point.

$$NH_4NO_3 \xrightarrow{\Delta} N_2O + 2H_2O$$

The main impurity of the product is nitrogen, although higher oxides of nitrogen, oxygen, carbon dioxide and ammonia may also be present which are formed as by-products.

Nitrous oxide is also formed by reducing nitric acid with stannous chloride and hydrochloric acid.

$$2HNO_3 + 8HCl + 4SnCl_2 \longrightarrow 4SnCl_4 + N_2O + 5H_2O$$

Characters : It is colourless, odourless and tasteless gas; heavier than air; it support combustion. One volume of gas dissolves in about 1.4 volumes of water at 20° at a pressure of 760 mm; freely soluble in alcohol; soluble in solvent ether and in oils. It liquefies under 50 atmospheres pressure at 15°.

It is supplied compressed in metal cylinders and kept under pressure in the cylinders. The whole cylinder should be painted blue; the name or chemical symbol of the gas should be stencilled in paint on the cylinder.

The critical temperature at which the gas can be liquefied by pressure is 36.5°. It is very stable and rather inert chemically at room temperatures. Its dissociation begins above 300° when the gas becomes a strong oxidizing agent.

$$2N_2O \longrightarrow 2N_2 + O_2$$

It is incommbustible but due to decomposition, it supports in combustion. Sulphur and phosphorus burn in an atmosphere of N_2O.

$$S + 2N_2O \longrightarrow SO_2 + 2N_2$$
$$P_4 + 10N_2O \longrightarrow P_4O_{10} + 10N_2$$
$$C + 2N_2O \longrightarrow CO_2 + N_2$$

When passed over red hot copper, it is reduced to nitrogen.

$$Cu + N_2O \longrightarrow CuO + N_2$$

Nitrous oxide is the only inorganic gas used as an anaesthetic. It is administered with oxygen in the ratio of 80 : 20. It does not have very rapid recovery time.

Tests for Purity : Tests for acidity or alkalinity; arsine; phosphine; carbon dioxide; carbon monoxide; halogens; hydrogen sulphide; nitric oxide; nitrogen dioxide; reducing substances; oxidizing substances; and water vapour.

Nitrogen may be present up to 10 per cent or more in the gaseous phase. In the liquid phase, the proportion is usually much smaller. Large proportion of nitrogen may cause asphyxia.

Arsine and phosphine are determined through a mercuric chloride paper attached to a glass tube, as in the limit test for arsenic. No visible stain in produced.

Carbon dioxide, carbon monoxide and halogens are detected as discussed under oxygen.

Nitric oxide and nitrogen dioxide are determined by passing nitrous oxide through an aqueous solution of potassium permanganate containing sulphuric acid. Then a mixture of sulphanilic in glacial acetic acid and N-(1-naphthyl) ethylenediamine hydrochloride is added and the extinction of the resulting solution is measured at 550 nm. The extinction should not be greater than that of the solution obtained by adding of a 0.00308% solution of sodium nitrite to the reagent mixture.

On passing the gas through aqueous solution of 2.1N potassium permanganate, the colour is not completely discharged indicating the absence of reducing substances.

On passing the gas through a freshly prepared aqueous solution of soluble starch and potassium iodide containing 1 drop of glacial acetic acid, no colour is developed indicating the absence of oxidizing substances.

The amount of water content is determined by passing the gas through an absorption tube containing magnesium perchlorate. The increase in weight of the tube does not exceed 2 mg per litre of gas.

Tests for Identification

1. A glowing splinter of wood bursts into flame on contact with the gas.
2. It is not absorbed by alkaline pyrogallol solution.

Assay : A quantity of about 50 ml of the gas drawn from a cylinder is measured into an evacuated vessel and immersed in liquid oxygen or liquid nitrogen for a suitable period. The uncondensed gas is then drawn off into a small eudiometer and measured which should not exceed 1 per cent v/v, showing the presence of not less than 99 per cent v/v of nitrous oxide.

Uses : Nitrous oxide has weak analgesic properties. A mixture with oxygen in 1 : 1 ratio is used for the relief of pain in childbirth and pain from myocardial infarction. It has strong analgesic properties, but produces little muscle relaxation. When administered without air or oxygen, nitrous oxide would produce deep anaesthesia in about 1 minute but the signs of hypoxia would occur.

CARBON DIOXIDE

CO_2; Mol. Weight = 44.01

Carbon dioxide contains not less than 99% v/v of CO_2.

Carbon dioxide is present in air in about 0.03% v/v. It is evolved from volcanoes decaying of dead bodies; during process of respiration, combustion and fermentation.

Preparation

1. It is prepared by treatment with acids or by heating carbonates of heavy metals or bicarbonates of alkali metals.

$$CaCO_3 \longrightarrow CaO + CO_2$$
$$2NaHCO_3 \longrightarrow Na_2CO_3 + CO_2 + H_2O$$
$$Na_2CO_3 + H_2SO_4 \longrightarrow Na_2SO_4 + CO_2 + H_2O$$
$$CaCO_3 + HCl \longrightarrow CaCl_2 + CO_2 + H_2O$$

2. On commercial scale carbon dioxide is manufactured from fuel gases which are passed under pressure over potassium carbonate to form the bicarbonate. Carbon dioxide is liberated by releasing the pressure and compressed into steel cylinders.

$$K_2CO_3 + CO_2 + H_2O \longrightarrow 2KHCO_3$$

3. When limestone is burnt in lime kilns, carbon dioxide is obtained as a by-product.

$$CaCO_3 \longrightarrow CaO + CO_2\uparrow$$
$$\text{Lime}$$

4. Fermentation of sugar produces alcohol and carbon dioxide as a by-product.

$$C_6H_{12}O_6 \longrightarrow 2C_2H_5OH + 2CO_2\uparrow$$

It is the normal end product of combustion of carbon materials. It is also formed in the metabolism of all aerobic organisms, and the reaction is catalyzed by the enzyme carbonic anhydrase.

5. Carbon dioxide is absorbed by plants in the presence of chlorophyll and sunlight to form carbohydrates (*photosynthesis*).

$$6CO_2 + 6H_2O \longrightarrow C_6H_{12}O_6 + 6O_2$$
Glucose

$$6_xCO_2 + 5_xH_2O \longrightarrow (C_6H_{10}O_5)_x + 6_xCO_2$$
Starch

Physical Characters : Carbon dioxide occurs as a colourless, odourless gas which does not support combustion; faint acid taste. It is supplied liquefied under pressure in metal cylinders.

It is about 1.5 times as heavy as air. It can be liquefied by pressure of 72 atmospheres at 31°. It is soluble in water (1 : 1) at normal temperature and pressure.

It is stored in cylinders painted grey or green in a cool place free from materials of an inflammable nature. The name of the gas or the chemical symbol 'CO_2' should be stencilled in paint on the shoulder of the cylinder and clearly and indelibly stamped on the cylinder valve.

Chemical Reactions

1. Carbon dioxide is neither combustible nor a supporter of combustion. But some active metals burn in the atmosphere of carbon dioxide.

$$CO_2 + 2Mg \longrightarrow 2MgO + C$$
$$CO_2 + 4Na \longrightarrow 2Na_2O + C$$

2. It dissolves in water to form an unstable carbonic acid which turns blue litmus red and neutralizes alkalies.

$$CO_2 + H_2O \longrightarrow H_2CO_3$$
$$2NaOH + CO_2 \longrightarrow Na_2CO_3 + H_2O$$
$$Na_2CO_3 + CO_2 + H_2O \longrightarrow 2NaHCO_3$$

The bicarbonate/carbonic acid ratio determines the body fluid pH. A decreased removal of carbon dioxide can cause respiratory acidosis while respiratory alkalosis is due to increased removal of the gas.

3. When passed through lime water, it first turns milky and is again clear. On boiling the clear solution, milkiness re-appears.

$$Ca(OH)_2 \xrightarrow[-H_2O]{+CO_2} CaCO_3 \xrightarrow[+H_2O]{+CO_2} Ca(HCO_3)_2$$

Lime water ··· Insoluble (milky) ··· Soluble

$$\downarrow \begin{array}{l} \text{heat} \\ -CO_2 \\ -H_2O \end{array}$$

$$CaCO_3$$

4. When passed through red-hot coke, it is reduced to carbon monoxide.

$$CO_2 + C \longrightarrow 2CO$$

Tests for Purity : Tests for acidity; phosphoric hydrides; hydrogen sulphide; organic reducing substances; carbon monoxide; ammonia; nitric oxide; nitrogen dioxide; sulphur dioxide.

For determing acidity, the gas is passed through a solution (1) diluted with water. Nitrogen is passed at a rate of 15-20 litres per hour. Another solution (2) is prepared containing hydrogen peroxide solution, hydrochloric acid and water. To each solution methyl orange solution is added. Any orange-yellow colour in solution (1) is not more intense than that in solution (2).

For detecting phosphoric hydrides, hydrogen sulphide and organic reducing substances the gas is passed through a mixture containing ammonical silver nitrate solution water and ammonia. The solution is not darker than a reference solution prepared at the same time and in the same manner but through which the gas has not been passed.

Carbon monoxide is detected by carrying out the limit test for carbon monoxide.

Tests for Identification

1. It extinguishes a flame.
2. When passed through barium hydroxide, a white precipitate is produced which dissolved, with effervescence, in 2M acetic acid.

Uses : Carbon dioxide is added to the oxygen in certain types of pump oxygenators to maintain the carbon dioxide content of the blood. It is used as a respiratory stimulant. Carbon dioxide and oxygen (95:5) is used in the treatment of carbon monoxide poisoning as CO_2 increases both the ventilatory exchange rate and the rate of dissociation of carbon monoxide from carboxyhaemoglobin.

Inhalation of carbon dioxide has been tried for the relief of intractable hiccups. Carbonated vehicles are useful for masking the unpleasant taste of saline aperients. Carbon dioxide is used for detoxifying heroin addicts without the painful withdrawal syndrome.

Solid carbon dioxide, or dry ice; has a temperature of-80° and is used to treat warts and naevi by cryotherapy, and skin conditions as acne, angiomas (blood tumour), corns, callus, eczema, moles and psoriasis.

Carbon dioxide is also used to prepare carbonated beverages in the soft drink industry. The most effervescent preparations contain sodium bicarbonate and an acid, usually citric acid.

$$NaHCO_3 + HA \longrightarrow Na^+ + A^- + H_2CO_3$$
$$H_2CO_3 \longrightarrow CO_2\uparrow + H_2O$$

Above a concentration of 6% carbon dioxide gives rise to headache, dizziness, mental confusion, palpitations, hypertension, dyspnoea, increased depth, rate of respiration and depression of central nervous system.

8

RESPIRATORY STIMULANTS

Respiratory stimulants (analeptics) are CNS stimulants and have a limited but useful role in the treatment of ventilatory failure in patients with chronic obstructive airways disease. They are effective only parenterally and have a short duration of action. These should be given only under expert medical supervision in hospital, except in a severe emergency and are best combined with active physiotherapy. Maintenance treatment with respiratory stimulant may be required in those patients who are unable to tolerate even a 24% inspired oxygen concentration without drowsiness or comatose and in patients with a long history of intolerance respiratory disability in contraindication to artificial ventilation. Respiratory stimulants may be harmful in patients where hypoxaemia is not associated with carbon dioxide retention, such as asthma or in respiratory failure due to neurological or muscular disease and drug overdose. They are occasionally used in the asphyxiated newborn infant but clearing the airways is the first essential and valuable time may be wasted in giving the respiratory stimulants. A few drops are placed on the tongue.

AMMONIUM CARBONATE

$[NH_4HCO_3]_m$ $[NH_2CO_2NH_4]_m$

It is a variable mixture of ammonium bicarbonate (NH_4HCO_3) and ammonium carbonate (NH_2CONH_4). It contains the equivalent of not less than 30.0 per cent of NH_3. It is manufactured by subliming a mixture of ammonium sulphate or chloride and calcium carbonate.

$$(NH_4)_2SO_4 + CaCO_3 \longrightarrow (NH_4)_2CO_3 + CaSO_4$$

The product is resublimed after adding a small amount of water to get a white semi-transparent fibrous mass of ammonium carbonate with an outer layer of white opaque powder of ammonium bicarbonate.

Characters : It occurs as translucent, hard, crystalline masses; odour is strongly ammonical; taste is pungent and ammonical. When exposed to air, it partially dissociates, and loses ammonia and carbon dioxide, becoming opaque and finally converted into porous lumps or a white powder of ammonium bicarbonate. It is freely soluble in water; partly soluble in alcohol yielding a residue of the bicarbonate. It is decomposed by hot water. A solution in water is alkaline to litmus. It volatilizes at about 60°.

$$NH_2CO_2NH_4 + H_2O \longrightarrow (NH_4)_2CO_3$$

Ammonium carbonate should be kept in a well-closed container at a temperature not exceeding 30° and protected from light.

Ammonium carbonate is readily converted into the normal carbonate by dissolving it in dilute ammonia water.

$$NH_4HCO_3 + NH_3 \longrightarrow (NH_4)_2CO_3$$

The decomposition of the salt is caused entirely by loss of ammonium carbonate yielding a white powder of ammonium bicarbonate.

$$(NH_4HCO_3)_m (NH_2CO_2NH_4)_n \longrightarrow nCO_2\uparrow + 2nNH_3 \uparrow$$
$$+ mNH_4HCO_3$$

Both ammonium carbonate and ammonium bicarbonate decompose to ammonia and carbon dioxide at 60°.

$$NH_4HCO_3 \longrightarrow NH_3\uparrow + CO_2\uparrow + H_2O$$
$$(NH_4)_2CO_3 \longrightarrow 2NH_3\uparrow + CO_2\uparrow + H_2O.$$

Tests for Purity : Tests for iron; chloride; sulphate; tarry matter; non-volatile matter.

For detecting tarry matter, the substance (5 g) is mixed with water (15 ml) and citric acid (7 g) and stirred until dissolved; no tarry odour is produced.

Incompatibility : Acids and acid salts, salts of iron, zinc; alkaloids, alum, calomel and tartar emetic.

Assay : The assay is based on the acidimetry and alkalimetry titration as discussed for sodium bicarbonate. A weighed amount (2 g) dissolved in N sulphuric acid (50 ml) is diluted with water (50 ml), boiled, cooled, and the excess of acid titrated with N sodium hydroxide, using methyl red solution as indicator. Each ml of N sulphuric acid is equivalent to 0.01703 g of NH_3

Uses : Ammonium carbonate is used as respiratory stimulant, expectorant and a pharmaceutical aid.

9

EXPECTORANTS AND EMETICS

Expectorant : The cough is a protective physiological reflex to clear the airway. Infections, chemical irritants, retained body secretion and the presence of foreign bodies block one's airway causing coughing by stimulating the nerve endings in the respiratory tract.

Irritative cough is dry cough, which may be produced by colds or by inhalation of irritating dust or gases and produces no sputum or other discharge. *Productive cough* is sputum or exudate producing cough and is often associated with asthma and bronchitis. Any cough that persists more than a week should be checked by a physician to detect its cause.

The drugs used in various combinations to alleviate cough are :

   (i) *Expectorants* : They reduce the viscosity of mucous and increase the secretions of the respiratory tract, e.g. ammonium chloride, sodium citrate, potassium iodide,

  (ii) *Bronchodilators* : They are used in cough associated with bronchospasm, e.g. ephedrine,

 (iii) *Cough sedatives/Suppressants/Antitussives* : They generally act on the cough centre in the brain to suppress cough, e.g. codeine;

  (iv) *Mucolytics* : They liquefy mucoprulent or tenacious sputum, e.g. acetylcysteine, and

   (v) *Anti-histamines* : They are often beneficial and are used in various combination products.

Since expectorants increase the volume of secretions in the respiratory tract and, therefore, facilitate their removal by ciliary action and coughing. The drugs are useful in the treatment of cough due to irritation of the respiratory conditions in which the secretion is thick and viscid, requiring liquefaction. Expectorants can stimulate the output of respiratory tract fluid. Agents used as expectorant are terpine hydrate, which has a direct effect on the bronchial secretory cells; ammonium chloride, glyceryl guaiacolate, potassium guaiacol-sulphonate, syrup of ipecac, iodinated glycerin, potassium iodide, and hydriodic acid syrup, which act with a reflex action by irritating the gastric mucosa and stimulate respiratory tract secretion.

Emetics : Nausea is a compulsive desire to vomit which may or may not culminate in vomiting. Vomiting is a complex physiological process that ultimately results in the forceful expulsion of the contents of stomach. The sensory stimuli causing vomiting reflex may have their orgin in the mucosa of the gastro-intestinal tract, the labyrinth of the inner ear, cerebral cortex or the brain area associated with emotional responses. The brain area which regulates the vomiting reflex is called the vomiting centre which is located in the medulla oblongata. Closely associated with this is the chemoreceptor trigger zone which is sensitive to many drugs and to certain metabolic disturbances. Stimulation of the vomiting centre also occurs following actions on other areas such as the vestibular apparatus of the ear in motion sickness. As a protective reflex, vomiting is frequently a symptom of disease and should not be treated until the cause has been found.

If vomiting is prolonged, dehydration, hypokalaemia and alkalosis may occur and replacement of fluid and electrolytes may be necessary.

Cancer chemotherapy can produce severe nausea and vomiting which will be difficult to treat. Post operative emesis may be caused by anaesthetic agents or opioid analgesics.

The drugs that produce vomiting are termed *emetics*. They may be :

(i) centrally acting by stimulation of the chemoreceptor trigger zone, (e.g. morphine);

(ii) peripherally acting (e.g. mustard, antimony and potassium tartrate and sodium chloride),

(iii) both peripherally and centrally acting (e.g. ipecacuanha).

The therapeutic use of emetics is limited to certain cases of poisoning, especially where facilities for gastric larvage are not available. If the ingested poison is a caustic, emesis may cause perforation of the stomach. Emetics should be avoided in children and in the elderly pregnant women and in patients suffering from cardiac decompensation, hypertension, hernia, peptic ulcer and pulmonary tuberculosis.

AMMONIUM CHLORIDE

NH_4Cl; Mol. Weight = 53.49

Ammonium chloride contains not less than 99.5 per cent of NH_4Cl.

Crude ammonium chloride is found is Karnal district of Haryana.

Preparation

1. It is prepared by purifying the crude product by sublimation or by boiling ammonium sulphate solution with sodium chloride in equivalent proportions.

$$(NH_4)_2SO_4 + 2NaCl \longrightarrow 2NH_4Cl + Na_2SO_4$$

2. Neutralization of hydrochloric acid with ammonia and evaporation of the solution to dryness yield ammonium chloride.

$$NH_3 + HCl \longrightarrow NH_4Cl$$

The product is purified by sublimation from an iron vessel or by recrystallization.

Characters : It occurs as a white, odourless crystalline powder or colourless crystals with a cooling saline taste; somewhat hygroscopic; strongly endothermic. It sublimes without melting. It is freely soluble in water and glycerol; more soluble in boiling water; sparingly soluble in alcohol. A 5% solution has a pH of 4.6 to 6.0; almost insoluble in acetone, ether and ethyl acetate. Hydrochloric acid and sodium chloride decrease solubility in water. It is stored in airtight containers.

Ammonium ion plays an important role in the maintenance of the acid-base equilibrium of the body, especially in acidosis. The diuretic effect of ammonium chloride is due to formation of a proton and a chloride ion, equivalent to hydrochloric acid. The hydrogen ion reacts with the body buffers, mainly bicarbonate, to form CO_2 and bicarbonate is displaced by a chloride ion.

The expectorant action of the ammonium salt may be due to local irritation. The salt forms thin and increases the quantity of the mucus.

Tests for Purity : Tests for arsenic; heavy metals; lead; iron; barium; sulphate; thiocyanate; sulphated ash; loss on drying and non-volatile matter.

When dilute sulphuric acid is added to an aqueous solution, no turbidity is produced within two hours indicating the absence of barium.

To an acidified solution with hydrochloric acid, few drops of ferric chloride are added. No red colour is produced indicating the absence of thiocyanate.

Incompatibility : Alkalies and their carbonates; lead and silver salts.

Test for Identification : It gives the reactions of ammonium salts and of chlorides.

Assay : The assay is based on indirect acid-base (acidimetry-alkalimetry) titration. An aqueous solution of the substance is treated with neutralized formaldehyde solution. This results in the liberation of hydrochloric acid equivalent to ammonium chloride. This is then titrated with a standard solution of sodium hydroxide using phenolphthalein as an indicator yielding pink colour at the end point.

$$4NH_4Cl + 4H_2O \longrightarrow 4NH_4OH + 4HCl$$
$$4NH_4OH + 6HCHO \longrightarrow (CH_2)_6N_4 + 10H_2O$$
$$\text{Hexamine}$$
$$4HCl + 4NaOH \longrightarrow 4NaCl + 4H_2O$$

To an aqueous solution, formaldehyde solution, previously neutralized to dilute phenolphthalein solution, is added. After two minutes the solution is titrated with 0.1 N sodium hydroxide using dilute phenolphthalein solution. Each ml of 0.1 N sodium hydroxide is equivalent to 0.005349 g of NH_4Cl.

Uses : Ammonium chloride is an expectorant, diuretic and systemic acidifying agent. It is used in the treatment of severe metabolic alkalosis, to maintain the urine at an acid pH in the treatment of some urinary-tract disorders or in forced acid diuresis; to potentiate mercurial diuretics.

Ammonium salts are irritant to the gastric mucosa and may produce nausea and vomiting.

ANTIMONY POTASSIUM TARTRATE

$$C_8H_4K_2O_{12}Sb_2 \cdot 3H_2O; \text{Mol. Weight} = 667.85$$

It contains not less than 99 per cent of $C_8H_4K_2O_{12}Sb_2 \cdot 3H_2O$. It occurs as odourless, colourless, transparent crystals or white powder. The crystals effloresce on exposure to air and do not readily rehydrate even when exposed to high humidity. It is soluble in water and glycerol; insoluble in alcohol. Solutions in water are acidic to litmus.

Tests for Purity : Test for arsenic; acidity or alkalinity; loss on drying.

Tests for Identification

1. When heated to redness, it chars, emits an odour resembling that of burning sugar, and leaves a blackened residue. This residue has an alkaline reaction, and when a small fragment of it is held in a nonluminous flame, the flame is tinted violet.

2. In a solution (1 in 20), acidified with hydrochloric acid, hydrogen sulphide produces an orange red precipitate, which is soluble in ammonium sulphide and in 1 N sodium hydroxide.

   The substance is preserved in well-closed containers.

Incompatibility : Tannic acid, alkalies and their carbonates, lead salts, astringent infusions (cinchona, rhubarb, etc), acacia, antipyrine, mercury bichloride, salts of heavy metals, albumin and soap.

Assay (U.S.P.) : The assay is carried out volumetrically by titration with a solution of iodine in the presence of sodium potassium tartrate and borax using solution of starch as an indicator. The end point is appeared as blue colour. This involves oxidation from the trivalent antimonious state to the pentavalent antimonic state. Iodine solution acts as an oxidizing agent.

$$Sb_2O_3 + 2H_2O + 2I_2 \longrightarrow Sb_2O_5 + 4HI$$

This oxidation is revesible and completed if the hydriodic acid is neutralized. Sodium hydroxide or sodium carbonate cannot be used for the removal of hydrodic acid since these alkalies themselves react with the iodine solution. These difficulties are overcome if the titration is carried out in the presence of sodium potassium tartrate and borax which yield an alkaline solution but which does not itself react with iodine.

$$2C_4H_4O_7 SbK + 3 H_2O + 2I_2 \longrightarrow 2C_4H_4O_6 KH + Sb_2O_5 + 4HI$$

An aqueous solution of antimony potassium tartrate (0.5 g) containing potassium sodium tartrate (5 g), sodium borate (2 g) and starch (3 ml), is immediately titrated with 0.1 N iodine to the production of a persistent blue colour. Each ml of 0.1 N iodine is equivalent to 16.7 mg of $C_8H_4K_2O_{12} Sb_2 . 3H_2O$.

Antimony potassium tartrate is a trivalent antimony compound with similar properties to antimony sodium tartrate. It is less soluble and more irritant than the sodium salt.

Uses : It is used in the treatment of cutaneous leishmaniasis.

POTASSIUM IODIDE

KI; Mol. Weight = 166.0

Potassium iodide contains not less than 99.0 per cent of KI. It is prepared by treating iron filing with iodine under water to get iodide which is then reacted with potassium carbonate.

$$K_2CO_3 + FeI_2 \longrightarrow 2KI + FeCO_3$$

Treatment of hydriodic acid with potassium bicarbonate also gives potassium iodide.

$$KHCO_3 + HI \longrightarrow KI + H_2CO_3$$

Characters : It occurs as odourless, colourless, transparent or somewhat opaque crystals or white granular powder; slightly hygroscopic; taste is saline and slightly bitter. On long exposure to air, it becomes yellow due to liberation of iodine, and small quantities of iodate may be formed; light and moisture accelerate the rate of decomposition. Aqueous solutions also become yellow in time due to oxidation, but a small amount of alkali prevents it.

Potassium iodine is soluble in water, alcohol and glycerol. Solutions in water are neutral or alkaline to litmus. Iodine readily dissolves in an aqueous solution of potassium iodide, forming a dark brown solution containing potassium tri-iodide.

Incompatibility : Potassium iodide is incompatible with alkaloidal salts, chloral hydrate, tartaric and other acids, calomel, potassium chlorate and metallic salts.

It is stored in well-closed containers, and protected from light.

Tests for Purity : Tests for alkalinity; arsenic; heavy metals; barium; lead; sodium; sulphate; cyanides, iodates; and loss on drying.

If no colour is produced on addition of phenolphthalein solution to an aqueous solution of potassium iodide containing a drop of 0.02 N sulphuric acid, the alkaline inpurities are absent. When no turbidity is developed within one minute on addition of dilute sulphuric acid to the solution, then barium is not present.

For the detection of cyanides, ferrous sulphate solution (1 drop) and sodium hydroxide solution (0.5 ml) are added to the aqueous solution of the substance. The reaction mixture is acidified with hydrochloric acid. If no blue colour is produced, cyanides are absent.

Iodates are determined by treating an aqueous solution with dilute sulphuric acid and then with starch solution; no blue colour is produced within two minutes when iodates are absent.

Tests for Identification : An aqueous solution (1 in 20) gives the reactions of potassium, and of iodides.

Assay : To an aqueous solution of the substance (0.5 g), hydrochloric acid and chloroform are added and the mixture is titrated with 0.05 M potassium iodate until the purple colour of iodine disappears from the chloroform. Each ml of 0.05 M potassium iodate is equivalent to 0.0166 mg of KI.

Uses : Potassium iodide is an antifungal, antitussive and expectorant agent; used as a source of iodine in pre-operative management of hyperthyroidism. Iodine is an essential element in the human diet; it is necessary for the formation of thyroid hormone. It is used for the prophylaxis and treatment of iodine deficiency disorders.

Prolonged use of iodine and iodides may cause metallic taste; increased salivation, pain and coryza.

10

ANTIDOTES

An antidote is an agent which counteracts as a poison. In the treatment of acute poisoning most patients require only supportive and symptomatic therapy. The active removal of poisons from the stomach by gastric lavage or emesis induction is done by the administration of substances like activated charcoal by mouth to reduce the absorption. However, emesis and charcoal are inadequate measures in corrosive poisoning, and aspiration should only be carried out with great care.

Techniques used to promote the elimination of poisons from the body such as forced diuresis, haemodialysis, or haemoperfusion are employed for a limited number of poisons. There are some specific antidotes and their use in appropriate circumstances can be life-saving. Such use does not preclude relevant supportive and symptomatic treatment.

Dipending on their action, antidotes are classified as :

(i) chemical antidotes which changes the chemical nature of poison, e.g. sodium thiosulphate which changes toxic cyanide to the non-toxic thiocyanate; sodium calcium edetate chelates agents used for heavy metal poison;

(ii) physiological antidote which acts by producing the effect opposite to that of poison, e.g. sodium nitrite convert haemoglobin into methaemoglobin in order to bind cyanide; and

(iii) mechanical antidotes which prevent the absorption of poison into the body. For example activated charcoal absorbs the poison prior to absorption across intestinal wall. Copper sulphate, magnesium sulphate and sodium monohydrogen phosphate inactivate and precipitate the toxic material as insoluble salts by chelation.

Antidote action occurs by counter acting the effects of a poison by producing other effects, e.g. sodium nitrite (a physiological antidote); by changing the chemical nature of the poison, e.g. sodium thiosulphate (a chemical antidote); and by preventing the absorption of the poison into the body, e.g. activated charcoal (a mechanical antidote). Sodium nitrite converts haemoglobin into methaemoglobin for binding cyanide; sodium thiosulphate; and activated charcoal adsorbs the poison prior to absorption across the intestinal wall. Other mechanical antidotes, e.g. cupric sulphate, magnesium sulphate, and sodium monohydrogen phosphate (Na_2HPO_4) inactivate and precipitate the toxic material as insoluble salt.

The cyanide poisoning may be due to inhalation of hydrocyanic acid and ingestion of soluble inorganic cyanide salts such as cyanamide, cyanogen chloride, seeds of apricot, bitter almond and choke-berry, peach; photographic chemicals and silver polishes. The adverse effects of cyanide poisoning include nausea, dizziness, headache, drowsiness, dyspnoea, hypotension, coma, convulsions and death. The death may occur within 15 minutes of inhalation hydrogen cyanide. Consumption of about 300 mg of potassium cyanide may cause death within several hours. Cyanide (CN^-) ions readily combines with ferric ions (Fe^{2-}) of cytochrome oxidase which prevents electron transfer and thus prevent cellular respiration or oxidation-reduction reactions.

Cyanide poisoning is treated by a combination of sodium nitrite and sodium thiosulphate. Sodium nitrite oxidizes ferrous (Fe^{2+}) ion of haemoglobin to the ferric ion of methaemoglobin, which then combines with the serum cyanide. The thiosulphate anion reacts with cyanide to form relative nontoxic thiocyanate ion which is excreted in the urine.

$$Na_2S_2O_3 + CN^- \xrightleftharpoons[\text{SCN}^-\text{ oxidase}]{\text{Rhodanese}} SCN^- + Na_2SO_3$$

SODIUM NITRATE

$NaNO_2$; Mol. Weight = 69.0

It contains 97 to 101 per cent of $NaNO_2$, calculated with reference to the substance dried over silica gel for four hours.

Its preparation, physical characters, chemical properties, tests for purity, assay and uses are described in the chapter on antioxidants (page 51).

11

ELECTROLYTES

Solutions of acids, bases and salts conduct electricity and when voltage is applied, they decompose into ions. This phenomenon of decomposition is called *electrolysis* and these substances are named *electrolytes*.

The concentration balances of the various inorganic and organic compounds of the body's fluids are maintained to have a constant environment of the cells and tissues. For this purpose there are regulatory mechanisms which control pH, ionic balances, osmotic balances, etc. Many products are used to correct an electrolyte imbalance due to a change in the composition of its fluid. These products include electrolytes, acids and bases, blood products, carbohydrates, amino acids and proteins.

The electrolyte concentration vary in intracellular fluid (45-50% of body weight), interstitial fluid (12-15%) and plasma or vascular fluid (4-5%). Besides plasma and interstitial fluid, the extracellular fluid also includes cerebrospinal fluid, lymph, peritoneal, pleural and synovial fluids. About 40% of the interstitial fluid (4 litres) is constituted of dense connective tissues such as bone and cartilage and does not take part in quick exchange with the remaining body fluid. The rest of the interstitial fluid (6.5 litres) and plasma (3.5 litres) comprise the active part of the extracellular fluid. These fluid compartments are separated from each other by membranes which are permeable to water and many organic and inorganic solutes. They are nearly impermeable to macromolecules (e.g. proteins) and selectively permeable to certain ions (e.g. Na^+, K^+, and Mg^{++}). Due to this permeablity mechanism each fluid compartment has a distinct solute pattern and the solution in each compartment is ionically balanced. Thus potassium, megnesium, and phosphate are found in the intracellular fluid and sodium and chloride are present in the plasma and interstitial fluids. The principal factors involved in fluid and electrolyte homoeostasis are maintenance of blood volume and osmotic equilibrium, acid-base balance, and the effects of specific ions. For electrical neutrality to exist in the extracellular fluid, the sum of the concentrations of cations must be equal to the sum of the concentrations of anions. Measurements of extracellular (plasma or serum) concentrations are usually limited to sodium, potassium, chloride, and bicarbonate. Assuming measurement only of sodium, bicarbonate, and chloride, the sum of the concentrations of sodium plus unmeasured cations (calcium, magnesium, potassium) equals the sum of the concentrations of bicarbonate and chloride plus unmeasured anions (phosphate, protein, sulphate and derivatives of organic acids). The difference between the concentrations of unmeasured anions and unmeasured cations is known as the anion gap. Variations in the anion gap are useful diagnostic indications to disorders of acid - base balance.

The electrolyte balance of the body is maintained by a regulation between the intake and output of water. The intake of water includes the fluid taken orally and release of water during the oxidation and mechanism of ingested food.

$$C_6H_{12}O_6 + 6H_2O \longrightarrow 6CO_2 + 6H_2O$$

Water is eliminated from the body by lungs (expiration), skin (perspiration), faeces and urine. Urine excretion is generally more in cold session to balance water losses by perspiration and respiration. Output of water is increased by diarrhoea and vomiting. The water intake is regulated by the thirst centre of hypothalamus gland. Excessive loss of water results into the concentration of the body fluid and rise in their osmotic pressure. This causes to draw out water from intracellular compartments causing dehydration of the cells.

When there is more water in the fluid compartments, osmetic pressure of the fluid is diminished. It promotes diuresis and loss of body water. Due to water loss, plasma is concentrated followed by concentration of extracellular and intracellular fluids. Along with water intracellular potassium also passes out into the extracellular fluid. It is compensated by passage of sodium from extracellular fluid into the cell. A 20% loss of water from the body may be fatal.

(A) MAJOR PHYSIOLOGICAL IONS

(i) **Calcium :** Calcium is an important constituent of bones and teeth and it is also concerned with the functioning of muscles and clotting mechanism of blood. Children, require higher amount of calcium as it is needed for growth of tissues and bones. Milk, milk-products and green vegetables are rich in calcium. Among the cereals, millet ragi, wheat, jowar and bajra are good source of calcium. Hypocalcaemia is resulted from hypoparathyroidism, vitamin D deficiency, bone cancer, fatty stool (steatorrhea), hyperactive adrenal cortex, acute pancreatitis, acute hyperphosphatemia and disorders in bone metabolism. Bone is also a storage tissue for calcium. At night, when a person sleeps or more without food intake, reabsorption of the bone occurs in order to maintain blood calcium levels.

(ii) **Magnesium :** Magnesium is the second most cation in concentration in the intracellular fluid compartment. Half amount of the total body magnesium (10-20 g) is combined with calcium and phosphorus in bone. It is used for protein synthesis and for the smooth functioning of the neuromuscular system. Low magnesium balance is resulted from malnutrition, dietary restriction, chronic alcoholism, faulty absorption, gastrointestinal diseases, medications and parathyroid hormone imbalances. Its deficiency causes personality changes, loss in body weight and cardiac disturbances.

(iii) **Sodium :** Sodium is the principal cation in the extracellular fluid compartments. This ion is required to maintain normal hydration and osmotic pressure. Sufficient amounts of sodium are present in the daily diet. Excess sodium is excreted by kidneys. About 80-95% of the sodium is reabsorbed in the glomerular filtrate by a hormonal control. Conditions causing low serum level (hyponatremia) are extreme urine loss as in diabetes, metabolic acidosis, addison's disease (decreased excretion of the hormone, aldosterone), diarrhoea, vomiting, and kidney damage. Increased serum sodium level (hypernatremia) is found in hyperadrenalism with increased aldosterone production, severe dehydration, certain type of brain injury, and excess treatment with sodium.

There is a correlation between sodium content of the tissue and hypertension. If sodium is not eliminated from the body, the concentration starts to increase, water is retained in the tissue to maintain osmotic balance and edema results.

(iv) **Potassium :** Potassium is the major intracellular cation, present in about 23 times higher than present in the extracellular fluid compartment. During transmission of a nerve impulse, potassium leaves the cell and sodium enters the cell and this mechanism is called the *sodium-potassium pump*. Potassium in the diet is readily absorbed. Excess of potassium is rapidly excreted by the kidney. Low serum potassium levels (hypopotassemia, hypokalemia) causes changes in myocardial function, flaccid and feeble muscles, and low blood pressure. It causes vomiting, diarrhoea, burns, haemorrhages, diabetic coma, intravenous infusion of solutions and alkalosis. High serum potassium levels (hyperpotassemia or hyperkalemia) is less common and usually occurs during kidney damage.

(v) **Chloride :** Chloride is the major extracellular anion of both interstitial and vascular fluids compartments and is required for maintaining proper hydration, osmotic pressure and normal cation-anion balance. Food is the main source of chloride, with the anion being almost completely absorbed from the intestinal tract. Chloride is removed from the body by glomerular filtration and is reabsorbed by the kidney tubules. Hypochloremia is resulted from salt-losing nephritis (inflammation of kidney), chronic pyelonephritis (inflammation of the kidney and its pelvis); metabolic acidosis causing either excessive production or diminished excretion of acids leading to the replacement of chloride by acetoacetate and phosphate; and prolonged vomiting with loss of chloride as gastric hydrochloric acid. Hyperchloremic conditions are observed in dehydration, decreased renal blood flow found with congestive heart failure, renal damage and excessive chloride intake.

(vi) **Bicarbonate :** Bicarbonate (HCO_3^-) is the second most prevalent anion in the extracellular fluid compartments. Along with carbonic acid it is utilized as the body's most important buffer system. A lack of bicarbonate causes metabolic acidosis and metabolic alkalosis.

(vii) **Phosphate :** Phasphate (HPO_4^{-2}) is the principal anion of the intracellular fluid compartment. It is an important buffer system; related to the utilization of calcium, carbohydrates and fats and is also present in the bones and teeth. Good sources of phosphorus are cereals, pulses, nuts and oil-seeds. In cereals they are in combination with phytates, a carbohydrate complex. Administration of ascorbic acid along with cereal-based diets improves the utilization of these minerals.

(viii) **Iron :** Iron forms an important component of haemoglobin which acts as a carrier of oxygen in the blood. Iron is necessary for growing children and pregnant women and deficiency of iron causes anaemia. Green leafy vegetables are rich in iron. Millets like bajra and ragi are also good sources of iron.

Copper is associated with the utilization of iron in the body. Iodine deficiency causes swelling of thyroid gland giving rise to the disease 'goitre'. While fluorine in concentration less than 1 ppm in drinking water prevents dental carries, it leads to a toxic condition known as fluorosis affecting teeth and bones in amounts greater than 2 ppm.

Electrolyte solutions are used to correct disturbances in fluid and electrolyte balance. The main functions of electrolytes are the maintenance of osmotic pressure and electroneutrality, the production of energy, in impulse transmission and maintenance of calcium in blood clotting and bone formations.

SODIUM CHLORIDE

NaCl; Mol. Weight = 58.44

Sodium chloride contains not less than 99.5 per cent of NaCl. It contains no added substances. In nature it is found in sea water, in salt wells, lakes (Sambhar in India; Lake Elton in Russia) and in deposits of rock salt, in Mandi (H.P.) and Khewra (Punjab, Pakistan).

Sodium chloride is prepared on commercial scale by evaporation of sea-water in shallow pans. It contains impurities of sodium carbonate, sodium sulphate, magnesium chloride, magnesium sulphate and calcium chloride. For removing impurities the common salt is dissolved in water in cemented tanks. Some lime and alum are added. The suspended impurities are settled down. The clear solution is decanted into iron pans and concentrated. The crystals of sodium chloride separate, settle down which are dried.

Rock salt is dug out or dissolved in water if present in deep places. The saturated solution is pumped out and evaporated to get the salt.

Physical Characters : It occurs as odourless, colourless crystals or white crystalline powder, transparent or translucent when in large crystals. It is soluble in water (1 in 3), glycerol (1 in 10); slightly soluble in alcohol and dehydrated alcohol. A 0.9% aqueous solution is iso-osmotic. Its solubility in water decreased by hydrochloric acid and it is almost insoluble in concentrated hydrochloric acid.

Solutions are sterilized by autoclaving or by filtration. Solutions, when stored, may cause separation of solid particles from glass containers and solutions containing particles must not be used.

It is stored in well-closed containers.

Tests for Purity : Tests for acidity or alkalinity; arsenic; iron; heavy metals; potassium; calcium and magnesium; barium; sulphate; phosphate; iodide or bromide; sodium ferrocyanide; loss or drying; clarity and colour of solution.

For determining acidity or alkalinity, an aqueous solution of the substance is titrated with sodium hydroxide or sulphuric acid using phenol red solution as indicator.

The amount of calcium is found out by adding hydrochloric acid (0.1 ml), strong ammonia-ammonium chloride solution (5ml) and erichrome black T solution (5 ml) to an aqueous solution (20 in 200) of the substance and the mixture is titrated with 0.005 M disodium ethylenediamine-tetraacetate (DETA) to a blue end point. Each ml of 0.005 M DETA is equivalent to 0.0002004 g of Ca.

If no tubidity is produced on addition of dilute sulphuric acid to an aqueous solution of the substance within two hours, then barium is absent.

Iodide and bromide are detected by digesting sodium chloride with alcohol. The reaction mixture is filtered, the filtrate dried, the residue is dissolved in water, and chloroform and dilute chlorine water solution are added. The chloroform layer does not acquire a violet yellow or orange colour.

The presence of sodium ferrocyanide is detected by addition of ferrous sulphate solution to the acidified solution of the substance. The solution is not more intensely coloured than a mixture of 2 ml of ferrous sulphate solution, 1 ml of dilute sulphuric acid acid and sufficient water to produce 100 ml.

Tests for Identification : It gives the reactions of sodium, and of chlorides.

Assay : The assay is dependent on the modified Volhard's method in which indirect volumetric precipitation titration is involved. An acidified solution of sodium chloride with nitric acid is treated with a measured excess amount of standard solution of silver nitrate in the presence of nitrobenzene. Some of the silver nitrate is consumed due to reaction with sodium chloride. The remaining unreacted silver nitrate is determined by titration with a standard solution of ammonium thiocyanate using ferric ammonium sulphate (ferric alum) as indicator

$$\underset{\text{(excess)}}{NaCl + AgNO_3} \longrightarrow \underset{\text{ppt}}{AgCl\downarrow} + NaNO_3 + \underset{\text{unreacted}}{AgNO_3}$$

$$\underset{\text{unreacted}}{AgNO_3 + NH_4SCN} \longrightarrow \underset{\substack{\text{silver} \\ \text{thiocyanate} \\ \text{precipitate}}}{AgSCN} + NH_4NO_3$$

$$3NH_4SCN + Fe^{3+} \longrightarrow \underset{\substack{\text{Ferric} \\ \text{thiocynate} \\ \text{(brick red colour)}}}{Fe (SCN)_3} + 3NH_4^+$$

The end point is obtained as a permanent brick red colour due to formation of ferric thiocyanate.

To an aqueous solution of the substance, 1N silver nitrate, nitric acid, nitrobenzene and ferric ammonium sulphate solution are added. The solution is titrated with 0.1N ammonium thiocyanate. Each ml of 0.1N silver nitrate is equivalent to 0.005844 g of NaCl.

Uses : Sodium chloride is an electrolyte replenisher, emetic; topical inflammatory. It is used in the treatment of extracellular volume depletion, dehydration and sodium depletion which may occur due to excessive diuresis, gastroenteritis or salt restriction. Solutions of sodium chloride (0.9%) may be used as eye-drops (as an irritating agent), as nasal drop (to relieve nasal congestion) and as a mouthwash (to remove debris; for throat infection). Sodium chloride has been included in dermatological preparations as a hydrating agent. It is also used in homoeopathic medicine.

General adverse effects of excess sodium chloride include nausea, vomiting, diarrhoea, sweating, abdominal cramps, fever, thirst, hypotension, tachycardia (rapid pulse rate), renal failure, oedema, respiratory arrest, irritability, weakness, convulsions, coma and death.

SODIUM CHLORIDE INJECTION
(Sodium chloride intravenous infusion)

Sodium chloride injection is a sterile, isotonic solution of sodium chloride in water for injection. It contains not less than 0.85 per cent and not more than 0.95 per cent w/v of NaCl. It contains no antimicrobial agents.

It is a clear, colourless solution. It is stored in single-dose containers of glass or plastic. On keeping, small solid particles may separate from a glass container. A solution containing such particles must not be used.

Tests for Purity : Tests for heavy metals; pyrogens; and pH (between 4.5 and 7.0).

Limit test for heavy metals is designed to determine the content of metallic impurities that are coloured by sulphide ion under specific conditions. The colour of an aqueous solution of the substance is matched with that standard lead solution after addition of hydrogen sulphide solution which is not darker in the test solution than that produced in the standard solution.

The test for pyrogens involves the measurement of the rise in body temperature of rabbits following the intravenous injection of a sterile solution of the substance. It is designed for products that can be tolerated by the test rabbit in a dose not to exceed 10 ml per Kg injected intravenously within a period of not more than ten minutes.

Assay : The assay is carried out as described under sodium chloride. Each ml of 0.1 N silver nitrate is equivalent to 0.005845 g of NaCl.

Labelling : The label on the container of the injection intended for intravenous infusion states

   (i) that the injection contains 150 millimoles of sodium and chloride ions per litre;

   (ii) that the injection should not be used if it contains visible solid particles.

Uses : It is used as fluid and electrolyte replenisher and as isotonic vehicle.

SODIUM CHLORIDE HYPERTONIC INJECTION

Sodium chloride hypertonic injection is a sterile solution of sodium chloride in water for injection. It contains not less than 1.52 per cent and not more than 1.68 per cent w/v of NaCl. It contains no antimicrobial agents.

It is a clear and colourless solution. It is stored in single-dose containers of glass or plastic. On keeping, small solid particles may separate from a glass container. A solution containing such particles must not be used.

Tests for Purity : Tests for arsenic; heavy metals; pyrogens; and pH (between 5.0 and 7.5).

Tests for Identification : It gives the reactions of sodium, and of chlorides.

Assay : The assay is carried out as described under sodium chloride. Each ml of 0.1 N silver nitrate is equivalent to 0.005845 g of NaCl.

Labelling : The label on the container of the injection intended for intravenous infusion states :

    (i) that the injection contains 270 millimoles of sodium and chloride ions per litre;

    (ii) the storage conditions;

    (iii) the date after which the injection is not intended to be used;

    (iv) that the injection should not be used if it contains visible solid particles.

Uses : It is used as fluid and electrolyte replenisher.

COMPOUND SODIUM CHLORIDE INJECTION

Compound sodium chloride injection contains NaCl (0.82-0.90% w/v), KCl (0.028-0.0315%) and $CaCl_2.2H_2O$ (0.03-0.036%). It contains no antimicrobial agents.

For its preparation the ingredients sodium chloride (8.6 g), potassium chloride (0.3 g), and calcium chloride (0.33 g) are mixed in water for injection sufficient to produce 1000 ml. The solution is filtered until clear, and sterilized by heating in an autoclave.

It is a clear and colourless solution; stored in single-dose containers of glass or plastic. When kept in glass containers for a long time, small solid particles may separate out. A solution containing such particles must not be used.

Tests for Purity : Tests for arsenic; heavy metals; pyrogens; and pH (between 5.0 and 7.5).

Tests for Identification : It gives the reactions of sodium, and of chlorides. When concentrated to one half of its volume, it gives the reactions of potassium and calcium.

Assay

1. **For NaCl :** The substance is diluted with water and determined by flame photometry measuring at 589 nm or by atomic absorption spectrophotometry using sodium solution I.P. Each g of sodium is equivalent to 2.54 g of NaCl.

2. **For KCl :** The substance is diluted and determined by flame photometry measuring at 767 nm or by atomic absorption spectrophotometry using potassium solution I.P. Each g of potassium is equivalent to 1.007 g of KCl.

3. **For CaCl$_2$. 2H$_2$O :** To the solution, 0.01 M magnesium sulphate and strong ammonia-ammonium chloride solution are added. The mixture is titrated with 0.01N disodium ethylenediametetraacetate (DETA) using mordant black 11 mixture as indicator. From the volume of DETA the volume of 0.01 M magnesium sulphate is substracted. Each ml of the remainder is equivalent to 0.001470 g of CaCl$_2$. 2H$_2$O.

Uses : It is used as a fluid and electrolyte replenisher.

COMPOUND SODIUM CHLORIDE SOLUTION

It is a sterile solution of sodium chloride (0.82-0.90%), potassium chloride (0.025-0.035%) and calcium chloride (0.03-0.036%) in purified water. It is a colourless solution. Its tests of purity, identification and assay comply with the requirements stated under compound sodium chloride injection. It is used as an irrigation solution (for external use).

SODIUM CHLORIDE AND DEXTROSE INJECTION

It is a sterile solution of sodium chloride (0.11-0.9%) and dextrose (2.5-25%). It is a clear, colourless or faintly straw-coloured solution; stored in single-dose containers in a cool place. On keeping, there may be separation of small solid particles.

Tests for Purity : Tests for 5-hydroxymethylfurfural and related substances; heavy metals; pyrogens; and pH (3.5-6.5).

5-Hydroxymethylfurfural and related substances are determined by measuring extinction at 284 nm which is more than 0.25.

Assay

1. **For Sodium Chloride :** The measured volume is titrated with 0.1 N silver nitrate using potassium chromate solution as indicator. Each ml of 0.1N silver nitrate is equivalent to 0.005845 g of NaCl.

2. **For Dextrose :** Dextrose is assayed by measuring optical rotation. The observed rotation in degrees multiplies by 0.9477 represents the weight in g of dextrose, $C_6H_{12}O_6$, in the volume taken for assay.

Uses : It is used as a fluid, nutrient, and electrolyte replenisher.

SODIUM LACTATE INJECTION

It contains not less than 1.75% and not more than 1.95% of sodium lactate. A 1000 ml contains lactic acid (14 ml), sodium hydroxide (6.7 g) and dilute hydrochloric acid in a sufficient quantity. It is prepared by dissolving the sodium hydroxide in water for injection (400 ml), adding the lactic acid and heating the solution in an autoclave at 115° to 116° for one hour. It is cooled, dilute hydrochloric acid added carefully until 0.15 ml of the solution gives a full orange colour with 0.05 ml of phenol red solution. Sufficient water for injection is added to produce 1000 ml, filtered and immediately sterilized by heating in an autoclave.

Physical Characters : It is clear colourless solution.

It is stored in single-dose containers of glass or plastic. On keeping there may be separation of small solid particles.

Tests for Purity : Tests for heavy metals; pyrogens; pH (between 5 and 7).

Tests for Identification

1. When warmed with potassium permanganate, acetaldehyde is formed which is recognisable by odour.

2. The residue on evaporation gives the reactions of sodium.

Assay : A measured amount (10 ml) is dried and ignited very gently until completely carbonized. The residue is boiled with 0.1 N sulphuric acid, filtered and washed thoroughly with hot water. The excess of acid is titrated in the combined filtrate and washings with 0.1 N sodium hydroxide using methyl orange solution as indicator. Each ml of 0.1 N sulphuric acid is equivalent to 0.01121 g of sodium lactate.

Uses : It is a fluid and electrolyte replenisher.

Official Preparations of Sodium Chloride

Sodium Chloride Injection, I.P.

Sodium Chloride Hypertonic Injection, I.P.

Compound Sodium Chloride Injection, I.P.

Compound Sodium Chloride Solution, I.P.

Sodium Chloride and Dextrose Injection, I.P., U.S.P.

Sodium Lactate Injection, I.P.

Sodium Chloride Eye Lotion, B.P.

Sodium Chloride Ophthalmic Ointment, U.S.P.

Sodium Chloride Inhalation Solution, U.S.P.

Bacteriostatic Sodium Chloride Injection, U.S.P.

Sodium Chloride Intravenous Infusion, B.P.

Sodium Chloride and Glucose Intravenous Infusion, B.P.

Sodium Chloride Irrigation, U.S.P.

Compound Sodium Chloride Mouthwash, B.P.

Sodium Chloride Tablets, B.P., U.S.P.

Sodium Chloride and Dextrose Tablets, U.S.P.

POTASSIUM CHLORIDE

KBr; Mol. Weight = 74.55

Potassium chloride contains not less than 99.0 per cent of KCl. In nature it is found as *sylvine* (KCl) and *carnallite*, $KCl.MgCl_2.6H_2O$ contaminated with magnesium sulphate and chloride.

Potassium chloride is prepared by fusing *carnallite* whereby the liquefied magnesium chloride hexahydrate is separated from the solid potassium chloride. Alternately, *carnallite* is dissolved by boiling with the mother liquor leaving other impurities undissolved. These are filtered off and the filtrate is crystallized to get cubic crystals.

Potassium chloride can also be prepared by reacting hydrochloric acid with potassium carbonate.

$$K_2CO_3 + 2HCl \longrightarrow KCl + H_2CO_3$$

Physical Characters : Potassium chloride occurs as odourless, colourless, cubical, elongated, or prismatic crystals or white crystalline powder; taste is saline. It is soluble in water (1 in 3), and glycerol (1 in 14); practically insoluble in alcohol and solvent ether. A solution is neutral to litmus. Hydrochloric acid, sodium or magnesium chlorides diminish its solubility in water.

Incompability : It is incompatible with amphotericin, amikacin sulphate, dobutamine hydrochloride, and fixed oil emulsions.

It is stored in well-closed containers.

Tests for Purity : Tests for acidity or alkalinity; clarity and colour of solution; bromides; iodides; heavy metals; sodium; calcium; magnesium; lead; arsenic; barium; iron; sulphate; and loss on drying.

Acidity or alkalinity is determined by titrating an aqueous solution with sodium hydroxide or hydrochloric acid using bromothymol blue solution. For detecting bromides and iodides, alcoholic soluble portion is treated with chlorine solution in the presence of chloroform. The organic layer does not acquire a violet, yellow or orange colour when bromides and iodides are absent.

Tests for Identification : A solution (1 in 20) gives the reactions of potassium, and of chlorides.

Assay : The assay is based on the Mohr's method of direct volumetric precipitation titration. An aqueous solution of the substance is titrated against a standard solution of silver nitrate using solution of potassium chromate as indicator.

$$NaCl + AgNO_3 \longrightarrow AgCl\downarrow + NaNO_3$$

When whole of sodium chloride has been precipitated as AgCl, addition of silver nitrate solution gives a brick red colour with the indicator. The end point is change of colour from yellow to red.

$$2AgNO_3 + K_2CrO_4 \longrightarrow Ag_2CrO_4 + 2KNO_3$$
$$\qquad\qquad\text{Pot} \qquad\qquad \text{Silver}$$
$$\qquad\quad\text{chromate} \qquad \text{chromate}$$
$$\qquad\quad\text{(yellow)} \qquad \text{(brick-red)}$$

An aqueous solution of the weighed substance is titrated with 0.1 N silver nitrate, using potassium chromate solution as indicator. Each ml of 0.1 N silver nitrate is equivalent to 0.007455 g of KCl.

Uses : Potassium chloride and its preparations are electrolyte replenisher and used in treatment of potassium deficiency, familial paralysis, myasthenia gravis (muscle weakness), Meniere's syndrome (disease of the inner ear) and as an antidote in digitalis intoxication.

In oral solution, fruit or vegetable juices are mixed to mask the saline taste.

Excessive use of the potassium leads to development of hyperkalaemia causing muscle weakness, paralysis, hypotension, heart block and cardiac arrest.

OFFICIAL POTASSIUM CHLORIDE PREPARATIONS

Potassium Chloride and Sodium Chloride Intravenous Infusion (B.P.)

It is a sterile colourless solution of potassium chloride and sodium chloride in water.

Potassium Chloride and Glucose Intravenous Infusion (B.P.)

It is a sterile colourless or faintly straw-coloured solution of potassium chloride and either anhydrous glucose or glucose in water.

Potassium Chloride, Sodium Chloride and Glucose Intravenous Infusion (B.P.)

It is a sterile solution of potassium chloride, sodium chloride and either anhydrous glucose or glucose in water.

Effervescent Potassium Chloride Tablets (B.P.)

Potassium Chloride Elixir, U.S.P.

Potassium Chloride Mixture, A.P.F.

Potassium Chloride Injection, U.S.P.

Potassium Chloride in Dextrose Injection, U.S.P.

Potassium Chloride Oral Solution, U.S.P.

Potassium Chloride Extended-release Capsules/Tablets, U.S.P.

Potassium Chloride, Potassium Bicarbonate, and Potassium Citrate Effervescent Tablets for Oral Solution, U.S.P.

(B) PHYSIOLOGICAL ACID-BASE BALANCE

Acids are constantly being produced during metabolism. Most metabolic reactions occur only within a very narrow pH range of 7.38-7.42. Therefore, the body utilizes several efficient buffer systems; two of them are bicarbonate-carbonic acid (HCO^{3-} : H_2CO_3) present in the plasma and kidney and monohydrogen phosphate-dihydrogen phosphate (HCO_4^{-2} : $H_2PO_4^-$) found in the cells and kidney. In red blood cells the haemoglobin (Hb) buffer system is present.

Carbon dioxide produced in the cells is diffused from the cells into the plasma. A small portion of CO_2 is dissolved in plasma and another small portion reacts with water to form carbonic acid, which is buffered by plasma protein. Most of the CO_2 enters the erythrocytes where it rapidly combines with haemoglobin or forms carbonic acid by reacting with carbonic anhydrase. The pH of the erythrocytes increased due to concentration of carbonic acid is compensated by haemoglobin. The bicarbonate anion then diffuses out of the erythrocyte and chloride anion diffuses in.

Carbonic anhydrase

$$H_2O + CO_2 \xrightarrow[\text{anhydrase}]{\text{carbonic}} H_2CO_3$$

$$H_2CO_3 + K^+ + HbO_2^- \longrightarrow K^+ + HCO_3^- + HHb + O_2$$

The bicarbonate and plasma carbonic acid acts as an efficient buffer system in plasma (pH 7.4). Oxygen combines with protonated deoxyhaemoglobin, releasing protons. These combines with bicarbonate yielding carbonic acid, which then dissociates to carbon dioxide and water. The CO_2 is liberated from the lungs.

(C) ELECTROLYTES USED IN ACID-BASE THERAPY

The sodium salts of bicarbonate, lactate, acetate and sometimes citrate and ammonium salts are used to treat metabolic acidosis. Supply of bicarbonate increases the HCO_3^-/H_2CO_3 ratio. Lactate, acetate and citrate ions are degraded to CO_2 and water by tricarboxylic acid cycle.

The various inorganic elements and ions associated with the body mechanism include Na^+, K^+, Ca^{2+}, PO_4^{3-}, Mg^{2+}, Fc^{2+}, Fe^{3+}, I^-, Zn^{2+}, Cu^{2+}, Co^{2+}, Mo, Cr^{3+}, Se, Cl^-, HCO^{3-}, F^- and SO_4^{2-}. Each ion has a definite concentration in various body fluids. The absorption and metabolism vary considerably. The major functions of electrolytes are to maintain electrolytic imbalance, including acid-base balance and osmotic equilibrium and to facilitate specific metabolic function through supply of specific ion to body fluids. The major physiological ions are Cl^-, PO_4^{3-}, HCO_3^-, Na^+, K^+, Ca^{2+} and Mg^{2+}.

SODIUM ACETATE

$CH_3COONa. 3H_2O$; Mol. Weight = 136.08

Sodium acetate contains not less than 99.0 per cent of $CH_3COONa. 3H_2O$. It is prepared by neutralization of acetic acid with sodium carbonate or sodium hydroxide, and then crystallizing the product.

$$2CH_3COOH + Na_2CO_3 \longrightarrow 2CH_3COONa + CO_2 + H_2O$$

Characters : It occurs as colourless, transparent crystals or a white granular powder or white flakes; odourless or with a slight odour of acetic acid; m.p. 58°; becomes anhydrous at 120°, decomposed at higher temperature. It effloresces in warm dry air. It is soluble in water (1 in 0.8), and alcohol (1 in 19). A 5% solution in water has a pH of 7.5 to 9.2. It is kept in airtight containers.

Tests for Purity : Tests for arsenic; calcium and magnesium; heavy metals; iron; chloride; sulphate; reducing substances; pH; clarity and colour of solution; loss on drying.

For determining calcium and magnesium, a mixture of dilute ammonia buffer solution, mordant black 11 mixture and zinc chloride is titrated with 0.05M disodium ethylene-diaminetetra-acetate (DETA) until the colour changes from violet-red to green. To this solution sodium acetate is dissolved and titrated with 0.05M DETA until the green colour is restored. Not more than 0.25 ml of 0.05 M DETA is required.

When reducing substances are absent, the pink colour is not entirely discharged on treatment of potassium permanganate with an acidified solution of the substance with dilute sulphuric acid.

Incompatibility : Aqueous solutions reacts with oxygen to produce slight pink colour. It can be prevented by addition of a solution of sodium metabisulphite.

Tests for Identification : It gives the reactions of sodium and of acetates.

Assay : To a weighed amount (0.25 g), dissolved in glacial acetic acid (50 ml), acetic anhydride (5 ml) is added and kept for 30 minutes. Additional glacial acetic acid (50 ml) is mixed and titrated with 0.1N perchloric acid, using 1-naphtholbenzoin solution as indicator. A blank determination is performed and any necessary correction is made. Each ml of 0.1N perchloric acid is equivalent to 0.01361 g of $CH_3COONa. 3H_2O$.

Uses : It is used as pharmaceutical aid (for peritoneal dialysis fluid); acidulant in food; and as an effective buffer in metabolic acidosis.

POTASSIUM ACETATE

CH_3COOK; Mol. Weight = 98.14

Potassium acetate contains from 99 to 101.0% of CH_3COOK. It occurs as colourless crystals or a white crystalline powder; odourless or with a faint acetic acid like odour. It is deliquescent in moist air. It is soluble in water and alcohol. A 5% solution in water has a pH of 7.5 to 9.5.

Potassium acetate should be kept in a well-closed container.

Tests for Purity : Tests for aluminium; arsenic; calcium; heavy metals; magnesium; sodium; chloride; nitrate; sulphate; readily oxidizable substances; loss on drying; and alkalinity.

For determining nitrate, an aqueous solution is treated with sodium chloride, indigo carmine solution and nitrogen-free sulphuric acid. A blue colour is produced which persists for at least 10 minutes.

Tests for Identification : It gives reactions characteristic of potassium salts and of acetates.

The presence of readily oxidizable substances is found out by treating an aqueous solution with sulphuric acid and potassium permanganate. The pink colour is not completely discharged.

The salt complies with the limit test for arsenic, calcium, heavy metals, magnesium and chloride.

Assay : Non-aqueous titration is carried out using perchloric acid and crystal violet solution as indicator. Each ml of 0.1N perchloric acid is equivalent to 9.814 mg of CH_3COOK.

Uses : It is used in solutions for haemodialysis and peritoneal dialysis and as an alkalizer. It is also used as a food preservative.

SODIUM CITRATE

$$CH_2COONa$$
$$|$$
$$HO—C—COONa;$$
$$|$$
$$CH_2COONa$$

$C_6H_5Na_3O_7.2H_2O$; Mol. Weight = 294.1

Sodium citrate is trisodium 2-hydroxy-propane-1,2,3-tricarboxylate dihydrate. It contains about 99% of $C_6H_5Na_3O_7$. It is prepared by mixing of calculated amounts of hot solution of citric acid and sodium carbonate and crystallizing the product.

$$3Na_2CO_3 + 2H_3C_6H_5O_7 \longrightarrow 2Na_3C_6H_5O_7 + 3CO_2 + 3H_2O$$

Characters : It occurs as white, granular crystals or a white crystalline powder; slightly deliquescent in moist air. It is freely soluble in water; practically insoluble in ethanol. It is stored in air-tight containers. Sterilized solutions of sodium citrate on keeping cause separation of small solid particles from a glass container. A solution containing such particles must not be used.

Tests for Purity : Tests for heavy metals; oxalate; sulphate; readily carbonizable substances; water; acidity or alkalinity; clarity and colour of solution.

Acidity or alkalinity is determined by neutralizing an aqueous solution with hydrochloric acid or sodium hydroxide using phenolphthalein as an indicator.

For determining oxalate zinc and phenylhydrazine are treated with acidified solution. Hydrochloric acid and potassium hexacyanoferrate solution are added. Any pink colour produced is not more intense than that obtained by treating at the same time and in the same manner a solution of oxalic acid.

Readily carbonisable substances are detected by heating the salt with sulphuric acid at about 90° for for one hour. On cooling the solution is not more intensely coloured than a reference solution.

Sodium citrate complies with the limit tests for chloride and sulphate.

Incompatibility : Aqueous solutions, owing to their alkalinity, may be incompatible with acidifying agents.

Tests for Identification : Aqueous solution gives reactions characteristic of sodium salts and citrates.

Assay : A solution of the substance in anhydrous acetic acid is titrated non-aqueously using 1-naphtholbenzein solution as indicator, until a green colour is produced. Each ml of 0.1 N perchloric acid is equivalent to 8.602 mg of $C_6H_5Na_3O_7$.

Uses : It is used as systemic alkalinizing substance. Sodium citrate has anti-clotting properties and is employed in mixtures as the acid citrate in the anticoagulation and preservation of blood for transfusion purposes. It is also used in dentifrices as a desensitising agent and added to the milk for infant feeding to prevent the formation in the stomach of large curds. It also has a diuretic effect due to increased body salt concentration.

POTASSIUM CITRATE

KOOC. CH_2. CH(OH) (COOK). CH_2COOK. H_2O; $K_3C_6H_5O_7.H_2O$;
Mol. Weight = 324.42

Potassium citrate is the monohydrate of tripotassium 2-hydroxy propane-1,2,3-tricarboxylate. It contains not less than 99.0 per cent of $K_3C_6H_5O_7$. It is prepared by mixing hot solutions of calculated amounts of citric acid and potassium carbonate, and crystallizing the product.

$$3K_2CO_3 + 2H_3C_6H_5O_7 \longrightarrow 2K_3C_6H_5O_7 + 3H_2O$$

Potassium citrate occurs as transparent, odourless, hygroscopic crystals or a white granular powder, taste is saline. It is soluble in water (1 in 1) and glycerol (1 in 2.5), practically insoluble in alcohol. Aqueous solutions are slightly alkaline and may be incompatible with acidifying agents. It is stored in airtight containers.

Tests for Purity : Tests for acidity or alkalinity; arsenic; heavy metals; lead; sodium; chloride; sulphates; oxalate; readily carbonisable substances; and water.

Acidity or alkalinity is determined by neutralizing aqueous solution with either 0.1N sulphuric acid or 0.1N sodium hydroxkide to thymol blue solution. A clear solution obtained after addition of potassium antimonate solution to the aqueous solution indicated the absence of sodium.

For determining oxalate, an aqueous mixture of the substance, hydrochloric acid, alcohol and calcium chloride remains clear. Readily carbonisable substances are detected by heating the substance with sulphuric acid for 30 minutes at 80-90°; the solution is not insensely coloured, than a mixture of ferric chloride, copper sulphate, cobalt chloride and hydrochloric acid.

Tests for Identification : A solution (1 in 20) gives the reactions of potassium, and of citrates.

Assay : A weighed amount (0.15 g) dissolved in glacial acetic acid is heated to 50°. It is cooled, 1-naphtholbenzein solution added and titrated with 0.1N perchloric acid until a green colour is obtained. A blank determination is performed. Each ml of 0.1 N perchloric acid is equivalent to 0.01021 g of $K_3C_6H_5O_7$.

Uses : It is used as systemic alkalizer and gastric antacid. It is used to relieve painful irritation caused by cystitis (inflammation of bladder).

SODIUM BICARBONATE INJECTION, U.S.P.

It is a sterile solution of sodium bicarbonate in water for injection, the pH of which may be adjusted by the addition of carbon dioxide; pH 7.0 to 8.5. It contains not less than 95% and not more than 105% of labelled amount of $NaHCO_3$.

It is preserved in single-dose containers.

Tests for Purity : Tests for pyrogen; pH (between 7 and 8.5).

Tests for Identification : It responds to the tests for sodium and for bicarbonate.

Assay : It is assayed by titrating the solution with 1N sulphuric acid and methyl red as indicator. Each ml of 1N sulphuric acid is equivalent to 84.01 mg of $NaHCO_3$.

AMMONIUM CHLORIDE INJECTION, U.S.P.

Ammonium chloride injection is a sterile solution of ammonium chloride in water for injection. It contains not less than 95% and not more than 105% of the labelled amount of NH_4Cl. Hydrochloric acid may be added to adjust the pH.

It is preserved in single-dose or in multiple-dose containers.

Tests of Purity : Tests for chloride content, pyrogen; pH (between 4 to 6).

Tests for Identification : It responds to the tests for ammonium and for chloride ions.

Assay : The distilled solution, obtained on addition of ammonium chloride and sodium hydroxide solution and heating, is titrated with 0.1 N sulphuric acid using methyl red. A blank determination is also performed. Each ml of 0.1 N sulphuric acid is equivalent to 5.349 mg of NH_4Cl.

(D) ELECTROLYTE COMBINATION THERAPY

In short-term therapy combination of glucose and saline solutions may be sufficient. In severe deficits, solutions containing additional electrolytes are usually required. The combination products are of two types-fluid maintenance and electrolyte replacement. Maintenance therapy with intravenous fluids is required to supply normal necessity of water and electrolytes to patents who cannot take them orally. All maintenance should contain at least 5% dextrose; the other ions are sodium (25-30 mEq/l), potassium (15-20 mEq/l), chloride (22m Eq/l), bicarbonate (20-33 mEq/l), magnesium (3 mEq/l) and phosphorus (3mEq/l).

Replacement therapy is required when there is excess loss of water and electrolytes caused by fever, severe vomiting, and diarrhoea. Two types of solutions are used in replacement therapy :

(i) a solution for rapid initial replacement, and

(ii) a solution for subsequent replacement.

The electrolyte concentrations in solutions for rapid initial replacement are almost similar to the electrolyte concentrations found in the extracellular fluids. The electrolyte concentrations of these solutions are given as hereunder.

Electrolytes	Concentration in 1, mEq/l	Concentration in 2, mEq/l
Na^+	130–150	40–121
K^+	4–12	16–35
Cl	98–109	30–103
HCO_3^-	28–55	16–53
Ca^{+2}	3–5	0–5
Mg^{+2}	3	3–6

(E) ORAL REHYDRATION THERAPY

In acute diarrhoea, loss of water and electrolytes can lead to significant dehydration and metabolic imbalance. Without appropriate treatment, this may cause fatal results, especially in infants. If a solution containing appropriate concentrations of both glucose and sodium chloride, 0.9% solution is administered orally, absorption of both sodium and water is greatly enhanced due to the action of glucose as a carrier molecule in the transport of one ion of sodium, together with water from the intestinal lumen. Sucrose and starches exert a similar effect as they release glucose in the intestine. The oral administration of fluid that contains a suitable combination of carbohydrates and electrolytes is known as *oral rehydration therapy* (ORT).

There are two basic treatment phases :

- (i) **Rehydration Phase :** It involves the replacements of fluid and electrolytes lost through diarrhoea and vomiting.
- (ii) **Maintenance Phase :** It is the replacement of losses due to continuing diarrhoea and vomiting, and of normal loss due to respiration, sweating, and urination which are especially high in infants.

Acute diarrhoea leads to loss of essential water and salts causing dehydration. Prevention of dehydration is, therefore, the first appropriate response to diarrhoea. An oral rehydration solution containing glucose and essential salts is adequately absorbed and replaces both previous and continuing fluid and salt loses. It does not stop the diarrhoea, but the diarrhoea usually continues for only a limited time. Glucose accelerates the absorption of sodium and water from the small intestine and this process is not impaired during acute diarrhoea. A rational response to diarrhoea involves prevention of dehydration using glucose-salt solution. House remedies used include coconut water, rice water, various soups, weak tea, and solutions consisting of different salts and sugars. Severe dehydration, in which loss of body weight is 10% or more, should be corrected by intravenous therapy.

The composition of carbohydrate-electrolyte mixtures used in ORT varies, principally in sodium content. Solutions for ORT contain 60 to 90 mmol/litre of sodium. Chlorine is required for maintenance of a normally expanded plasma compartment and is an essential constituent of oral rehydration salts preparations for replacement of faecal losses. Significant losses of potassium can occur in children with diarrhoeal illness. Most oral rehydration solutions contain 20 to 25 mmol/litre of potassium. A base in oral rehydration solution is required to correct or prevent the acidosis which often accompanies dehydration. Acidosis is resulted from faecal loss of bicarbonate and decreased renal excretion of acid. Bases such as lactate (except citrate and bicarbonate) are used in some proprietary rehydration preparations.

Glucose is used as the carbohydrate in almost all currently available oral rehydration preparations. Sucrose, which is cheaper and more readily available, is equally effective in promoting the absorption of sodium and water. Optimal ranges of concentrations of glucose in oral rehydration preparations have been reported as 56 to 140 mmol/litre, 80 to 120 mmol/litre, are 2.0% to 2.5%. If concentration of glucose is very high, the resultant fluid will be hypertonic; this will result in osmotic diarrhoea due to unabsorbed carbohydrate, with no further enhancement of sodium absorption.

Rice-based solutions are not only as effective as glucose-base solutions in rehydration and maintenance of hydration but also offer the advantage of reduced duration and volume of diarrhoea.

(F) SALT INTAKE AND HYPERTENSION

The effect of individual salt intake on individual blood pressure is difficult to study. It is suggested that weight reduction and reduced sodium intake each make an independent contribution to the lowering of the blood pressure and enhance the effect of drug treatment of high blood pressure. With a reduction of 5 g in the average daily salt intake, average diastolic pressure can be lowered by 4 mm Hg. It is recommended that populations should be encouraged to reduce the consumption of salt 5 g daily or less.

(G) MULTIPLE ELECTROLYTE POWDERS

Oral Rehydration Salt (Electral) : Each packet (35 g) contains sodium chloride (1. 25 g), potassium chloride (1.50 g), sodium citrate (2.90 g), anhydrous dextrose (27 g) and excipients which is dissolved in 1 litre of water and supplies electrolytes (mEq/l) as sodium (51), potassium (20), chloride (41), citrate (30 g) and dextrose (150 mmole/l). The solution should be used in recommended dilution within 24 hours for the replacement of fluid and electrolytes loss and maintenance of hydrogen in diarrhoea due to organisms like Rota viruses, *E. coli.* and in vomiting in patients of all age groups. It is also useful in muscle weakness, muscle cramps and prostration due to exhaustion, for athletes and industrial workers and to replace fluid losses.

The powder is stored in a dry place. The sachet wall should be closed after use and keep away from moisture.

Oral Rehydration Salts (WHO; UNICEF) : It contains sodium chloride (3.5 g), potassium chloride (1.5 g), sodium bicarbonate (2.5 g) or sodium citrate dihydrate (2.9 g), and anhydrous glucose (20g); for solution in 1 litre of water.

(H) MULTIPLE ELECTROLYTE SOLUTIONS

Oralyte Ready-P Oral Solution : A sterile solution containing sodium chloride (117 mg), sodium acetate (136 mg), potassium acetate (196 mg), magnesium chloride (30 mg), calcium chloride (37 mg) and anhydrous dextrose (2 g) in 100 ml solution. Once the bottle is opened, the contents have to be consumed within 48 hours.

Paediatric Solution for Intravenous Use : A sterile solution containing dextrose (5 g), sodium acetate (0.3 g), potassium chloride (0.10 g), magnesium chloride (0.03 g), dibasic potassium phosphate (0.025 g), and sodium metabisulphate (0.02 g); the pH adjusted with hydrochloric acid.

Elliott's B Solution : A sterile solution containing sodium chloride (730 mg), potassium chloride (30 mg), calcium chloride dihydrate (20 mg), magnesium sulphate (30 mg), sodium phosphate heptahydrate (20 mg), glucose (20 mg), sodium bicarbonate (190 mg), phenol red (10 µg), water for injection to 100 ml.

Ringer's Injection (U.S.P.) : A sterile solution containing sodium chloride (860 mg), potassium chloride (30 mg), calcium chloride dihydrate (33 mg) and water for injection to 100 ml).

(I) DIALYSIS SOLUTIONS

Dialysis solutions are solutions of electrolytes formulated in concentrations similar to those of extracellular fluid. Glucose may be added as an osmotic agent. Dialysis solutions are used in the management of renal failure and poisoning. They allow the selective removal of toxic substances, electrolytes, and excessive body fluid from the blood. In haemodialysis, the exchange of ions between the solution and the patient's blood is made across a synthetic semi-permeable membrane. In peritoneal dialysis, the exchange is made across the membranes of the peritoneal cavity.

In dialysis, bicarbonate is best given as acetate or lactate in order to avoid the release of carbon dioxide into solution.

Intraperitoneal Dialysis Fluid (I.P.) : It consists of sodium chloride (5.56 g), sodium acetate (4.76 g), calcium chloride (0.22 g), magnesium chloride (0.152 g), sodium metabisulphite (0.15 g), dextrose (anhydrous) (17.0 g) and purified water sufficient to produce (1000 ml).

12

OFFICIAL COMPOUNDS OF CALCIUM, IRON AND IODINE

CALCIUM CHLORIDE

$CaCl_2 . 2H_2O$; Mol. Weight = 147.02

Calcium chloride contains not less than 97.0 per cent of $CaCl_2.2H_2O$. It occurs in sea water.

Preparation

1. It is prepared by adding pure calcium carbonate in slight excess to hot, diluted hydrochloric acid. The reaction mixture is filtered, concentrated and crystallized at 10°. The crystals are filtered by vacuum and transferred in a well-closed container.
2. It is also obtained as a by-product of the ammonia-soda (Solvay) process and as a joint product from natural salt brines.

Physical Characters : It occurs as white, hygroscopic, odourless, crystalline powder or granules; m.p. 772°. It is freely soluble in water (with liberation of much heat) and alcohol; very soluble in boiling water. A 5% solution in water has a pH of 4.5 to 9.2. The crystals deliquesce in moist air, effloresce in dry air and melt in their water of crystallization when gently warmed.

Tests for Purity : Tests for arsenic; heavy metals; lead; sulphate; aluminium and phosphate; magnesium and alkali salts; iron; clarity and colour of solution; acidity or alkalinity; hydrochloric acid -insoluble matter; and alcohol-insoluble matter.

For detecting acidity or alkalinity, an aqueous solution is titrated with hydrochloric acid or sodium hydroxide using phenolphthalein solution as indicator.

The concentration of magnesium and alkali salts is determined by treating solution of the substance with ammonium oxalate solution and then with sulphuric acid. The mixture is dried, the residue heated to redness, cooled and weighed.

For determining aluminium and phosphate to the acidified aqueous solution with dilute hydrochloric acid containing phenolphthalein, a solution of ammonium chloride-ammonium hydroxide is added until the solution is faintly pink and then heated. No turbidity or precipitate is produced.

Incompatibility : Calcium salts are incompatible with oxidizing agents, citrates, soluble carbonates, bicarbonates, phosphates, tartrates, and sulphates. Physical incompatibility has also been reported with amphotericin, cephalothin sodium, cephazolin sodium, novobiocin sodium, tetracyclines, etc.

Tests for Identification : A solution (1 in 10) gives the reactions of calcium, and of chlorides.

Assay : An acidified aqueous solution is titrated with 0.05 M disodium ethylenediaminetetraacetate whose each ml is equivalent to 0.007351 g of $CaCl_2$. $2H_2O$.

Uses : Calcium salts are used mainly as calcium replenisher, i.e., in the treatment of calcium deficiency; as diuretic, urinary acidifier and antiallergic agent. It is also used for preparing solutions for intravenous or intramuscular injection. The anhydrous salt is commonly used as a desiccant (drying and dehydrating agent) for organic compounds.

Administration of some calcium salts by mouth can cause gastro-intestinal irritation and constipation. Excessive use of calcium salts leads to hypercalcaemia; the symptoms are anorexia (loss of apetite), nausea, vomiting, constipation, abdominal pain, muscle weakness, mental disturbances, polydipsia (excessive thirst), polyuria, bone pain, nephrocalcinosis, renal calculi, and in severe cases, cardiac arrhythmias and coma. It is irritating to the veins and should be injected slowly. Rapid injection may cause cutaneous burning sensation, peripheral vasodilation, and fall in blood pressure.

CALCIUM LACTATE

$CaC_6H_{10}O_6$. xH_2O; Mol. Weight = 218.22 (anhydrous)

Calcium lactate is the hydrated calcium salt of 2-hydroxy propionic acid. It contains not less than 98.0 per cent of anhydrous calcium lactate.

It is prepared by adding a slight excess of calcium carbonate to a hot, dilute solution of lactic acid, and boiling the mixture for half an hour.

$$2CH_3CH(OH)COOH + CaCO_3 \longrightarrow (CH_3CH(OH)CO_2)_2Ca + CO_2 + H_2O$$

The hot solution is filtered, the filtrate concentrated and crystallized.

Physical Characters : It occurs as a white, odourless, crystalline or granular powder; the pentahydrate is slightly efflorescent; becomes anhydrous at 120°. It is soluble in water (1 in 20); readily soluble in hot water; almost insoluble in alcohol. It is stored in airtight containers.

Tests for Purity : Tests for arsenic; iron; heavy metal; chloride; sulphate; reducing sugars; water; acidity or alkalinity.

If not more than a slight brick-red precipitate is produced on heating an aqueous solution of calcium lactate with potassium cupri-trartrate solution, then reducing sugars are absent.

Tests for Identification

1. A solution (1 in 20) gives the reactions of calcium.
2. A solution acidified with sulphuric acid and warmed with potassium permanganate develops the odour of acetaldehyde.

Assay : A weighed amount (0.3 g) is dissolved in water (50 ml) and the assay is completed as described under calcium gluconate. Each ml of the remainder is equivalent to 0.01091 g of $CaC_6H_{10}O_6$.

Uses : Calcium lactate has similar actions and uses to calcium chloride. It is also used as a preservative in foods and beverages and in dentifrices.

CALCIUM AMINOSALICYLATE

$Ca^{2+}.H_2O$; Mol. Weight = 398.38

Calcium aminosalicylate is the trihydrate of calcium 4-amino-2-hydroxybenzoate. It contains not less than 98.0 per cent of $CaC_{14}H_{12}N_2O_6$.

Characters : It occurs as a white or cream-coloured, odourless, hygroscopic, crystalline powder. It is soluble in water (1 in 7) and slightly soluble in alcohol. A 2% solution in water has a pH of 6 to 8. Aqueous solutions are unstable and darken in colour. The U.S.P. directs that solutions should be prepared within 24 hours of administration and that a solution must not be used if it is darker in colour than a freshly prepared solution. It is stored in airtight containers and protected from light.

Tests for Purity : Tests for 3-aminophenol; 5-aminosalicyclic acid; chloride; sulphide; sulphate; lead; arsenic; iron; heavy metals; calcium; water; clarity of solution; acidity or alkalinity; colour of solution; alcohol and acetone.

For detecting alcohol and acetone, a solution is partially distilled, and the iodoform test is performed in the distillate.

For determining the percentage of 3-aminophenol, its diazonium salt is prepared by treating with sodium nitrite and the extinction is measured at the maximum at about 430 nm. The percentage is calculated from the formula, (A-032 / 1.09).

Formation of purple colour on addition of resorcinol and iodine solution to the aqueous solution indicates the presence of 5-aminosalicylic acid.

Hydrogen sulphide and sulphur dioxide are detected by treating the aqueous solution with dilute hydrochloric acid. No odour of hydrogen sulphide or of sulphur dioxide is detectable and the vapour does not darken moistened lead acetate paper.

The concentration of calcium is found out by titrating the solution of the substance with disodium ethylenediamine tetraacetate (DETA). Towards the end of the titration, sodium hydroxide and calcon mixture are added and the titration is continued until the colour of the solution changes from pink to blue colour. Each ml of 0.05 M DETA is equivalent to 0.002004 g of Ca.

Tests for Identification

1. To an aqueous solution few drops of ferric chloride are added. A purple-red colour is produced which persists on addition of acetic acid or alcohol.
2. To an aqueous solution, dilute hydrochloric acid, sodium

nitrite and α-naphthylamine solution are added. A red colour is produced. When sodium hydroxide solution is added till alkaline, the red colour changes to orange.

3. A solution (1 in 20) gives the reactions of calcium.

Assay : The assay is based on the diazotization (nitrite) titration. To an aqueous solution, hydrochloric acid and potassium bromide are added. It is titrated with 0.1 M sodium nitrite solution. Each ml of 0.1 M sodium nitrite is equivalent to 0.1722 g of $CaC_{14}H_{12}N_2O_6$.

Uses : It is an antibacterial (tuberculostatic) agent.

CALCIUM GLUCONATE

$CaC_{12}H_{22}O_{14}.H_2O$; Mol. Weight = 448.40

Calcium gluconate contains not less than 98.0 per cent of $CaC_{12}H_{22}O_{14}. H_2O$.

It is prepared by heating a solution of gluconic acid with a slight excess of calcium carbonate. The reaction mixture is filtered and the filtrate crystallized.

Physical Characters : It occurs as a white, tasteless, odourless, crystalline or granular powder. It does not lose its water on drying without some decomposition. It is soluble in water (1 in 30), boiling water (1 in 5); insoluble in alcohol and other organic solvents; pH of aqueous solution is 6 to 7. More concentrated aqueous solutions (20 to 30%) are easily obtained by the addition of boric acid. Calcium salts can form complexes with many drugs; this may result in the formation of a precipitate.

Tests for Purity : Tests for arsenic; lead; heavy metals; chloride; sulphate; sucrose and reducing sugars; acidity or alkalinity; clarity and colour of solution; completeness of solutions.

For determining sucrose and reducing sugars, to an aqueous solution dilute hydrochloric acid is added, boiled for 2 minutes, cooled and neutralized with sodium carbonate solution. It is filtered, potassium cupri-tartrate added, and heated; no red precipitate is formed indicating the absence of sugars.

Tests for Identification

1. To an aqueous solution, ferric chloride test solution is added; a yellow colour is produced.
2. An aqueous mixture of the substance containing glacial

acetic acid and phenylhydrazine is heated. White crystals of phenylhydrazide are formed melting at 200° (dec).

3. A solution (1 in 10) gives the reactions of calcium.

Incompatability : It is incompatible with oxidizing agents (gluconic acid is oxidized). Aqueous solutions of calcium gluconate are precipitated with borates, oxalates, tartrates, carbonates, phosphates, sulphates, and citrates due to insolubility of calcium salts of the above anions.

Assay : The assay is based on complexometric type titration forming a well defined simple complex between calcium and disodium ethylenediamine titraacetate (EDTA) using mordant black 11 as an indicator. The end point is a change of colour from red to blue. In this assay, a solution of magnesium sulphate is added before the titration to make the end point sharp. Magnesium also forms a similar complex with EDTA. But these titration have to be carried out in the presence of a buffer such as strong ammonia-ammonium chloride solution.

$$Ca^{2+} + H_2Y^{2-} \longrightarrow CaY^{2-} + 2H^+$$

An aqueous solution of the substance containing magnesium sulphate and strong ammonia-ammonium chloride solution is titrated with 0.05 M disodium ethylenediamine tetra acetate, using mordant black 11 mixture as indicator. From the volume of 0.05 M disodium ethylenediaminetetraacetate required, the volume of 0.05 M magnesium sulphate is substracted. Each ml of the remainder is equivalent to 0.022420 g of $CaC_{12}H_{22}O_{14}.H_2O$.

Uses : Calcium gluconate has similar actions, uses and adverse effects to calcium chloride. It is also used in the treatment of burns from hydrofluoric acid as a gel or injected as a solution.

CALCIUM LEVULINATE

$(CH_2COCH_2CH_2COO^-)_2$ $Ca^{2+}.2H_2O$;
$CaC_{10}H_{14}O_6.2H_2O$; Mol. Weight = 306.33

Calcium levulinate is the dihydrate of calcium 4-oxopentanoate containing not less than 97.5 per cent of $CaC_{10}H_{14}O_6$.

It occurs as a white crystalline or amorphous powder with burnt sugar-like odour; m.p 125°; loses one water molecule on drying in vacuum at room temperature and all water at 50°. It is freely soluble in water; slightly soluble in alcohol; insoluble in chloroform and ether. A 10% solution in water has a pH of 7 to 8.5.

Tests for Purity : Tests for arsenic; heavy metals; reducing sugars; melting range (119-125°); loss on drying; pH (7-8.5 of 10% solution).

Tests for Identification

1. To an aqueous solution, sodium hydroxide solution is added and filtered. To the filtrate iodine solution is added; a precipitate of iodoform is produced.
2. To an aqueous solution dinitrophenylhydrazine solution is added. A precipitate is formed which is filtered (m.p. 198°).
3. A solution (1 in 10) gives the reactions of calcium.

Assay : A weighed amount (0.6 g) is dissolved in water (50 ml) and the assay completed as described under calcium gluconate. Each ml of the remainder is equivalent to 0.01351 g of $CaC_{10}H_{14}O_6$.

Uses : Calcium levulinate has similar actions and uses to calcium chloride.

CALCIUM PANTOTHENATE

$[HOCH_2C (CH_3)_2 CONHCH_2CH_2COO^-]_2 Ca^{2+}$;
$CaC_{18}H_{32}O_{10}N_2$; Mol. Weight = 497.54

Calcium pantothenate is the calcium salt of the dextrorotatory isomer (R)-3-(2,4-dihydroxy-3,3-dimethyl butyramido) propionic acid cantaining not less than 90.0 per cent of dextrorotatory calcium pantothenate.

It occurs as a white, odourless, slightly hygroscopic powder; taste is sweet with slightly bitter afterwards; m.p. 195-196° (dec). It is freely soluble in water; soluble in glycerin; practically insoluble in alcohol, chloroform and solvent ether. The U.S.P. specifies that the physiological activity of racemic calcium pantothenate is nearly one-half that of calcium pantothenate. It is stored in airtight containers. Solutions are most stable at pH 5-7. Rate of hydrolysis is a function of pH and is catalyzed by the presence of electrolytes. Solutions are not stable to autoclaving.

Tests for Purity : Tests for calcium; nitrogen; heavy metals; loss on drying; pH (7-9 of 5.0% solution); specific rotation (+ 25.0 to + 27.5°).

For determining concentration of calcium assay is carried out as described under calcium gluconate. Each ml of the remainder is equivalent to 0.00204 g of Ca.

Tests for Identification

1. A solution (1 in 20) gives the reactions of calcium.
2. The substance is boiled with 1 N sodium hydroxide, cooled, 1 N hydrochloric acid and ferric chloride solution are added; a strong yellow colour is produced.
3. To a solution of the substance in 1 N sodium hydroxide, copper sulphate solution is added. A blue colour is produced.

Assay :

1. Assay for calcium is carried out as described under calcium gluconate. Each ml of the remainder is equivalent to 0.002004 g of Ca.
2. For the assay of nitrogen a weighed amount of the substance, anhydrous sodium sulphate, copper sulphate, nitrogen free sulphuric acid and hydrogen peroxide are digested. Sodium hydroxide solution is added and steam distilled. The distillate is collected in 0.01 N sulphuric acid, titrated with 0.01 N sodium hydroxide using methyl red-methylene blue solution as indicator. A blank experiment is performed, the difference between the titration represents the ammonia liberated by the substance. Each ml of 0.01 N sulphuric acid is equivalent to 0.0001401 g of N.

Uses : Pantothenic acid is a vitamin B substance. It is a component of coenzyme A which is essential in the metabolism of carbohydrate, fat, and protein. Therefore, calcium pantothenate is used as a dietary supplement.

Pantothenic acid is reported to be generally nontoxic.

TRIBASIC CALCIUM PHOSPHATE

$CaO. 3P_2O_5. H_2O$; $Ca_3(PO_4)_2. H_2O$. Mol. Weight = 328.2

Tribasic calcium phosphate consists of a variable mixture of calcium phosphates having the approximate composition of $10CaO.3P_2O_5.H_2O$. It contains not less than 34.0 per cent and not more than 40.0 per cent of calcium, and an amount of phosphate equivalent to not less than 90 per cent of calcium phosphate, calculated with reference to the ignited substance.

The B.P. specifies that it consists mainly of tricalcium diortho-phosphate, $Ca_3(PO_4)_2$, together with calcium phosphates of more acidic or basic character. It occurs in nature as the minerals *oxydapatit*, *voelicherite* and *white lockite*. The technical product is known as "bone ash".

Preparation

1. It is manufactured from bones which are calcined until white, powdered and digested with sulphuric acid. The insoluble tribasic calcium phosphate is converted into soluble phosphoric acid and insoluble calcium sulphate.

$$Ca_3(PO_4)_2 + 3H_2SO_4 \longrightarrow 2H_3PO_4 + 3CaSO_4$$

The solution is filtered and the filtrate is treated with calcium hydroxide to precipitate calcium phosphate.

$$2H_3PO_4 + 3Ca(OH)_2 \longrightarrow Ca_3(PO_4)_2 + 6H_2O$$

2. Decomposition of calcium chloride and sodium phosphate in the presence of aqueous ammonia at high temperature yields calcium phosphate. The white precipitate is filtered, washed to free from chlorides and dried.

$$3CaCl_2 + 2Na_2HPO_4 + 2NH_4OH \longrightarrow$$
$$Ca_3(PO_4)_2 + 4NaCl + 2NH_4Cl + 2H_2O$$

3. Commercially it is prepared from phosphate rock.

Physical Characters : It occurs as a white, odourless, tasteless amorphous powder; practically insoluble in water, alcohol or acetic acid; soluble in dilute hydrochloric or nitric acid.

Tests for Purity : Tests for arsenic; heavy metals; iron; barium; dibasic salt and calcium oxide; water; loss on ignition; sulphate; chloride; fluoride; carbonate; water-soluble substances; and acid-insoluble substances.

Water-soluble substances are determined by dissolving the salt in water. The solution is filtered, the filtrate evaporated and the residue dried at 105° to constant weight. When effervescence is produced on treating the salt with hydrochloric acid, then carbonate is present. Test of chloride is carried out by dissolving the salt in nitric acid. The solution complies with the limit test for chloride. An acidified solution with hydrochloric acid complies with the limit test for sulphates. If citric acid is added to the acidified solution, then the solution complies with the limit test for iron. The acidified solution is titrated with N sodium hydroxide for detecting the presence of dibasic salt and calcium oxide.

Tests for Identification

1. An aqueous solution acidified with dilute hydrochloric acid gives the reactions of calcium.
2. A solution in dilute nitric acid gives the reactions of phosphates.

Assay :

(a) **For Calcium :** The assay for calcium is performed as described under dicalcium phosphate.

(b) **For Phosphate, PO_4 :** An aqueous solution of the substance (0.2 g) is acidified with dilute nitric acid, filtered, and strong ammonia solution is added to produce a slight precipitate. The precipitate is dissolved in dilute nitric acid, ammonium molybdate solution added, precipitate filtered, washed with potassium nitrate solution, the precipitate dissolved in 1 N sodium hydroxide, phenolphthalein solution added and excess alkali titrated with 1 N sulphuric acid. Each ml of 1 N sodium hydroxide is equivalent to 0.006743 g of $Ca_3(PO_4)_2$.

Uses : Calcium phosphate has similar actions and uses as calcium chloride and calcium gluconate. It may be of use in patients requiring both calcium and phosphorus supplementation. It is a useful non-hygroscopic diluent for powders and vegetable extracts, and in fine powder as an abrasive in toothpastes. It is also used in homoeopathic medicine.

CALCIUM CARBONATE

(See page 61)

CALCIUM HYDROXIDE

(See page 24)

DICALCIUM PHOSPHATE

(Sée page 135)

OFFICIALS OF CALCIUM

Calcium Disodium Edetate (U.S.P.). $C_{10}H_{12}CaN_2Na_2O_8 \times H_2O$; Mol. Weight (anhydrous 374.28). used to treat heavy metal poisoning.

Calcium Ipodate (N.F.), Organoiodine Radiopaque compounds.

Calcium Stearate (N.F.), $Ca[O_2C\ (CH_2)_{16}CH_3]_2$; is used as a lubricant in the tableting process.

Calcium Sulphate, (N.F.). $CaSO_4$; Mol. Weight 134.14; is used as a pharmaceutical agent.

Calcium Acetate, B.P.

Calcium Aminosalicylate, I.P.

Calcium Aminosalicylate Tablets, I.P.

Calcium Carbonate Tablets, I.P., B.P., U.S.P.

Calcium Chloride Injection, I.P., B.P., U.S.P.

Calcium Gluconate/Injection/Tablets, I.P., B.P., U.S.P.

Calcium Hydroxide, Solution, I.P., B.P.

Calcium Lactate/Tablets, I.P., B.P., U.S.P.

Calcium Levulinate/Injection, I.P., U.S.P.

Calcium Pantothenate, I.P., B.P.

Calcium Phosphate, B..P.

Dibasic Calcium Phosphate/Tablets, I.P., U.S.P.

Tribasic Calcium Phosphate, I.P.

Effervescent Calcium Gluconate Tablets, B.P.

Calcium Hydrogen Phosphate, B.P.

Calcium Sodium Lactate, B.P.

Dried Calcium Sulphate, B.P.

Calcium and Magnesium Carbonate Tablets, U.S.P.

Plaster of Paris Bandage, B.P.

FERROUS SULPHATE

$FeSO_4.7H_2O$; Mol. Weight = 278.0

Ferrous sulphate contains not less than 98.0 per cent of $FeSO_4.7H_2O$

Its hydrates occur in nature as the minerals : *melanterite, siderotil, szomolnikite* and *tauriscite.*

Preparation : Ferrous sulphate is prepared by adding a slight excess of iron to dilute sulphuric acid. When the effervescence of hydrogen is ceased, the liquid is concentrated and cooled to get crystals.

$$Fe + H_2SO_4 \longrightarrow FeSO_4 + H_2$$

Commercially ferrous sulphate is obtained by exposing moist iron pyrites to air when slow oxidation takes place.

$$2FeS_2 + 2H_2O + 7O_2 \longrightarrow 2FeSO_4 + 2H_2SO_4$$

Physical Characters : It occurs as odourless bluish - green crystals or granules or a pale green crystalline powder; taste-metallic and astringent. It is efflorescent in dry air; on exposure to moist air it is oxidized and becomes brown in colour due to the formation of basic ferric sulphate. It forms tetrahydrate at 56.6° and monohydrate at 65°. It is completely soluble in water (1 in 5); practically insoluble in alcohol. Aqueous solutions are oxidized slowly by air when cold; rapidly when hot; rate of oxidation increased by addition of alkali or exposure to light. It is stored in tightly-closed containers.

Chemical Reactions

1. Light green crystals of ferrous sulphate lose water and turn brown when exposed to air oxidation and ferric sulphate is formed.

$$4FeSO_4 + 2H_2O + O_2 \longrightarrow 4Fe(OH)SO_4$$
Ferric sulphate

2. On heating it decomposes into ferric oxide, sulphur dioxide and sulphur trioxide.

$$2FeSO_4 \longrightarrow Fe_2O_3 + SO_2 + SO_3$$

3. With nitric oxide, ferrous sulphate forms black-coloured nitroso ferrous sulphate, $FeSO_4.NO$.

4. Ferrous sulphate is a reducing agent. It decolourizes acidified potassium permanganate and turns acidified potassium dichromate green. Nitrogen dioxide is reduced to nitric oxide and black nitroso ferrous sulphate is formed.

$$2FeSO_4 + H_2SO_4 + NO_2 \longrightarrow Fe_2(SO_4)_3 + H_2O + NO$$

5. It forms double salts with sulphates of alkali metals, represented as $R_2SO_4.$ $FeSO_4.6H_2O$. With ammonium sulphate, it gives ferrous ammonium sulphate, $FeSO_4.(NH_4)_2SO_4.6H_2O$ (Mohr's salt).

Tests for Purity : Tests for arsenic; copper; zinc; lead; manganese; oxysulphate; pH (3 to 4 of 5% solution).

Copper is determined by treating an acidified solution (A) in hydrochloric and nitric acids with citric acid. The solution is made alkaline with ammonia, sodium diethyldithiocarbonate solution added and extracted with carbon tetrachloride. The colour of the resulting solution is not greater than that of a solution prepared by treating dilute copper sulphate solution in the same manner.

Zinc is determined by treating the solution (A) with citric acid and resorcinol and neutralizing it with ammonia solution. It is extracted with dithizone solution and hydrochloric acid added. Ammonium chloride and potassium ferrocyanide are added to the acidified layer. Any turbidity produced is not greater than that developed by addition a potassium ferrocyanide solution to a freshly prepared mixture of dilute zinc sulphate, hydrochloric acid, ammonium chloride and water.

Lead is determined by treating solution (A), made alkaline with ammonia solution, with potassium cyanide and sodium sulphide solution. The solution is not more intensely coloured than a mixture of hydrochloric acid, nitric acid, standard lead solution and sodium sulphide solution diluted with water.

For determining manganese to the aqueous solution, nitric acid and ammonium persulphate are added and heated. Any colour developed is decolourized with sodium sulphite. Phosphoric acid and sodium periodate are added, boiled and cooled. The colour of the solution should not be deeper.

For detecting oxysulphate, an aqueous solution on boiling forms a clear solution which is not more than faintly turbid.

Tests for Identification : A solution (1 in 20) gives the reactions of ferrous salts, and of sulphates.

Incompatibility : Alkalies, carbonates, gold acid, silver salts, lead acetate, lime water, potassium iodide, potassium and sodium tartrate, sodium borate, tannin, vegetable astringent infusion and decoctions.

Assay : The assay is based on oxidation reduction (redox) titration. An acidified solution of the substance is titrated with ceric ammonium sulphate in the presence of sulphuric acid using ferroin sulphate solution as an indicator. Ceric ammonium sulphate is a strong oxidizing agent. It oxidizes the divalent ferrous sulphate to the trivalent ferric sulphate.

A weighed amount (1 g), dissolved in water (30 ml) and dilute sulphuric acid (20 ml), is titrated with 0.1 ceric ammonium sulphate using ferroin sulphate solution as indicator. Each ml of 0.1 N ceric ammonium sulphate is equivalent to 0.0278 g of $FeSO_4 \cdot 7H_2O$.

DRIED FERROUS SULPHATE

Dried ferrous sulphate is ferrous sulphate deprived of part of its water of crystallization by drying at 40°. It contains from 80 to 90 per cent of $FeSO_4$. It is a greyish-white to buff-coloured powder; taste is metallic and astringent. Its aqueous solution gives the reactions of ferrous salts and of sulphates. It is slowly but completely soluble in freshly boiled and cooled water; practically insoluble in alcohol; stored in tightly closed containers. It is tested for copper, zinc, lead, manganese and oxysulphate. Assay is carried out as for Ferrous sulphate.

Uses : Ferrous sulphate is a haematinic agent. Compounds of iron are used in the treatment of iron deficiency, e.g. anaemia.

The oral administration of iron preparations sometimes produces gastro-intestinal irritation and abdominal pain with nausea, vomiting, diarrhoea, or constipation.

FERROUS FUMARATE

$(\overline{O}OC\text{-}CH\text{=}CH\text{-}COO^-)\ Fe^{2+}$; Mol. Weight = 169.91
$C_4H_2FeO_4$ $FeC_2H_4\ (CO_2)_2$

Ferrous fumarate contains not less than 93.0 per cent of $C_4H_2FeO_4$. It is a fine reddish-orange to reddish-brown powder, tasteless or slightly astringent; odourless or with a slight odour; slightly soluble in water; very slightly soluble in alcohol. It is prepared by mixing hot aqueous solution of ferrous sulphate and sodium fumarate and separating the resulting slurry by filtration. The hot solution of sodium fumarate is preferably added to the ferrous sulphate solution. The commercial material contains a minimum of 31.3% total Fe and not less than 2.0% ferric iron.

It is stored in well-closed containers.

Ferrous fumarate dissolves in dilute hydrochloric acid with the precipitation of fumaric acid.

$$FeC_2H_2(CO_2)_2 + 2HCl \longrightarrow Fe^{-2} + 2Cl^- + C_2H_2\ (COOH)_2$$

Tests for Purity : Tests for arsenic; heavy metals; lead; sulphate; ferric iron; and loss on drying (1%).

For determining heavy metals, the salt is ignited, dissolved in hydrochloric acid and nitric acid, extracted with solvent ether and heated. Citric acid is added and the reaction mixture made alkaline with ammonia. Potassium cyanide solution and sodium sulphide solution are added. Any brown colour produced is not more intense than that produced by treating standard lead solution in a similar manner.

The acidified solution of the salt with hydrochloric acid complies with the limit test for sulphates. Ferric iron is determined by adding potassium iodide to the acidified solution and titrating the liberated iodine with 0.1 N sodium thiosulphate, using starch solution as indicator. The experiment is repeated without the ferrous fumarate. The difference between the titration represents the amount of iodine liberated by the ferric iron. Each ml of 0.1 N sodium thiosulphate is equivalent to 0.005585 g of ferric iron.

Tests for Identification

1. An acidified aqueous solution is precipitated and filtered. The filtrate gives the reactions of ferrous salts.
2. The precipitate from test 1 when treated with sodium carbonate and potassium permanganate solutions, the permanganate is decolourized and a brownish solution is formed.
3. When a mixture of the substance, resorcinol and sulphuric acid is heated, a deep-red, semisolid mass is formed. The mass is added to a large volume of water, an orange yellow solution without any fluorescence is obtained.

Assay : The assay is based on oxidation reduction titration. A weighed amount (0.3 g) is dissolved in dilute sulphuric acid, heated, cooled and water is added. The mixture is titrated with 0.1 N ceric ammonium sulphate, using ferroin sulphate solution as indicator. Each ml of 0.1 N ceric ammonium sulphate is equivalent to 0.01699 g of $C_4H_2FeO_4$.

Uses : Ferrous fumarate has the actions and uses of iron salts and is given by mouth for the treatment of iron-deficiency.

FERROUS GLUCONATE

$[HOCH_2(CHOH)_4COO^-]_2$ Fe^{2+}. $2H_2O$'; Mol. Weight = 482.17. $FeC_{12}H_{22}O_{14}$. $2H_2O$.

Ferrous gluconate contains not less than 95.0 per cent of $FeC_{12}H_{22}O_{14}$. It is prepared by double decomposition in solution between barium gluconate and ferrous sulphate. The precipitated barium sulphate is removed and the solution is dried.

It occurs as greenish-yellow to grey powder or granules. It may have slight odour resembling that of burnt sugar. It is slowly soluble in water (1 in 10) producing a greenish-brown solution, but more readily soluble on warming; practically insoluble in alcohol. Aqueous solutions are stabilized by the addition of glucose. It is stored in airtight containers and protected from light.

Tests for Purity : Tests for arsenic; barium; lead; ferric iron; heavy metals; chloride; sulphate; oxalic acid; reducing sugars; loss on drying; clarity and colour of solution; acidity.

For determining oxalic acid an aqueous solution of the substance containing hydrochloric acid is extracted with solvent ether. The ether layer is dried, the residue dissolved in water; acetic acid and calcium chloride are added, no turbidity is produced when oxalic acid is absent.

Sulphuric acid is added to an aqueous solution of the salt. If no turbidity of $BaSO_4$ is produced within five minutes, then barium is absent. Ferric iron and heavy metals are determined as mentioned under ferrous fumarate. For detecting reducing sugars, hydrogen sulphide is passed into the alkaline solution. The solution is filtered, the filtrate acidified with hydrochloric acid and the solution boiled until the vapours no longer darken lead acetate paper. Sodium carbonate solution is added, filtered, potassium cupri-tartrate solution added to the filtrate and boiled. No red precipitate is formed within one minute when the reducing sugars are absent.

Tests for Identification

1. A solution (1 in 20) gives the reactions of ferrous salts.
2. An aqueous solution containing a little of glacial acetic acid and phenylhydrazine is heated for 30 minutes. The crystals of gluconic acid phenylhydrazide are separated which melted at about 202°.

Assay : The assay is based on oxidation reduction titration. To a weighed amount (1.5 g) dissolved in water and 2N sulphuric acid, zinc powder is added, kept for 20 minutes, filtered and the filter is washed with water. To the combined filtrate and washings ferrous sulphate solution is added and titrated with 0.1 N ceric ammonium sulphate until the colour is changed from orange to green. A blank determination is performed. Each 0.1 N ceric ammonium sulphate is equivalent to 0.04461 of $FeC_{12}H_{22}O_{14}$.

Uses : It has the actions and uses of Ferrous sulphate.

IRON AND AMMONIUM CITRATE
(Ferric Ammonium Citrate)

Iron and ammonium citrate is a complex ammonium ferric citrate containing from 20.5 to 22.5 per cent of Fe. For its preparation ferric hydroxide is precipitated by addition of a ferric salt (e.g. ferric sulphate) to an alkali solution with stirring. The ferric hydroxide is filtered, washed and stirred with sufficient amount of citric acid to dissolve it. A slight excess of ammonia is added and undissolved ferric hydroxide is removed by filtration. The clear, reddish-brown filtrate is concentrated to a syrup with addition of small amount of ammonia during the period of concentration process. The syrup is spread on glass plates, dried below 40°, and scraped off as scales. Green scales can be prepared by varying the method of preparation and using excess of citric acid.

$$Fe_2(SO_4)_3 + 6NaOH \longrightarrow 2Fe(OH)_3 + 3Na_2SO_4$$

Characters : It occurs as thin, transparent, dark red scales or granules or a brownish-red granular powder; odourless; taste is astringent. It is deliquescent in moist air and is affected by light. It is highly soluble is water; almost insoluble in alcohol. It is stored in tightly-closed, light resistant containers.

Solutions of ferric ammonium citrate sometimes form a precipitate of unknown composition on standing. The typical brownish-red colour of ferric ammonium citrate is due to basic complexes of variable composition, $FeC_6H_5O_7 . xFe(OH)_3$. In acid solutions these complexes are present mainly as true electrolytes; in alkaline solutions they are decomposed with the formation of colloidal basic hydrosols. The formation of these complexes is observed by the change in colour from brownish red on addition of alkali to a yellow-green solution of ferric citrate. Further addition of alkali gives colloidal ferric hydroxide, which flocculates on standing; but hydrogen-ion concentration of the solution is not changed when ammonia is added. Therefore, the compound is not decomposed.

Tests for Purity : Tests for arsenic; lead; zinc; chloride; free ferric compound; and sulphate.

For determining free ferric compound an aqueous solution is treated with potassium ferrocyanide solution. No blue precipitate is formed unless acidified with hydrochloric acid.

Lead is determined by dissolving the substance in hydrochloric acid. The solution is extracted with solvent ether, heated and made alkaline with ammonia solution. Potassium cyanide and sodium sulphide solutions are added. Any colour produced is not darker than that produce by mixing the calculated amounts of hydrochloric acid, nitric acid and standard lead solution, making alkaline with ammonia solution and adding potassium cyanide and sodium sulphide solution.

Zinc is detected by dissolving the substance in hydrochloric acid. Nitric acid is added, boiled, extracted with solvent ether and warmed. Citric acid and resorcinol are added, neutralized with ammonia solution and extracted with dithizone solution. The dithizone layer is extracted with hydrochloric acid and then with chloroform. To the acid layer, hydrochloric acid, ammonium chloride and potassium ferrocyanide are added. After fifteen minutes any turbidity produced is not more than that produced by the addition of potassium ferrocyanide solution to a freshly prepared mixture of calculated amount of zinc sulphate, hydrochloric acid, ammonium chloride and sufficient water.

Tests for Identification

1. The substance is ignited and the residue dissolved in hydrochloric acid; the solution gives the reactions of ferric salts.
2. When warmed with sodium hydroxide solution; ammonia is evolved and the solution gives the reactions of citrates.

Assay : A weighed amount (0.5 g) is dissolved in water and sulphuric acid and warmed until the dark brown colour becomes yellow. 0.1N potassium permanganate is added to get pink colour, then hydrochloric acid and potassium iodide also added. The reaction mixture is diluted and titrated with 0.1 N sodium thiosulphate using starch solution as indicator. Each ml of 0.1 N sodium thiosulphate is equivalent to 0.005585 of Fe.

Uses : Ferric ammonium citrate is a haematinic agent. It has the actions and uses of ferrous sulphate.

IRON DEXTRAN INJECTION

Iron dextran injection is a sterile colloidal solution containing a complex of ferric hydroxide with dextrans of low molecular weight in water for injection. It contains from 4.75 to 5.25 per cent w/v of iron. The molecular weight is between 5000 and 7500.

It occurs as a dark brown solution. It is stored in single-dose or multiple-dose containers.

Iron dextran injection does not give reactions for ferric iron. However, hydrolysis of the injection with hydrochloric acid yields ferric chloride which is removed with hydrogen sulphide. The dextran is then hydrolyzed to glucose which is detected by reduction of Fehling's solution.

Tests for Purity : Tests for copper; zinc; arsenic; chloride; heavy metals; pyrogens; undue toxicity; absorption from injection site; acidity; non-volatile residue; pH (between 5.2 and 6.2); content of dextrans (between 17 and 23 per cent); molecular size of dextrans.

Non-volatile residue is determined by evaporating the content on a water bath.

For determining undue toxicity, the content is injected into a tail of each of ten mice. Not more than three mice die within five days of injection.

Copper, zinc, chloride and heavy metals are determined as mentioned for ferrous sulphate.

Absorption from injection site is determined by injecting the semitendinosus muscle of one leg of rabbits, sacrificing the animals after seven days, and dissecting the treated legs to examine the muscles; no heavy deposit of unabsorbed iron compounds is observed, and the tissue is only slightly coloured.

For molecular size of dextrans the solution is diluted and the ferric hydroxide is precipitated by autoclaving which is separated by filtration. The filtrate is concentrated and the optical rotation determined. The specific rotation of the dextrans is calculated by both total solids and sodium chloride. The viscosity ratios of various dilutions are then determined. The exact dextran contents are calculated from the optical rotations and the specific rotations already measured. The intrinsic viscosity is then deduced from there viscosity ratios.

Content of dextrans is determined by treating the diluted solution with anthrone and sulphuric acid and then measuring extinctions of the solution at wave length 625 nm. The operation is repeated with water. From the difference between extinctions, the content of dextrose is calculated.

Identification

1. When dilute ammonia solution is added to a few drops of the injection; no precipitate is produced.

2. An acidified solution is heated and precipitated by adding excess of strong ammonia solution. The precipitate is filtered, washed with water and dissolved in dilute hydrochloric acid. The resulting solution gives the reactions of ferric salts.

3. The acidified solution is heated, cooled and basified with strong ammonia solution. Hydrogen sulphide gas is passed, boiled to remove hydrogen sulphide and filtered. The filtrate is boiled with potassium cupri-tartrate solution and then with hydrochloric acid. It is neutralized with sodium hydroxide solution, potassium cupri-tartrate solution is re-added and re-boiled; a red precipitate is produced.

Assay : A dilute solution of the injection containing sulphuric acid is passed through activated zinc amalgam 'reductor' column. The eluates are titrated with ceric ammonium sulphate, using ferroin sulphate solution as indicator. Each ml of 0.1 N ceric ammonium sulphate is equivalent to 0.005585 g of Fe.

Uses : Iron dextran is used in the treatment of iron-deficiency anaemia where oral therapy is ineffective.

Severe anaphylactoid reactions may occur after iron dextran therapy. Patients may feel delayed reactions such as arthralgia, myalgia (pain in muscle), and fever.

Officials of Iron

Ferrous Fumarate/Tablets; I.P., B.P., U.S.P.

Ferrous Fumarate Oral Suspension, B.P.

Ferrous Glyconate/Tablets/Capsules/Elixir I.P., B.P., U.S.P.

Ferrous Sulphate/Tablets/Oral solution/Syrup, I.P., B.P., U.S.P.

Dried Ferrous Sulphate, I.P.

Iron and Ammonium Citrate, I.P.

Iron Dextran Injection, I.P., B.P., U.S.P.

Iron Sorbitol Injection, B.P.

Iron Sorbitex Injection, U.S.P.

Ferrous Succinate Capsules/Tablets, B.P.

Paediatric Ferrous Sulphate Oral Solution, B.P.

Ferrous Succinate/Capsules/Tabletes, B.P.

Green Ferric Ammonium Citrate, N.F.

Ferric Cocodylate, N.F.

Ferric Chloride, N.F.

Ferric Hypophosphite, N.F.

Soluble Ferric Phosphate, N.F.

Ferric Pyrophosphate, N.F.

Ferric Glycerophosphate, N.F.

Saccharated Ferric Oxide, N.F.

Ferrous Carbonate, N.F.

IODINE PRODUCTS

Iodine products such as Lugol's solution (Strong Iodine Solution, 5% iodine and 10% potassium iodide), sodium iodide, potassium iodide, etc. are used adjunctively with antithyroid drugs in hyperthyroid patients in preparation for thyroidectomy and to treat thyrotoxic crisis or neonatal thyrotoxicosis. They are also used for thyroid blocking in a radiation emergency.

AQUEOUS IODINE ORAL SOLUTION (B.P.)

Potassium iodide (100 g) and the iodine (50 g) are dissolved in 100 ml of the purified water and sufficient of the purified water is added to produced 1000 ml. It contains content of iodine from 4.75 to 5.25% w/v and contents of potassium iodide from 9.5 to 10.5% w/v.

Assay : The solution (25) is diluted to 100 ml with water.

For iodine : The solution is titrated with 0.1N sodium thiosulphate. Each ml of 0.1N sodium thiosulphate is equivalent to 12.69 mg of I.

For Potassium Iodide : Aqueous acidified solution is titrated with 0.5N potassium iodate until the dark brown solution, which is produced, becomes pale brown. Amaranth solution (1 ml) is added and the titration continued until red colour just changes to pale yellow. From the number of ml of 0.05 N potassium iodate required substract one quarter of the number of ml of 0.1 N sodium thiosulphate required in the assay for iodine. Each ml of the remainder is equivalent to 16.60 mg of KI.

Storage : Aqueous iodine oral solution should be kept in a well-closed container, the materials of which are resistant to iodine.

Labelling : The label states that the material should be well diluted before use.

The solution contains about 130 mg of total iodine, free and combined.

The solution is intended to be diluted before use.

—

ALCOHOLIC IODINE SOLUTION (B.P.)

Potassium iodide (25 g) and iodine (25 g) are dissoled in the purified water and sufficient ethanol (90%) added to produced 1000 ml. It contains the content of iodine from 2.4 to 2.7%, content of potassium iodide from 2.4 to 2.7% and ethanol content from 83 to 88%.

Assay for Iodine : 10 ml of the solution is dissolved in water (20 ml) and titrated with 0.1 N sodium thiosulphate. Each ml of 0.1N sodium thiosulphate is equivalent to 12.69 mg of I.

Assay for Potassium Iodide : Assay is carried out as for aqueous iodine solution. Each ml of the remainder is equivalent to 16.60mg of KI.

The solution should be kept in a well-closed container, the materials of which are resistant to iodine.

The Label States

1. The date after which the solution is not intended to be used.
2. The conditions under which it should be stored.

IODIZED OIL FLUID INJECTION (B.P.)

Iodized oil fluid injection is a sterile iodine addition product of the ethyl esters of the fatty acids obtained from poppy-seed oil. It contains content of combined iodine from 37.0 to 39.0% w/w.

Characters : It is a straw-coloured or yellow, oily liquid; odour, not more than slightly alliaceous. It is practically insoluble in water; soluble in chloroform, ether and petroleum spirit.

Tests for Identification : The substance (0.05 ml) is boiled with glacial acetic acid (2 ml) and zinc powder (0.1 g) for 2 minutes; water added, shaked, decanted from any undissolved zinc and hydrogen peroxide solution (1 ml). Iodine vapour is evolved.

Tests for Purity : Acidity; weight per ml; free iodine.

Assay : The substance (1 g) is refluxed with glacial acetic acid (10 ml) and zinc powder (1 g) for 1 hour. Hot water (30 ml) is added, the solution is filtered, washed, hydrochloric acid (25 ml) and potassium cyanide solution (8 ml) added and titrated with 0.05 N potassium iodate until the dark brown solution, which is produced, becomes light brown. Starch mucilage (5 ml) is added and the titration continued until the blue colour disappears. Each ml of 0.05 N potassium iodate is equivalent to 12.69 mg of combined iodine.

Storage : The injection should be kept in an atmosphere of carbon dioxide or nitrogen and protected from light.

Uses : The injection is used as radio-opaque agent.

Officials of Iodine

Iodine, I.P., B.P.

Povidone-Iodine Solution, B.P.

Aqueous Iodine Oral Solution, B.P., U.S.P.

Alcoholic Iodine Solution, B.P.

Iodised Oil Fluid Injection, B.P.

Iodine Tincture, U.S.P.

Iodine Topical Solution, U.S.P.

Strong Iodine Tincture, U.S.P.

13

RADIOPHARMACEUTICALS

Radiopharmaceutical preparations are the preparations containing one or more radionuclides. Radioactive compounds are used in medicine as sources of radiation for radiotherapy and for diagnostic purposes. These compounds may be considered as sealed radioactive sources that are bonded or encapsulated to prevent the escape of the radioactive material.

Unsealed sources are radioactive materials usually in liquid or gaseous form that are removed from their containers for application. Radiopharmaceuticals come within this category.

(A) RADIOACTIVITY

A nuclide is a species of atom characterized by the number of protons and neutrons in its nucleus and also by its nuclear energy state. Isotopes of an element are nuclides with the same atomic number but different mass numbers. These isotopes differ in some of their physical properties. Some isotopes may be stable, the differences between them arising solely from their difference in mass. There are a number of isotopes which are unstable and, therefore, radioactive; e.g. uranium 235. In addition, artificial radionuclides are prepared by converting stable nuclei into unstable form. Radionuclides are radioactive and transform spontaneously into other nuclides.

The symbol used for a nuclide is the chemical symbol of the atom, with the mass number as a superscript and the atomic number as a subscript. Thus the symbols for the 3 hydrogen isotopes – common hydrogen, deuterium, and tritium – are $^1_1$H, $^2_1$H, and $^3_1$H, and the symbols for the 3 naturally occurring uranium isotopes are $^{234}_{92}U$, $^{235}_{92}U$, and $^{238}_{92}U$, as the atomic number can be inferred from the chemical symbol–it is the usual practice to omit the subscript. It is also common practice to write out the full name of the element followed by the superscript, e.g. chromium - 51 for ^{51}Cr.

Disintegration Constant and Units

Radioactive disintegration is independent on the temperature, pressure and the state of chemical combination of the disintegrating atom. Each radionuclide disintegrates at a particular rate depending on the number of atoms, by the emission of a typical particle or electromagnetic radiation of characteristic energy. Radionuclides are identified by half-life, disintegration constant, type and energy of the radiation emitted. Radioactive disintegration is an spontaneous process and every radionuclide has the same probability of disintegrating within unit time. This probability is a fundamental constant known as *disintegration* or *decay* constant, denoted as 1. The unit of radioactivity is the *curie*, in short Ci. The other units are :

1. **Milli-curie (mc) :** It is equal to 1×10^{-3} curie.
2. **Micro-curie (µc) :** It is equal to 10^{-6} curie.
3. **Becquerel (Bq) :** It is equal to 2.7×10^{-11} curie.
4. **Electron volt (ev) :** It is ionizing radiation form of energy. It is the kinetic energy acquired by an electron during accleration through a potential difference of 1 volt.
   (1 ev $= 1.60 \times 10^{-19}$ joule).
5. **Roentgen (R) :** It is unit of exposure ($1R = 2.58 \times 10^{-4}$ Ckg^{-1}, where C = coulomb).
6. **Rad :** It is unit of absorbed dose.
   (1 Rad $= 10^{-2}$ JKg^{-1})
7. **Rem :** It is unit of dose equivalent.
8. **Exposure Rate constant :** It is the dose rate in roetgen per hour at 1 m distance from curie.

The disintegration rate of a radionuclide is equal to the rate of emission of particles. The minimum detectable weight of a radionuclide depends on its half-life and mass number. The specific activity of a radioactive substance is the activity associated with unit weight expressed in any convenient units such as counts per minute per gram.

Emissions from Radioisotopes

Three main types of emission from radioactive substances are *alpha* (α) particles, *beta* (β) particles, and *gamma* (γ)-rays. Most sources emit more than one type of radiation.

Alpha particles are positively charged particles (helium nuclei of mass number 4), each consisting of 2 protons and 2 neutrons. All the α-particles emitted from a particular radionuclide have the same energy and consequently the same range in a given medium.

Beta particles (β⁻ or β⁺) are identical with electrons or positrons but arise from the nucleus. They are emitted with great velocity and their energies are spread over spectrum. Positrons are similar to electrons, having a similar mass but a positive charge. In β-emission the energy is shared between the β-particles and neutrons in varying amounts and so the β-particles emitted by a radionuclide do not all have the same energy and range. The fraction of the particles that can penetrate on absorbing medium decreases with the thickness of the absorber. Therefore, absorption of β-particles is described in terms of 'half-thickness' (in mg/cm²) of the absorber necessary to absorb half of the particles.

Gamma-rays are electromagnetic radiations with a wave length much shorter than those of light. These emissions of gamma - rays may be partly replaced by the ejection of electrons known as internal conversion of electrons. This phenomenon, like the process of electron capture, causes a secondary emission of x-rays due to reorganization of the electrons in the atom. For example, in chromium-51, electron capture (EC) occurs, an electron from an inner shell being absorbed by the nucleus with the production of an x-ray. This secondary emission may itself be partly replaced by the injection of electrons known as Auger electrons, β⁺-particles are annihilated on contact with matter, the process is accompanied by the emission of γ-rays with an energy of 511 KeV.

The penetrating power of each radiation varies considerably according to its nature and its energy. Alpha particles are completely absorbed in a thickness of a few micrometers to some tens of micrometres of solid or liquid. Beta particles are completely absorbed in a thickness of several millimetres to several centimetres. Gamma rays are not completely absorbed but only attenuated. The denser the absorbent, the shorter the range of alpha and beta particles and the greater the attenuation of gamma rays.

Decay of Radionuclides

A radionuclide will consist of unstable atoms which will at some time undergo an energy change with the emission of ionizing radiation. In quantitative terms this transition occurs at a rate which is characteristic of the radionuclide and it is expressed as its half-life, the time required for the activity to fall by one-half. Many radionuclides have complex decay characteristics with several possible energies of emitted particles and radiation. Some radionuclides may be in an excited or metastable state denoted by the suffix m attached to the mass number (e.g. Technetium - 99 m) and undergo *isomeric transition* with the release of γ-rays.

Each radionuclide is characterized by an invariable half-life, expressed in units of time, and by the nature and energy of its radiation (s). The energy is expressed in electron volts (eV), keloelectronvolts (KeV) or mega-electron volts (MeV).

The radioactivity of a preparation is the number of nuclear disintegrations or transformations per unit time.

The type of emission from a radionuclide largely determines it usefulness in medicine. Those emitting α-particles are very less used because detection and measurement are difficult. Positron-emitters, e.g. carbon-11, nitrogen-13 and oxygen-15, have become more popular and are used in positron-emission tomography, where the radiation is measured within the body. Gamma-rays emitting radionuclides are most accessible and are the most common radiation source in radiopharmaceuticals. Positrons on contact with matter release gamma rays.

Biological Effects and Uses of Radiation

The effect of radioactive particles passing through biological tissues depends upon a number of factors such as :

  (a) the ability of the radiation to penetrate tissue,
  (b) the energy of the radiation
  (c) the particular tissue and surface area exposed, and
  (d) the dose rate of the radiation.

The destructive effect of radioactivity is directly related to its interaction with molecules present in the tissue to produce abnormal ions. These chemical species change the local pH or initiate free radical chain reactions forming peroxides and other toxic compounds, causing necrosis and destruction of the tissues or an organ. Water is the predominant chemical compound present in most tissues. It forms free radicals which abstract radicals from other molecules and produce different types of potentially toxic species. These species change the DNA in cells and form crosslinking between certain amino acids in protein.

Different types of radiation differ significantly in their abilities to penetrate tissue. Alpha particles have a potential to produce an excess amount of free radicals. The range and penetration of these particles are very low and would not penetrate the surface even if they are very close to the skin. But the ionizing power of gamma rays is relatively low, their range and penetrating ability are quite high to produce significant damage at distances of several meters from the source. They collide with atoms of the tissues and damage them.

Radiation in general is harmful to all living cells. In radiotherapy the aim is to destroy diseased tissue without destroying healthy tissues. α-Radiation is not sufficiently effective due to less penetration. β-Radiation is used to treat surface lesions, e.g. on the eye. γ-Radiation is the most penetrating and used to treat deep-seated tumours. X-Radiation is generally used for external therapy. In internal therapy the radionuclide is placed in a natural or surgical cavity of the body or ejected into the body. Sometimes reliance is placed on the selective uptake of an element by an organ; e.g. γ-emitter iodine-131 is used to destroy diseased thyroid tissue orally and arrives naturally to the thyroid. Short-live radionuclide (e.g. iodine-131 and gold-198) may be left in the body permanently, but long-lived sources (e.g. radium-226) must be removed when the treatment is finished.

Radium-226 is a reactive element chemically, and when used internally, soluble radium compounds will form, diffuse throughout the body and eventually deposit in the bones with chemically similar compounds. There they would remain since radium has a long half-life of 1,622 years, and cause great damage. Artificial γ-emitters (e.g. cabalt-60 and iridium-192) have many advantages over radium. They are cheap, their disintegration products are harmless, they are unreactive chemically, and they can be prepared in many shapes.

Many materials are opaque to visible light, but are transparent to γ-and X-radiations. These radiations are used to record radiographs of these materials. γ-Emitters are portable and independent of electrical supply. These emitters are used for radiographing objects whose radiographs can not be recorded by X-rays instrument. In medical diagnosis, X-rays are excessively used since there is no important difference in the absorption of high-energy γ-rays.

Radioisotopes are used for diagnostic purposes. The quantities of isotopes for diagnostic procedures are very small than required in radiotherapy, sometimes a mere fraction of a microgram. The function of a particular organ may be studied by administrating a particular radio isotope, e.g. iodine-131 for thyroid gland. Radionuclides can be used to trace the location of objects with which they are mixed and the site of the radioactivity with the help of a radiation detector. The radiotracer may be chemically different from the material (a physical tracer) it is tracing or identical with it (a chemical tracer). Iodine - 131, when used as a physical tracer in the form of di-iodofluorescein, can be given to map out a brain tumour. The labelled dye is injected into the patient where it is preferentially absorbed by the diseased brain tissue. It emits γ-radiation which can be detected through the skill. This helps to learn the site and extent of tumour before operating. To determine the site of blockage in a blood vessel or capillary, a radioisotope is administered into the body. The hinderance of the blood supply due to blockage at a particular site is detected with the help of γ-radiation.

Measurement of Radioactivity

The absolute measurement of the radioactivity of a given sample may be carried out only if the decay scheme of the radionuclide is known. The measurement is usually based on the coincidence method in which, for example, a beta emission and a gamma emission are counted separately and in coincidence using special apparatus. The three count rates are sufficient to determine the efficiencies of the counters and the absolute disintegration rate. In practice many corrections are required to obtain accurate results.

The efficiency of radiation detectors varies greatly with the type and energy of the radiation measured. In most counting apparatus the geometrical efficiency for counting particles or photons leaving the source is much less than 100 per cent. The counting apparatus is calibrated by measuring absolute activity carefully using a source prepared from a standard radioisotope solution.

Geiger - Muller Counter : It consists of sensing unit to indicate the intensity of radioactivity by counting the number of subatomic particles emitted by a radionuclide. The equipment is sensitive for detection of b-and g-particles. It contains a positively charged wire mounted coaxially and serving as an anode. The wire is surrounded by a negatively charged cylinder of stainless steel or of glass silvered on the inner surface. The cylinder serves both as the body of the tube and as the cathode. A special gas mixture is filled inside the cylinder in between the anode and the cathode.

Construction

The counter consists of a 1-2 cm diameter cylinder of glass coated with silver on the inner side or stainless steel. The cylinder acts as a cathode. A mounted fine wire located coaxially inside the tube works as an anode. The space inside the cylinder is filled with a mixture of ionizing gas such as argon (Ar) and helium (He) and a smell proportion of quenching vapour, e.g. chlorine, bromine, ethyl alcohol and ethyl formate. Quenching vapour prevents the false pulses that may be produced due to positive ions approaching the cathode and absorbs the photons emitted by excited atoms returning to their ground state. Radiation entering the tube through the window, a thin section of outer wall, ionizes atoms of the gas. In the presence of high voltage (300 - 1300 V) the electrons are attracted by the anode and positively charged particles towards the cathode along with constituting a flow of current. Each particle of radiation generates a pulse of current which can be recorded by a scaler. All pulses from a Geiger-Muller counter possess the identical amplitude for any incident radiation and different radiation types and their energy cannot be distinguished.

An electron, especially a β-particle, passing through the cylinder collides another electron of the gas molecules to ionize few of them. If a high voltage of about 800-1300 volts is applied between the electrodes, the process of ionization continues until an 'avalanche' of negatively charged electrons falls to the positively charged wire. In the same way, an avalanche of positively charged ions to the negatively charged cylinder falls within a fraction of second along the whole length of the anode. Due to the passage of these ions through the G.M. tube, a flow of current is maintained. Each β-particle causes a brief pulse of current to flow, which is recorded by a device called as *scaler*. It accumulates and indicates the total number of pulses. The radiations enter through a very thin section of the outer wall, known as *window*, or through the end of the tube.

The positive ions are much heavier than the electrons. They acquire lower velocity and move relative more slowly towards the cathode than the movement of electrons towards the anode. Hence, an interval of time elapses before the heavier positive ions which are left as a sheath surrounding the anode. Though the collection of the electrons at the anode is completed in a fraction of a microsecond, a fresh discharge cannot take place until the sheath of positive particles has moved sufficiently away from the anode. The counter, therefore, will not respond to any further ionizing radiation. The interval of time, during which the counter is inactive; is called *dead time* or *paralysis* for which the counter is to be corrected. In addition this, the positive ions, in the absence of a quenching agent, produce secondary electrons on reaching the cathode (cylinder wall), which in turn generate another pulses. Each such pulse must be quenched. The quenching agent, consists of polyatomic organic molecules or halogen molecules, is introduced into the counter. It has a lower ionization potential than the ionizable gas. During the movement of the positive ions towards the cathode, their energy is dissipated on collision with the molecules of the quenching agent which are then neutralized by secondary elections.

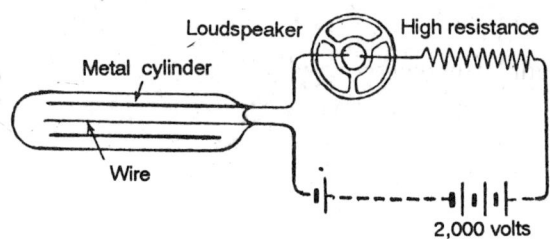

Fig. 13.1 : Schematic representation of Geiger Muller Counter.

Comparative measurements are generally carried out against a standard source using a Geiger-Muller (G.M.) counter, a proportional counter, a scintillation counter or an ionization chamber. A G.M. Counter is used to measure β-and β,γ-emitters. The scintillation and semiconductor counters are used for measuring γ-rays. Low-energy β-emitters are measured by a liquid-scintillation counter.

For measuring radioactivity it is essential to work under well-defined geometrical conditions so that the radioactive source is always at the same position in the apparatus and its distance from the measuring device is constant and remains the same when the sample being measured is replaced by the standard preparation. Solutions of radiopharmaceutical preparations may be measured directly by using an ionization chamber or a well-crystal scintillation detector. The G.M. counter or a flat crystal scintillation counter is preferred to measure radioactivity of the residue. It is advisable to cover the dry residue with a strip of adhesive cellulose acetate the mass per unit area so that its absorption of radiation is negligible. The residue on evaporation of the standard solution should be nearly identical with that of the solution being examined. The two solutions should contain the same substances in the same conditions on surfaces of identical size of the same material. When these precautions are taken, the results obtained are satisfactory, whatever the measuring apparatus used. The efficiency of the measuring apparatus remains constant during the time of measuring by using a secondary source consisting of a radionuclide of long half-life. Low-energy β-emitters may be measured by liquid scintillation counting. The sample is dissolved in a solution containing one or more organic fluorescent substances, which convert part of the energy of disintegration into photons of light, which are detected and converted into electrical impulses by a photo-multiplier.

All measurements of radioactivity must be corrected by substracting the background activity due to radioactivity in the environment and to spurious signals generated in the equipment itself. When counts are made at high levels of activity, a correction may be required for loss by coincidence due to the finite resolving time of the detector. With some equipment this correction is made automatically. Corrections for loss by coincidence must be made before the correction for background radiation.

Determination of radioactivity show statical variations because they are related to the probability of nuclear disintegration. A sufficient number of count must be registered to compensate for variations in.

Adverse Effects of Radionuclides

When radionuclides are administered, the internal irradiation of tissues carries similar dangers to exposure to ionizing radiation from an external source. Local high irradiation doses may arise if these nuclides are specially localized in a tissue. The most serious danger is genetic damage prior to and during the reproductive period. Tissues whose cells are in a continuous state of multiplication are particularly sensitive to the effects of radiation.

Untoward effects of exposure to the larger doses of irradiation include leucopenia, anaemia, inflammation of the skin, radiation sickness (reduction of white corpuscles in blood), and neoplasms (new formation or tumor). The effects might arise from the carrier or from contaminants the number of disintegrations per unit of time. At least 10,000 counts are necessary to obtain a standard deviation of not more than 1 per cent.

General Uses of Radioactive Materials

Radiopharmaceuticals are used widely in madicine and surgery, mainly for the diagnosis and sometimes for the treatment of diseases. They can offer facilities not provided by other diagnostic techniques such as contrast media, ultrasound, computerized tomography or other external irradiation. In many cases radionuclides or labelled compounds are administered and the radioactive concentrations are subsequently measured in organs, tissues, blood, urine, or faeces. The quantities used are always the smallest which will give the desired accuracy of image or of measurement.

Storage

Radiopharmaceutical preparations should be kept in an airtight container in a place sufficiently shielded to avoid irradiation of personnel by primary or secondary emissions. These preparations are stored with the national and international regulations concerning the storage of radioactive substances. They are intended for use within a short time. During storage containers and solutions may darken due to the emitted radiation. Such darkening does not necessarily involve deterioration of the preparations. Thus effects of temperature and light should be considered. Radiopharmaceuticals are liable to decomposition by self-irradiation effects which may cause degradation of solvent, preservatives, or other compounds. There can also be a continuous formation of oxidizing and reducing chemical species due to the effect of the radioactivity on any chemical substances present in the radiopharmaceutical, even in minute amounts.

Exposure to radiation can lead several complicated disorders such as leukaemia (blood cancer), change in body pH, initiation of free radical chain reactions, necrosis, destruction of the tissues, etc. Therefore, persons working with radioisotopes, detectors, tracer experiments, radio-assay and production of radioactive materials should take certain precautions. Radioactive materials must not be touched and they are handled with forceps. Protective coverings must be used while working with the radioisotopes. These materials should be preserved in suitable labelled containers. The areas where radioactive substances are present should be restricted and these are destroyed carefully. Foods materials should not be carried in the radioactive laboratory since food contaminated with radioactive material can damage internal organs.

Official Preparations

Calcium-47 ($^{47}_{20}$Ca) is supplied as calcium chloride in the form of an injection. Its half-life is short, i.e., 4.54 days. Calcium - 47 has been used as a urinary and faecal marker.

Chromium–51($^{51}_{24}$Cr) is supplied as sodium chromate solution or injection. It is used to label red blood cells so that red-cell survival and red-cell volume can be measured. Chromium–51 activity in the faeces can be used to estimate gastro-intestinal blood losses. Cobalt -57, cobalt -58 and cobalt-59 are usually supplied as cyanocobalamin in the form of aqueous solutions. Co-57 and Co-58 are used for the measurement of absorption of vitamin B$_{12}$ in the diagnosis of pernicious anaemia.

Erbium-169 is supplied as erbium citrate (^{169}Er) in the form of an injectable suspension. It is used in the treatment of arthritic conditions of small joints.

Fluorine-18 ($^{18}_{9}$F) is a position-emitting radionuclide. Fluorine-18-labelled analogues of glucose, principally 2-fluoro-2-deoxy-D-glucose, have been clinically used in the assessment of regional cerebral and myocardial metabolism and for the detection of tumours in the lungs and liver. Fluorine-18 - labelled amino acids have also been used for pancreatic scintigraphy.

Gallium-67 ($^{67}_{31}$Ga) is supplied as gallium citrate in the form of a carrier-free injection. It is used for the diagnosis of various infections, sarcoidosis, and other inflammatory lesions.

Gold-198($^{198}_{79}$Au), used in the treatment of rhuematoid arthritis, is supplied as sterile colloidal suspensions of metallic gold stabilized with gelatin and glucose. Indium -11, supplied as a complex of indium with bleomycin in the form of a carrier free injection, is used for the detection of tumours, in cerebrospinal fluid studies, cisternography and ventriculography.

Iodine-125 ($^{125}_{53}$I) is not very suitable for the external counting of radioactivity in the thyroid gland because its γ-energy is weak and tissue absorption is high. Many labelled compounds of iodine-125 are available for *in vitro* assay to detect and estimate drugs and hormones in body fluid. Iodine-131 ($^{131}_{53}$I) is mainly used in studies of thyroid function, for tests on the function of the heart, kidney and liver, and on fat absorption or protein loss from the gastro-intestinal tract.

Iron-59 is supplied as ferric chloride (^{99}Fe) in the form of a solution or as ferric citrate in the form of an injection. It is used in the measurement of iron absorption and utilization. Krypton-81 m is a daughter of rubidium-81 and is prepared immediately before use. It is used as a gas in lung ventilation studies or as an intravenous infusion in perfusion studies of the lung, heart and brain.

Phosphorus-32 is supplied as sodium phosphate in the form of an injection and used in the treatment of polycythaemia vera and in the diagnosis of malignant neoplasms. Potassium-42 is supplied as potassium chloride (^{42}K) in the form of an injection. It is used to measure exchangeable potassium and for myocardial scanning. Selenium-75 ($^{75}_{34}$Se) is supplied as L-selenomethionine (^{75}Se) in the form of an injection. Malignant lymphomas is located with its help. Sodium-22 ($^{22}_{11}$Na), supplied as sodium chloride in the form of an injection, is used in the determination of body's exchangeable sodium. Strontium-85, mainly used for bone scanning, is available as strontium chloride in the form of an injection. Sulphur-35 ($^{35}_{16}$S) is marketed as sodium sulphate in the form of a carrier-free injection and is used for the estimation of the extracellular fluid volume.

Technetium-99 m ($^{99m}_{43}$Tc) is a daughter of molybdenum-99. Due to its short-half life (66.2 hours), it is normally prepared just before use. Because it has a short half-life, its administration in relatively large doses and detection of its γ-emission readily, technetium-99 m is very widely used for scanning bone and organs such as brain, gall-bladder, kidney, liver, lung, spleen and thyroid. It may also be used to measure cerebral blood flow and for scintography of the salivary glands, stomach, heart and joints. Allergic reactions have been reported with technetium-99m preparations.

Thallium-201 is supplied as thallous chloride (^{201}Tl) in the form of an injection and employed for scanning the myocardium in the investigation of coronary artery disease, acute myocardial infarction and for post-surgical assessment of coronary artery. Xenon-133 is available as an injection and used for measurements of lung perfusion and regional blood flow. Yttrium-90, marketed as a colloidal aqueous suspension with silicate, is used in the treatment of arthritic conditions of joints.

(B) RADIOPAQUE CONTRAST MEDIA

Radiopaque contrast media are chemical compounds of elements of high atomic number. They hinder the passage of x-rays and used as diagnostic aid in radiology or roentgenology (use of x-ray in the imaging or shadowing of various internal organ structures). X-rays pass through most soft tissue. When special photographic film or a photosensitive plate is placed on the side of the patient, the film or plate darkens in an amount proportional to the number of x-rays passing through it. Bone and teeth interfere the passage of x-rays, appear light on exposed to the film and allows their visualization for the diagnosis of fractures and malformations. The ability to stop this type of radiation by the bone and teeth is due to their chemical constituents, calcium and phosphorus, present in significant concentration. They occur in close-packed structures providing excess localizations of electron density. Passage of x-rays is interfered due to the excess electrons in an atom or molecule. Soft tissues are made up of carbon, hydrogen, and oxygen. They are relatively low in atomic number and do not provide a dense electron barrier.Therefore, skin and soft organs appear only as shadow on x-ray film. The iodine compounds are covalently bonded organic iodides.

The most radiopaques contain barium and iodine and are used for x-ray examinations of the kidney, liver, blood vessels, heart and brain. Although they do not have the highest atomic numbers, they are the most easily incorporated into molecules exhibiting relatively low toxicity. They become concentrated in the organ to be studied, thus producing opacity to x-rays and as contrast media in the diagnosis of soft tissues by x-rays.

BARIUM SULPHATE

$BaSO_4$; Mol. Weight = 233.4

Barium sulphate contains not less than 97.5 per cent of $BaSO_4$. In nature it is found as *barite;* also as heavy spar. It may be prepared by adding any soluble sulphate to a soluble barium salt; for example, addition of sodium sulphate to a solution of barium chloride precipitates barium sulphate.

$$BaCl_2 + Na_2SO_4 \rightleftharpoons BaSO_4 + 2NaCl$$

Barium sulphate occurs as a fine, heavy, white, odourless, tasteless, bulky powder free from grittiness. It is practically insoluble in water and organic solvents; in dilute acids and alkalies; soluble in hot concentrated sulphuric acid forming the soluble bisulphate salts.

$$BaSO_4 + H_2SO_4 \longrightarrow Ba(HSO_4)_2$$

Tests for Purity : Tests for acidity or alkalinity; phosphate; arsenic; heavy metals; copper; lead; mercury; tin; zinc; sulphide; oxidizable sulphur; acid-soluble substances; soluble barium salts; bulkiness or sedimentation; and loss on drying.

Acidity or alkalinity is determined by heating barium sulphate with water. The solution is filtered, bromothymol blue solution is added to the filtrate and neutralized with 0.01N hydrochloric acid or 0.01N sodium hydroxide.

For detecting the presence of phosphate, ammonium molybdate solution is added to an acidified solution of barium sulphate with nitric acid. No yellow precipitate is formed.

An acidified solution of the salt with hydrochloric acid is boiled. A lead acetate paper is exposed to the vapour. The paper does not darken when sulphide is absent.

For determining acid-soluble substances, an acidified solution, prepared by boiling the substance in dilute hydrochloric acid, is filtered. The filtrate is evaporated, the residue dried and weighed. The presence of soluble barium salts is found out by digesting the residue obtained in the test for acid-soluble substances with water. The solution is filtered, dilute sulphuric acid added to the filtrate and set aside for thirty minutes; no turbidity is produced.

Bulkiness is determined by allowing to stand an aqueous suspension of the substance in a graduated cylinder. The barium sulphate does not settle down below the 15 ml mark.

Tests for Identification

1. The substance is boiled with sodium carbonate solution,

diluted with water, filtered and the filtrate acidified with dilute hydrochloric acid. The solution gives the reactions of sulphates.

2. The residue of test 1 is washed with water; dilute hydrochloric acid added to the residue, filtered and to the filtrate dilute sulphuric acid added. A white precipitate is formed which is insoluble in dilute hydrochloric acid.

Assay : A mixture of the substance (0.6 g), sodium carbonate, and potassium carbonate is heated to 1000° for 15 minutes. It is cooled, water added, filtered by decantation and the residue washed with sodium carbonate solution. Dilute hydrochloric acid, ammonium acetate, potassium dichromate and urea are added to the residue, heated in an oven at 80-85° for 16 hours, filtered, the precipitate washed with potassium dichromate and finally with water and dried at 105°; 1.0 g of the residue is equivalent to 0.9213 g of $BaSO_4$.

Uses : Barium sulphate is a diagnostic aid (radio-opaque medium) used as a contrast medium for x-ray examination of the gastro-intestinal tract. It is not soluble in acidic gastric juice and hence does not produce the systemic effects of soluble toxic barium salts. It is given in the form of a suspension.

Constipation may occur after oral or rectal barium sulphate administration, Barium ion will produce a stimulation of all muscles. It stimulates smooth muscles causing vomiting, severe cramps, diarrhoea and haemorrhage : stimulation of the heart muscle can produce cardiac arrest and causes death.

14

QUALITY CONTROL OF DRUGS AND PHARMACEUTICALS

Quality of any goods is the essence which characterizes its usefulness and which distinguishes its image. The quality of drugs is determined by their conformance to the standards as detailed in the second schedule of drugs and cosmetic act for various types and categories of pharmaceutical products. Drugs which do not comply to the led standards, are considered as substandard. The products which, for reasons of being misleading in any of their particulars are called 'Misbranded drugs' and 'Adulterated drugs'. Spurious drugs are the preparations which may be camouflaging the genuine ones or of fictitious nature. Such products are not only substandard but also amounting to an act of crime for which any severe punishment is less. Drugs also become of substandard due to faulty formulation, faulty processing, unsatisfactory packaging and due to unfavourable conditions of handling during transportation or storage. For drugs, because their usage in human beings, their quality assurance is essential.

Quality has its own cost which can be measured by taking into consideration the price of conformance which includes prevention cost; and the price of nonconformance which is caused by product failure, rejection, re-work, down time, etc.

The manufactured drug should attributes of efficacy, safety and stability of the investigated formulation. These attributes have to be maintained throughout the shelf life of the manufactured product until it is administered to a patient. In order to attain this objective the manufacturing process has to be as accurate as reproducible as possible.

Quality assurance program is the devise and implement systems and procedures that provide a high probability that each dose or package of a pharmaceutical product will have homogenous characteristics and properties to insure both safety and efficacy of the formulation.

The high quality of pharmaceutical products are manufactured by following written procedures in carrying out operations. Raw materials must be characterized and purchased from reputable suppliers so that uniform, stable product could be prepared. Facilities must be designed, systems installed and the proper equipment selected to eliminate cross contamination of one product by another, the material flow and personnel movements are planned to reduce the potential for product mix-ups and the air and water should be adequate in amount and quality for the particular operations being performed.

Production personnel must be trained properly to perform their jobs, and the directions they follow must be written.

Shipping department are responsible for seeing that the products are protected from adverse handling and environmental conditions during transit.

Almost all drug substances dispensed in the oral solid-dosage form are stable under ordinary conditions. The essential qualities of a good compressed tablet are characterized by a number of specification given in the monographs. These specifications includes the appearance, size, shape, thickness, dissolution time, and disintegration time.

The appearance, size, shape, and thickness of the tablet are generally used to distinguish and identify the active ingredients which they contain. The remaining specifications assure that the products do not vary from allowable limits within the same lot or from one production lot to another. All such qualities of drugs and pharmaceuticals are designed to ensure a safe, therapeutically effective oral solid-dosage form.

Quality Control System

Quality control can be defined broadly as the regular control of quality within a company, a department staffed with scientists and technicians responsible for the acceptance or rejection of incoming raw materials and packaging components, for the myriad of in-process tests and inspections, to assure that systems are being controlled and monitored and, finally, for the approval or rejection of completed dosage forms.

Quality control, therefore, includes not only the analytical testing of the finished product, but also the assessment of all operations beginning with the receipt of raw materials and continuing throughout the production and packaging operations, finished product testing, documentation, surveillance and distillation.

Since a company produces the drugs, it should have main responsibility for quality results. Quality assurance must establish control points to monitor the quality of the product. The control points located during production process include raw materials, in-process, complete processing, packaging line, finished product, and stability monitoring.

The quality control system can vary in details, but not in principle, from company-to-company. It depends on the nature and size of the manufacturing facility and on the types of oral solid-dosage forms produced.

1. Good Manufacturing Practice (GMP) Requirements

Most of the governments issue regulations from time to time according to its own needs governing the manufacture, processing, packaging, and distribution of finished pharmaceuticals. The regulations extend into the area of finished pharmaceuticals, buildings, equipments, personnel, components, master production and control records, batch production, production and control procedures, product containers and their components, laboratory controls, distribution records, stability, expiration dating, and complaint files. Regulations for good manufacturing practices during drug manufacturing are aimed as assuring that only those tablets which have met the established specifications and are packed and labelled under proper controls are distributed for sale.

Specifications published in the official compendia are designed to assure a pharmaceutically elegant and therapeutically effective dosage form. The acceptable limits may vary due to special problems associated with the production of the particular tablet.

2. Environmental Control and Sanitation

To assure high standards of quality and purity of drugs, an effective sanitation program of an industry is required. The unit is protected from insects and rodents. Personal cleanliness, proper hair covering and clothing with appropriate pockets should be needed. Floors, walls, ceilings should be resistant to external forces, easily cleanable and in good repair. Adequate ventilation, proper temperature, and proper humidity are other important factors. Ventilation is usually designed to absorb and remove dust. Air filters, dust collectors and scrubbers to clean the air should be checked on a routine schedule. The water supply may be potable, distilled, or deionized and under adequate pressure to keep the water flowing clean.

Quality assurance must review and check, based on written procedures that specify the details of the testing procedures and schedules for sanitation, cleaning records, ventilation system and water system.

3. Manufacturing Working Formula Procedures

These procedures include documentation of the component materials, processing steps, production operation specifications and equipments to be used. A working formula procedure should be prepared for each batch size. Quality assurance must review and check the working formula procedures for each production batch before, during and after production operation for : signed and date of issuing person, proper identification, calculations of both active and inactive materials, re-assay dates, processing period, equipments to be used and proper labelling.

4. Raw Materials

Quality assurance must check the released raw material taken in the production department. Most raw materials are weighed in an environmental control weighing area where they are transferred to a secondary container properly labelled with a sticker bearing all the information of the original container label. Raw materials should be properly identified with name, dosage form, item number, lot number, weight and signatures.

The storage conditions of raw materials, particularly hygroscopic substances, are important. The drugs are contaminated by different type of foreign materials. Therefore, a suitable store or plant warehouse is an absolute necessity which should be inspected periodically for quality assurance.

Excessive microbial flora is usually associated with raw materials from natural sources, e.g., gum arabic and tragacanth.

Synthetic raw materials are normally free or low in microbial contamination.

Samples of raw materials should be collected in clean containers under disinfected and aseptic conditions for microbiological analysis or clean container and clean technique for analytical analysis. Samples should be labelled as to lot number, receiving number, supplier, container size and type, name of raw material, and date of receipt.

Chemical, physical, and biological characteristics of raw materials are determined for assuring reproductibility from batch - to - batch production. The test methods, and supplier's ability are established.

5. Manufacturing Equipment

Quality assurance must ensure that manufacturing equipment be designed, placed, and maintained to facilitate thorough cleaning, be suitable for its intended use, and minimize any contamination of drugs and their containers during manufacture. The equipments should be thoroughly cleaned to remove drug residues from the previous operations and maintained in accordance with specific written directions. Adequate records of procedures and tests should be maintained by quality assurance.

Prior to the start of any production step, the quality assurance personnel should ascertain that the proper equipment and tooling for each manufacturing stage are being used. Equipment must be identified by labels bearing the name, dosage form, item number, and lot number. Equipment used for special batch production should be completely separated in the production department and all dust - producing operations should be provided with adequate exhaust system.

Weighing and measuring equipments, e.g. disintegration apparatus, friability testers, and balances, should be calibrated and checked at suitable intervals by appropriate methods; records of such tests should be maintained by quality assurance.

6. Analytical Control

The Analytical Control Laboratory is responsible for testing and approving raw materials, work in-process and finished products. Laboratory most be staffed with trained persons to perform the complex analyses required to evaluate the acceptability of a product. Equipment is required to allow timely and accurate analysis.

Detailed specifications must be available. Good raw material specifications must be written in precise terminology. Details of test methods, type of instruments to use, manner of sampling, and proper identification should be provided. Raw material name includes structural formula, molecular weight, chemical name (s), item number, dates of issue and superseded and signature. Description, solubility, identity by specific chemical tests, IR and UV absorption, melting range, congealing and boiling points, and chromatographic techniques, purity and quality by general completeness of solutions, pH, specific rotation, nonvolatile residue, ash, acid-insoluble ash, residue on ignition, loss on drying, water content, heavy metals, arsenic, lead, mercury, selenium, sulphate, chloride, carbonates, acid value, iodine value, saponification value, special quality tests, particle size, crystallinity characters, polymorphic forms, special purity tests, ferric in ferrous salts, peroxides and aldehydes in ether and related degradation products, assay and microbial limits are mentioned under specifications.

7. Inspection Control

Sampling and inspection of incoming raw materials, packaging and labeling components, physical inspection of product at various intermediate stages, packaging line inspection and the control of shipping are the part of Inspection Control. Depending on the organizational structure, additional or different responsibilities will be assigned to this unit.

The manufacturer should physically inspect and assign lot numbers for all raw materials received. Each raw material is sampled according to standard sampling procedures and is sent to the quality control laboratory for testing. If acceptable, it is moved to the release storage area and properly labelled to indicate the item number, name of material, lot number, date of release, reassay date, and signature of a quality assurance inspector. The raw material is retested to assure that it still conforms to specifications at time of use. Quality assurance should reserve samples from active and inactive raw materials required to determine whether the material meets the established specification. These reserve samples should be retained for at least 5 years.

Any raw material not meeting specifications must be separated from the acceptable materials, labelled as rejected, and returned to the supplier or disposed of promptly. Generally the raw materials should be classified as active or therapeutic ingradients and as inactive, inert materials.

8. Sampling Procedure

The finished drug products should be inspected to assure the quality. The sample procedures used are variables sampling, switching procedures, for large lot sizes, the smaller sample size, etc.

Production control includes packaging carrying the name of the tablet product, item number, lot number, number of labels, inserts, operations to be performed, the quantity to be packaged, etc. Since labels may be spoiled during the packaging operation, a definite number in excess is issued.

Container is a device that holds the drug and is in direct contact with the drug. The immediate container remains in direct contact with the drug at all times. The container components should not interact physically or chemically with tablet product to alter the strength, quality or purity beyond the specified requirements. The specifications and test procedures mentioned are as well-closed, tightly-closed, and four different types of glass containers. The features to be considered in designing for containers according to specifications and test methods are : properties of container tightness; moisture and vapour tightness; toxicity, chemical and physical characteristics of materials needed in container preparation; physical or chemical changes of container upon prolonged contact with drug; and compatibility between container and tablet.

Plastics are generally used in rigid containers, and tablet packaging. Polyethylenes, polypropylenes, cellulose plastics, polystyrene and polyvinylchloride are the polymers used as plastics. The additives such as stabilizers, plasticizers, lubricants, colourants, fillers, impact modifiers and processing aids are added to most of the plastics. Polyethylene is one of the most thermally stable plastic which offers the best protection from breakage and is used for dry drug packaging. Drugs are protected from adverse moisture conditions by the use of a seal adhesive such as a synthetic resin and emulsion-based material.

Tamper-resistant package is used in blister package, strip package, bubble pack, foil pouches, bottle seals, shrink seals or bands and film wrapppers. Blister package provides users with convenience, pleasing appearance, and tamper resistance. It is composed of a semirigid thermoplastic resin blister filled with drugs in tablet form lided with a heat sealable backing material like aluminium foil.

9. Documentation

During the course of producing a pharmaceutical product, numerous documents and records are generated. Each batch is assigned a specific code or lot number which include data on each significant phase of production, control and distribution. The batch record provides a historical blueprint of every step, starting from the receipt of chemical raw materials and packaging components. Recording charts or computer printouts of significant operations such as autoclaving, drying, air-particulate monitoring, lyophilizing, etc; all are the part of the batch history. Each required document must be checked for completeness and accuracy. When the batch is released, accurate shipping records must be maintained.

10. New advances

Statistics and trend analysis are tools used to determine the proper sample size required for testing, for measuring the uniformity of solid dosage forms, etc. Electronic data processing is useful for assessing process and test parameters and for analyzing the data collected during production. The control of many operations by computers and microprocessors provides the capability for producing products of further improved uniform quality. Robotics is applied in pharmaceutical production, packaging and laboratory operations.

11. Drug Control Administration

In view of the importance of quality in the case of pharmaceutical products for the society, there are statutory legal provisions to ensure their quality. In India, this function is performed by the Drugs Standard Control Organisation of the Ministry of Health at the Centre and the Drug Control Administrations in different States. Although the Drug Control Administration at the Centre and the States have been in existence for a long time but still their strength and size is much too inadequate to enable them perform the functions expected of a progressive Drug Control Administration. The current status of the capabilities of Drug Control Administration in India is listed below :

Functions Capability

- Formulate drug laws to   Adequate
  regulate the usage of drugs

- Regulate the introduction and
  registration of new drugs
    - Herbal products   Inadequate
    - Modern drugs including
      Antibiotics & Biological   Adequate
    - Biotechnology based products   Inadequate
- Control pharmaceutical production
  to ensure observance of GMP   Inadequate
- Ensure the quality of marketed   Most
  drugs and drug surveillance   Inadequate

The reasons for the inadequacies of the drug control administration both at the Centre and in the States are listed below;

- Size of the directorates are very small and scientifically weak.
- Number of Drug Control testing laboratories are very few and very poorly equipped.
    - Most of the laboratories are not equipped to test biological products.
    - No testing laboratory established for biotechnology based products.
- Staff members inadequate to enforce/ensure observance of drug control laws.
- In most States there is not even one Drug Inspector per district.

15

IMPURITIES IN PHARMACEUTICALS

Chemical compounds manufactured on commercial scale contain different types of impurities, although the proportion of total impurities may be very small. These impurities include the raw materials, dust particles, moisture, etc.

The impurities commonly present in pharmaceutical preparations are of the following types :

 (i) Toxic impurities, e.g. lead and asrenic salts.

 (ii) Activity depressing impurities, e.g. presence of water in hard soap.

 (iii) Impurities due to which the substance becomes incompatible with other substances.

 (iv) Impurities causing technical difficulties in the use of the substance; e.g. presence of potassium iodate (KIO_3) in potassium iodide (KI) or presence of carbonate in solutions of ammonia.

 (v) Impurities due to colouring or flavouring substances, e.g. sodium salicylate is discoloured due to phenolic compounds; sodium chloride becomes damp due to the presence of magnesium salts.

 (vi) Impurities due to humidity, e.g. presence of traces of moisture may cause many substances to lose their free flowing qualities or they may be easily oxidizable.

 (vii) Impurities which change the physical and chemical properties of the substances and making them unfit for medicinal use.

 (viii) Impurities decreasing the shelf-life of a compound.

The pharmaceutical preparations should be free from toxic and other impurities. Pharmacopoeias prescribe limits for harmful compounds present in the substances.

In some cases, the impurities may add to the therapeutical value of substances, e.g. presence of traces of copper adds medicinal value of iron preparations which helps in the formation of haemoglobin due to its catalytic action.

SOURCES OF IMPURITIES

Following are the important sources of impurities in pharmaceutical preparations :

1. Raw Materials

Raw materials are usually present in final products as impurities from which the substances are prepared. For example, all sodium compounds may contain traces of chloride which are usually prepared from sodium chloride. In bismuth salts silver, copper and lead are present and these materials are used in the process of manufacture of bismuth.

Zinc metal contains arsenic, aluminium, copper, iron, magnesium, manganese and nickel as impurities. If these metals are present in trace amounts in the raw materials, e.g. zinc metal, then these impurities are added during production process in appreciable amounts to the final product like zinc sulphate. Copper may contain iron and arsenic as impurities which may be derived to the final products, e.g. copper sulphate.

2. Process used in the Manufacture

When a solvent reacts with the metallic container in which the reaction is carried out, traces of metallic impurities are added to the compound. The equipment used in the manufacturing process of drugs is constructed from glass, silica, earthenware, wood, rubber, silver, copper, lead, iron, steel, aluminium, nickel, tin and different alloys. Most of these metallic substances react with some organic compounds and mineral acids and contaminate the final products. The water and steam pipe may contain lead which is added in the drug. Sulphuric acid is manufactured by lead chamber process and when this acid is used, lead may be added as an impurity.

Tap water is used in different processes. It generally contains chloride, calcium and magnesium which may be added to the final products. Some specific impurities may be due to a particular process used in the manufacturing of some chemical compounds. For example, potassium iodide is manufactured from iodine which is obtained from a sea weed 'kelf. When nitrogenous organic matter is burnt with alkalies, cyanides are formed. Therefore, the pharmacopoeia prescribes a limit test for cyanide in potassium iodide.

If reagents used for the production of drugs are not removed completely by washing, they may be present in the final products as impurities. For example, ammoniated mercury is synthesized by reacting mercuric chloride ($HgCl_2$) with ammonia solution. If the precipitated ammoniated mercury is not washed properly to remove ammonium hydroxide, the end-product may contain ammonium hydroxide as impurity. Similarly, calcium carbonate should be washed to remove excess of sodium carbonate and sodium chloride.

Sometimes intermediate products may be added to the final products. For example, potassium is synthesized by treating potassium hydroxide with iodine. The resulting mixture is evaporated to dryness and the residue heated with charcoal to yield potassium iodide and carbon monoxide. Sometimes the intermediate products, potassium iodate, is not completely converted into potassium iodide and may be present in the final product as impurity.

$$6KOH + 3I_2 \longrightarrow 5KI + KIO_3 + 2H_2O$$
$$KIO_3 + 3C \longrightarrow KI + CO$$

Improper concentration of reactants and incomplete reactions may produce compounds containing impurities. For example, if calcium carbonate is not completely reacted with hydrochloric acid during preparation of calcium chloride due to imperfect combination, then any unreacted substance will be in the final product. Similarly, zinc metal is not completely converted into the zinc oxide when it is burnt in the presence of oxygen. Therefore, a small amount of zinc metal may be present in the final product.

Atmospheric impurities, e.g. dust particles containing aluminium oxide, silica glass, porcelain and plastic particles, sulphur dioxide, hydrogen sulphide and black smoke may be added as impurities to the product during manufacturing process. Sodium hydroxide readily absorbs carbon dioxide from the atmosphere producing sodium carbonate.

$$2NaOH + CO_2 \longrightarrow Na_2CO_3 + H_2O$$

3. Impurities Due to Storage Conditions

Storage conditions affect the stability of every drug. If a drug is not stored properly, its deterioration takes place due to which impurities in the drug are added and all types of properties changed. These changes may affect the therapeutic values of a medicament or increase its toxicity. Environmental conditions such as temperature, atmospheric gases, moisture contents, light and microorganisms are the worst enemy of drugs. Certain chemical reactions always take place inside the drug molecules whether it is in tablet, powder, syrup or liquid form. Chemical reactions tend to take place more rapidly in liquid system than in the dry state. Therefore, solutions are less stable than suspensions which in turn are less stable than solid dosage forms. Most of the drugs have a tendency to deteriorate.

The most common decomposition reactions in medical products are oxidation and phytochemical reactions proceeded by absorption of light by the molecules. Atmospheric oxygen can initiate oxidation of a medicament even present in low concentration. Such reactions are catalyzed by traces of metals and ultraviolet radiation from light sources. Chloroform, ether, volatile oils, fats, vitamin A, vitamin C, vitamin D, and many other organic drugs are deteriorated by the action of oxygen. The photo-oxidation of tablet coatings is particularly important to the pharmaceutical industries.

Ferrous sulphate is converted into insoluble ferric oxide by air and moisture. Surgical solution of chlorinated soda rapidly deteriorates when exposed to light and heat. Solution of potassium hydroxide absorbs atmospheric carbon dioxide and exerts a solvent action on lead containing glass. Therefore, it should be preserved in lead-free air-tight bottles of green glass. Ether and chloroform decompose in the presence of air and light.

Iodine reacts with rubber corks and some metals, Therefore, it should be preserved in glass bottles fitted with glass stoppers. Iodine may contain metals or rubber as impurities with which it reacts. Potassium iodide is liquified in the presence of moist air for long time. Similarly, potassium and sodium hydroxides and calcium chloride absorb moisture from the atmosphere.

All chemicals should be stored in well-closed containers made of metal or dark glass and extremes of temperatures are avoided, as inorganic are not much effected by ordinary temperatures. Sunlight does not influence many inorganic compounds.

solvents, determination of melting points, boiling points, optical rotation, refractive index, viscosity for liquids, specific gravity, freezing point, weight per ml, specific gravity, chromatographic behaviour, e.g. Rf values and retention time, photometric determinations, e.g. colourimetry, nephelometry, flame photometry, spectrophotometry, e.g. ultra-violet, infra-red, nuclear magnetic resonance (NMR), electron skin resonance (ESR), mass spectra, etc. Quantitative determination of acid, esterification, hydroxyl, acetyl, ester, iodine and saponification values for vegetable oils helps to find out quality of vegetable oils. Some other parameters for determination of purity are swelling powder (e.g. bentonite), soluble matter (kaoline), adsorption power (kaolin), fine particles (light kaolin), coarse particles (light kaolin and bentonites), setting properties (plaster of paris) and stability of solution (sodium antimony gluconate).

3. **Acidity, Alkalinity and pH :** When a compound is synthesized using acids and alkalies, then some amount of the acid or alkali may be present as an impurity. Aqueous solutions of many substances have an specific pH value and any change in the pH value indicates the presence of impurity.

4. **Insoluble Residue :** A compound may be completely soluble in a given amount of a solvent at a specific temperature. If insoluble ingredients are present, the solution becomes turbid or opalescence. These insoluble matters are separated by filtration and their amount can be determined by weighing the dried filter paper.

5. **Anions and Cations :** Certain anions or cations are added to a pharmaceutical compound by adsorption and co-precipitation. Chloride, sulphate, iron, lead, arsenic, heavy metals, ammonium, etc. are the general impurities. General quantitative or limit tests with necessary variation are given in individual monograph. For other anion or cation special tests are prescribed.

6. **Ash Value :** Ash value is determined by igniting crude vegetable drugs, organic compounds, and some inorganic compounds to a constant weight. In some cases water-insoluble ash, hydrochloric-insoluble ash and sulphuric acid-insoluble ash are determined. The ash contains impurities such as chloride, sulphate, iron, heavy metals, lead, etc.

7. **Loss on Drying and Ignition :** Certain compounds are

dried or ignited on a specific temperature and then loss in weight is determined. The weight of water is found out by drying the substance.

8. **Organic and Carbonisable Substances :** Purity of some specified substances is also determined by separating, drying and weighing organic compounds and readily carbonisable substances as mentioned in the monographs.

9. **Assay :** Assay is the chemical determination of a compound to assess whether it conforms to the prescribed standard or not. The common assay procedures include gravimetric, volumetric, gasometric, photometric, alkaloidal, radiochemical, radio-immuno, esterification methods, etc.

Gravimetric methods are based on the quantitative transformation of substances into a definite chemical compound by a suitable chemical reaction. The product is separated in pure state and weighed. The methods involved in the gravimetric analysis are precipitation, volatilization, adsorption, extraction, fractional distillation, filtration, washing, drying or ignition, weighing and repeated drying or ignition till constant weight. Magnesium sulphate, zinc sulphate and bismuth oxychloride are compounds estimated gravimetrically.

Volumetric methods are based on titrimetric and gas-methods. Titration methods involve the determination of the volume of a standard solution (titrant) required to react quantitatively with a solution of the substance to be analyzed (titrate) to get an end point. The various titrimetric methods involved are :

1. Acidimetry and alkalimetry for sodium bicarbonate, ammoniated mercury, ammonium chloride and boric acid.

2. Oxidation reduction (redox) titrations for potassium permanganate, sodium oxalate, hydrogen peroxide, ferrous sulphate, and antimony potassium tartrate.

3. Iodometric and iodimetric titrations for copper sulphate, chlorinated lime and iodine.

4. Precipitation type for sodium chloride, ammonium chloride and yellow mercuric oxide.

5. Complexometric type carried out with ethylenediamine tetra-acetate for calcium gluconate, magnesium sulphate and zinc sulphate.

6. Diazotization (nitrite) titration and

7. Non-aqueous titration.

16

LIMIT TESTS

In limit tests opalescence, turbidity or colour is compared with the fixed standards as prescribed in the pharmacopoeias. The extent of opalescence, turbidity and colour is affected by the presence of other impurities present in the substance, variation in time and method of performance of the tests. Therefore, no numerical values for the limits in these tests are prescribed in the pharmacopoeias. Generally an aqueous solution of the substance is prepared. Sometimes a solution of the substance is prepared by dissolving in an acid, or if the solution is alkaline, it is neutralized with nitric or hydrochloric acid.

LIMIT TEST FOR ARSENIC

In the limit test for arsenic, the amount of arsenic present is expressed as arsenic, As.

Basis of the Test : The pharmacopoeial test of arsenic, which is a toxic component in medicinal substances, is based on the fact that arsenic in the arsenious state can be readily reduced to arsine (AsH_3) gas which passing over mercuric chloride paper develops a yellow to brown stain, the intensity and length of which are proportional to the amount of arsenic. A standard stain, prepared from a definite amount of arsenic, expresses the limit. Reduction of the arsenic to arsine, both in the sample and the standard, is done by the combined action of zinc, acid, stannous chloride and potassium iodide. The arsine is carried over along with hydrogen to the mercuric chloride or bromide paper supported in the test apparatus. The rate of evolution of hydrogen is controlled which is dependent on the quantity and surface area of zinc, concentration of hydrochloric acid, salt in the reaction mixture, temperature and dimension of the apparatus. Rapid evolution produces a long and diffuse stain while a short and intense colour is developed by a slow evolution.

Chemically, the arsenic impurity is converted in acidic medium into arsenious acid or arsenic acid depending upon the valency state of arsenic :

$$As^{3+} \longrightarrow As(OH)_3 \text{ or } H_3AsO_3$$
$$\text{Trivalent} \qquad \text{Arsenious acid}$$

$$As^{5+} \longrightarrow O = As(OH)_3 \text{ or } H_3AsO_4$$
$$\text{Pentavalent} \qquad \text{Arsenic acid}$$

This solution is reacted with a reducing agent like stannous chloride or sulphurous acid to convert the pentavalent arsenic acid into the trivalent arsenious acid which is converted into gaseous arsenious hydride (arsine gas) with the help of nascent hydrogen produced by the action of zinc with hydrochloric acid.

$$H_3AsO_4 \longrightarrow H_3AsO_3 \xrightarrow[3H]{Zn + HCl} AsH_3 + 3H_2O$$
$$\text{Arsenic} \qquad \text{Arsenious} \qquad \text{Arsine}$$
$$\text{acid} \qquad \text{acid} \qquad \text{gas}$$

Arsine gas is carried out through the tube with the help of hydrogen to the mercuric chloride paper. Reaction of arsine with mercuric chloride produces a yellow coloured stain. The intensity of the colour is dependent on the quantity of arsenic.

$$2AsH_3 + HgCl_2 \longrightarrow Hg\begin{cases} AsH_2 \\ AsH_2 \end{cases} + 2HCl$$
$$\text{Yellow}$$

Apparatus

A wide-mouthed flask or bottle capable of holding about 120 ml is fitted with a rubber bung through which passes a glass tube. The latter, made from ordinary glass tubing, has a total length of 200 mm and an internal diameter of exactly 6.5 mm (external diameter about 8 mm). It is drawn out at one end to a diameter of about 1 mm and a hole not less than 2mm in diameter is blown in the side of the tube, near the constricted part. When the bung is inserted in the bottle containing 70 ml of liquid, the constricted end of the tube is above the surface of the liquid, and the hole in the side is below the bottom of the bung. The upper end of the tube is cut off square, and is either slightly rounded or ground smooth.

Two rubber bungs (about 25 mm × 25 mm), each with a hole bored centrally and tube, exactly 6.5 mm in diameter, are fitted with a rubber band or spring clip for holding them tightly together. Alternatively the two bungs may be replaced by any suitable contrivance satisfying the conditions.

During the test, the liberated gases pass through the side hole; the lower hole acts as an exit for water which condenses in the tube.

General Method of Testing

By a variable method of procedure, suitable to the particular needs of each substance, a solution is prepared from the substance being examined which may or may not contain that substance, but contains the whole of the arsenic (if any) originally present in that substance. This solution, referred to as the 'test solution', is used in the actual test.

General Test : The glass tube is lightly packed with cotton wool, previously moistened with *lead acetate solution* and dried, so that the upper surface of the cotton wool is not less than 25mm below the top of the tube. The upper end of the tube is then inserted into the narrow end of one of the pair of rubber bungs, either to a depth of about 10 mm when the tube has a rounded off end, or so that the ground end of the tube is flush with the larger end of the bung. A piece of *mercuric chloride paper* is placed flat on the top of the bung and the other bung placed over it and secured by means of the rubber band or spring clip in such a manner that the borings of the two bungs (or the upper bung and the glass tube) meet to form a true tube 6.5 m in diameter interrupted by a diaphragm of *mercuric chloride paper*.

Instead of this method of attaching the *mercuric chloride paper*, any other method may be used provided (i) that the whole of the evolved gas passes through the paper; (ii) that the portion of the paper in contact with the gas is a circle 6.5 mm in diameter; and (iii) that the paper is protected from sunlight during the test. Thé test solution prepared as specified, is placed in the wide-mouthed bottle, 1 g of *potassium iodide AsT* and 10 g of *zinc AsT* are added, and the prepared glass tube is placed quickly in position. The action is allowed to proceed for forty minutes. The yellow stain which is produced on the *mercuric chloride paper* if arsenic is present is compared by daylight with the *standard stains* produced by operating in a similar manner with known quantities of *dilute arsenic solution AsT*. The comparison of the stains is made immediately at the completion of the test. The *standard stains* used for comparison are freshly prepared; they fade on keeping.

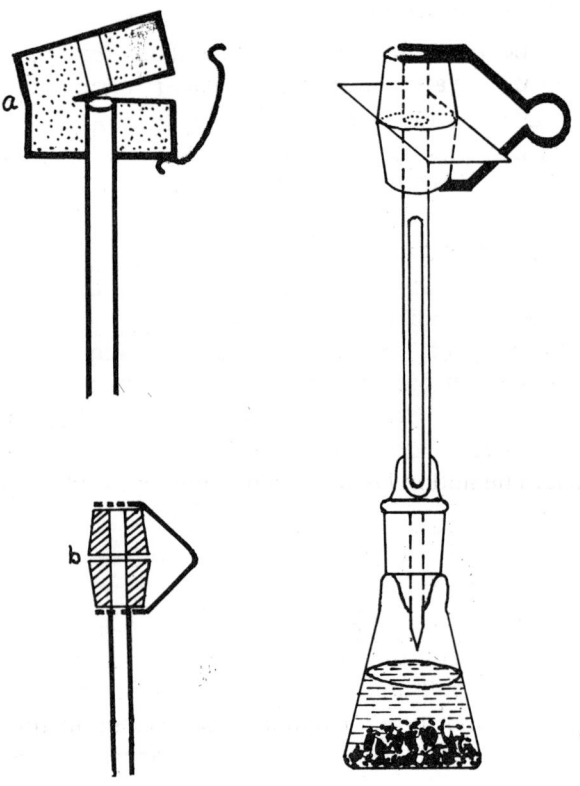

Fig. 16.1 : Regular arsenic apparatus with alternate devices (a) and (b) for fixing mercuric chloride paper.

By matching the depth of colour with *standard stains*, the proportion of arsenic in the substance may be determined. A stain equivalent to the 1-ml *standard stain* produced by operating on 10 g a substance indicates that the proportion of arsenic is 1 part per million.

Notes

1. The action may be accelerated by placing the apparatus on

a warm surface, care being taken that the mercuric chloride paper remains dry throughout the test.

2. The most suitable temperature for carrying out the test is generally about 40°, but because the rate of evolution of the gas varies somewhat with different batches of zinc AsT, the temperature may be adjusted to obtain a regular, but not violent, evolution of gas.

3. The tube must be washed with hydrochloric acid AsT, rinsed with water, and dried between successive tests.

4. The stains may be preserved by dipping in hot melted paraffin or placing over phosphorus pentoxide protected from light. Potassium iodide blackens the stains and makes the comparison easier.

5. Lead acetate papers are used to trap any hydrogen sulphide evolved together with arsine. Hydrogen sulphide reacts with mercuric chloride paper developing a dark stain, thus interfering with the formation of the required mercuric arsenide stain. Metallic zinc may contain traces of sulphide which on reaction with the acid yields hydrogen sulphide.

6. Stannous chloride is required for the complete evolution of arsine. The action between pure zinc and hydrochloric acid is slow and the presence of other metals accelerates the formation of hydrogen. Stannous salts reduce arsenic to arsenious state.

Standard Stains : Solutions are prepared by adding to 50 ml of *water*, 10 ml of *stannated hydrochloric acid AsT* and quantities of *dilute arsenics solution AsT* varying from 0.2 ml to 1 ml. The resulting solutions, *when treated as described in the* **General test**, yield stains on the *mercuric chloride paper* referred to as the standard stains.

Preparation of the Test Solution

In the various methods of preparing the test solution, the quantities are so arranged, unless otherwise stated, that when the stain produced from the solution to be examined is not deeper than the 1-ml standard stain, the proportion of arsenic present does not exceed the permitted limit.

MODIFICATION OF THE GENERAL TESTING METHOD

Some substances require special treatment for performing limit test for arsenic. All the arsenic present in the sample should be present in the final solution in a readily reducible form and the interfering substances should be removed from test sample.

Carbonates, Hydroxides and Oxides

Treatment of carbonates with hydrochloric acid produces carbon dioxide and some hydrochloric acid gas with effervescence and the reaction is exothermic. Oxides and hydroxides on treatment with hydrochloric acid form hydrogen gas with effervescence and evolution of heat. Arsenious chloride $(AsCl_3)$ is evolved with hydrochloric acid. If a sample of these substances is treated with hydrochloric acid as such, a part of arsenic may be lost as $AsCl_3$. Therefore, carbonates, oxides and hydroxides are first treated with excess of brominated hydrochloric acid. The bromine oxidizes arsenious to arsenic to the pentavalent form which is not volatile with hydrochloric acid. To perform the test, the arsenic should again be reduced to arsenious state by removing excess of bromine with a few drops of stannous chloride solution.

Sodium Carbonate, Anhydrous, AsT : *Anhydrous sodium carbonate* which complies with the following additional test :

5 g are dissolved in 50 ml of water, 20 ml of brominated hydrochloric acid AsT are added; the excess of bromine is removed with a few drops of **Stannous chloride solution AsT,** and the **General test** applied; no visible stain is produced.

Organic Compounds

Most of the organic compounds are insoluble in acid and in water. When gas is evolved in the liquid containing such compounds, undesirable frothing occurs. Therefore, any interfering organic compound should be removed by igniting with anhydrous sodium carbonate before performing the test. Some organic compounds are destroyed by wet oxidation with nitric and sulphuric acids.

Ammonium Oxalate AsT : Ammonium oxalate which complies with the following additional test:

5 g are heated with 15 ml of water, 5 ml of nitric acid AsT, and 10 ml of sulphuric acid AsT in a narrow-necked, round-bottomed flask until frothing ceases, cooled and the General test is applied; no visible stain is produced.

Nitric Acid and Nitrates

Nitric acid and nitrates prevent the reduction of arsenic which are removed by heating the substance with concentrated sulphuric acid and evaporating nitric acid off. Arsenic is left in the sulphuric acid. The remaining traces of nitric acid are removed by diluting residual sulphuric acid with water and re-evaporating the mixture. Now the nitrosyl sulphuric acid formed during first evaporation is decomposed and the sulphuric acid becomes free from nitric acid. Solution of ferric chloride also contains some nitric acid which is also removed by the similar treatment.

Nitric Acid AsT : Nitric acid which complies with the following additional test :

20 ml are heated in a porcelain dish with 2 ml of sulphuric acid AsT until white fumes are given off. It is cooled, 2 ml of water are added and again heated until white fumes are given off; cooled 50 ml of water and 10 ml of stannated hydrochloric acid AsT added and the General test is applied; no visible stain is produced.

Boric Acid and Borax

Boric acid is slightly soluble in hydrochloric acid, but it is dissolved along with citric acid. Borax is converted into boric acid on treatment with hydrochloric acid. Therefore, citric acid is added to dissolve boric acid and borax before addition of stannated hydrochloric acid.

Ammonia Solution

Solutions are heated on a water bath to remove the free ammonia. Arsenic is left as ammonium arsenate and arsenite in the solutions which are acidified with brominated hydrochloric acid and stannous chloride is added.

Liquid Glucose and Potassium Acid Tartrate

Liquid glucose often contains traces of sulphur dioxide as preservative while sulphites are present in potassium acid tartrate. These substances are treated with brominated hydrochloric acid to oxidize the sulphurous acid. Excess of bromine is removed by adding few drops of stannous chloride solution.

Hypophosphorus Acid

Reduction of hypophosphorus acid yields phosphine which interacts with mercuric halide papers. Hence, it is oxidized to phosphoric acid by treating with potassium chlorate and hydrochloric acid. Excess of chlorine formed by the reaction of chlorate and hydrochloric acid is removed by boiling and then by treating with stannous chloride.

Oxidizing Agents

The oxidizing agents such as potassium chlorate should be completely reduced, otherwise, whole of the hydrogen will be utilized to reduce the substance and arsine would not be evolved.

Potassium Chlorate AsT : Potassium chlorate which complies with the following additional test :

5 g are mixed in the cold with 20 ml of water and 22 ml of hydrochloric acid AsT are added; when the first reaction has subsided, heated gently to expel chlorine, the last traces removed with a few drops of stannous chloride solution AsT, 20 ml of water added, and the General test applied; no visible stain is produced.

Compounds of Copper, Bismuth, Antimony and Iron

Copper deposits on zinc forming a zinc-copper mixture which interfere in the steady evolution of hydrogen and all the arsenic will not convert into arsine. Bismuth deposits on zinc forming a solid sponge-like mass preventing evolution of hydrogen. Antimony compounds form antimony hydride with nascent hydrogen which produces a dark stain on mercuric chloride paper interfering with the stain developed due to arsine. Iron also reduces the rate of evolution of hydrogen and arsenic is not reduced completely to arsine:

Copper, bismuth and iron salts are treated with dilute hydrochloric acid (20%) and distilled. Whole of the arsenic present in the substance distils in the first 75% of distillate. Sufficient stannous chloride is added to reduce ferric salts to ferrous state.

A double distillation is required to perform the test of antimony compounds since antimony is slightly volatile in hydrochloric acid.

Sulphur

Sulphur is present as arsenic sulphide which is soluble in ammonium sulphide and ammonia. Therefore, sulphur is digested with ammonia to form ammonium polysulphides in which arsenic sulphide is soluble. The mixture is filtered to separate undissolved sulphur and the filtrate dried. The residue containing arsenic and some sulphur is treated with anhydrous sodium carbonate and water. Sodium polysulphide is formed in which arsenic sulphide is soluble. The solution is boiled and bromine added to oxidize arsenic to arsenate and sulphide to sulphate. The solution is acidified, boiled and treated with stannous chloride to perform the general test. ⎯

The other test solutions are prepared as described following

Bromine Solution AsT : Bromine (30 g) and potassium bromic˙ (30 g) are dissolved in water (sufficient to produce 10 ml). Tₓ solution complies with the following test:

10 ml are evaporated on a water-bath nearly to dryness, ſ ml of water, 10 ml of hydrochloric acid AsT and sufficient stannous chloride solution AsT are added to reduce the remaining bromine and the **General test** is applied; the stain produced is not deeper than a 1-ml standard stain, showing that the proportion of arsenic present does not exceed 1 part per million.

Potassium Iodide AsT : Potassium iodide which complies with the following additional test :

10 g are dissolved in 25 ml of hydrochloric acid AsT and 35 ml of water, 2 drops of stannous chloride solution AsT added; and the **General test** is applied; no visible stain is produced.

Citric Acid AsT : Citric acid which complies with the following additional test : 10 g are dissolved in 50 ml of water, 10 ml of stannated hydrochloric acid AsT added and the **General test** is applied, no visible stain is produced.

Hydrochloric Acid AsT : Hydrochloric acid diluted with water to contain about 32 per cent w/w of HCl and complying with the following additional tests :

(i) 10 ml are diluted with sufficient water to produce 50 ml, 5 ml of ammonium thiocyanate solution added and stirred immediately; no colour is produced.

(ii) To 50 ml, 0.2 ml of bromine solution AsT is added, evaporated on a water-bath until reduced to 16 ml, adding more bromine solution AsT, if necessary, in order that an excess, as indicated by the colour, may be present throughout the evaporation; 50 ml of water and 5 drops of stannous chloride solution AsT are added and the **General test** is applied; the stain produced is not deeper than a 0.2 mˡ standard stain prepared with the same acid, showing that the proportion of arsenic present does not exceed 0.05 part per million.

Hydrochloric Acid (constant-boiling composition) AsT : Hydrochloric acid AsT is heated to constant boiling composition in the presence of hydrazine hydrate, using 1 ml of a 10 per cent w/v solution in water per litre of the acid.

Mercuric Chloride Paper : Smooth white filter paper, not less than 25 mm in width, soaked in a saturated solution of mercuric chloride, pressed to remove superfluous solution, and dried at about 60° in the dark. The grade of the filter paper is such that the weight is between 65 and 120 g per sq. mm; the thickness in mm. of 400 papers is approximately equal, numerically, to the weight in g per sq. m.

Note : Mercuric chloride paper should be stored in a stoppered bottle in the dark. Paper which has been exposed to sunlight or to the vapour of ammonia affords a lighter stain or no stain at all when employed in the limit test for arsenic.

Stannated Hydrochloric Acid AsT

Stannous chloride solution AsT	1 ml
Hydrochloric acid AsT	100 ml

Stannous Chloride Solution AsT : Prepared from stannous chloride solution by adding an equal volume of hydrochloric acid, boiling down to the original volume, and filtering through a fine-grain filter paper.

It Complies with the following Test :

To 10 ml, 6 ml of water and 10 ml of hydrochloric acid AsT are added, distilled and collected 16 ml. To the distillate 50 ml of water and 2 drops of stannous chloride solution AsT are added and the **General test** is applied; the stain produced is not deeper than a 1 ml standard stain, showing that the proportion of arsenic present does not exceed 1 part per million.

Sulphuric Acid AsT : Sulphuric acid which complies with the following additional test :

10 g are diluted with 50 ml of water, 0.2 ml of stannous chloride solution AsT is added and the **General test** applied; no visible stain is produced.

Zinc AsT : Granulated zinc which complies with the following additional tests :

Stannated hydrochloric acid AsT (10 ml) is added to 50 ml of water, and the **General test** applied, using 10 g of the zinc and allowing the action to continue for one hour; no visible stain is produced (limit of arsenic). The test is repeated with the addition of 0.1 ml of dilute arsenic solution AsT; a faint but distinct yellow stain is produced (test for sensitivity).

LIMIT TEST FOR LEAD

Lead is a toxic substance present in pharmaceutical preparations. The main sources of this impurity are sulphuric acid and the lead apparatus. The I.P. and U.S.P. method is based on the reaction between lead and dithizone (diphenylthiocarbazone). In chloroform solution dithizone extracts lead from an alkaline aqueous solution as lead dithizone which has red colour in chloroform solution. Since dithizone itself imparts a green colour in chloroform, the resultant colour of dithizone and lead dithizone is violet. The colour produced by a given amount of the sample is compared with that produced by a known volume of a standard solution of lead. If the colour is intense than that produced by the standard, it contains lead in excess of the prescribed limit. For the test, the lead present as impurity is separated by extracting an alkaline solution of the substance with dithizone extraction solution which removes all the lead in the form of its complex in chloroform layer.

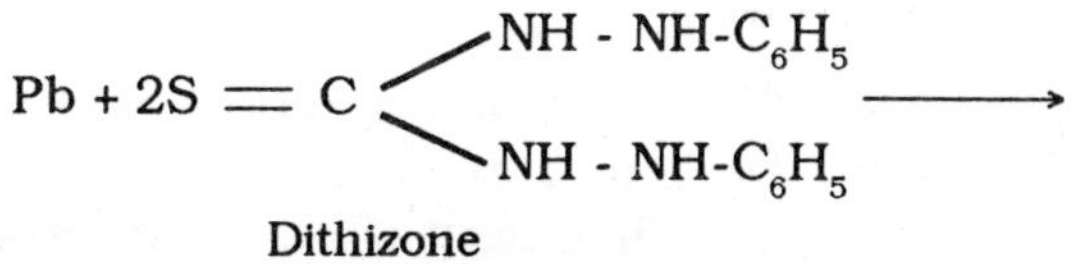

$$Pb + 2S = C \Big\langle \begin{matrix} NH\text{-}NH\text{-}C_6H_5 \\ NH\text{-}NH\text{-}C_6H_5 \end{matrix} \longrightarrow$$

Dithizone

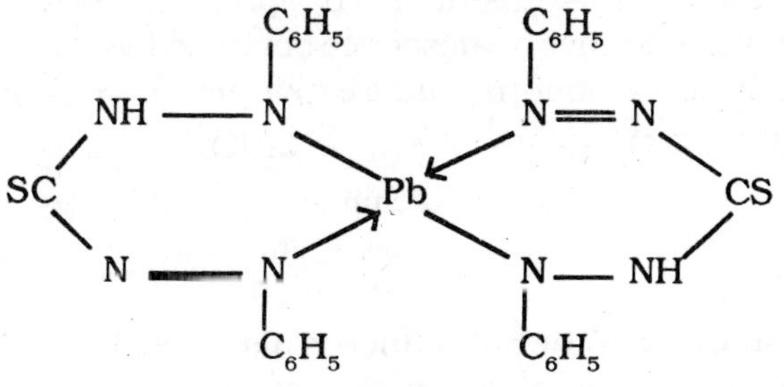

Lead dithizonate

Method

The volume of the prepared sample in a separator is transferred and unless otherwise directed in monograph, 6 ml of ammonium citrate solution Sp., and 2 ml of hydroxylamine hydrochloride solution Sp. are added (For the determination of lead in iron salts use 10 ml of ammonium citrate solution Sp.). Two drops of phenol red solutin are added and the solution made just alkaline (red in colour) by the addition of strong ammonia solution. The solution is cooled, if necessary, and 2 ml of potassium cyanide solution Sp. are added. Immediately the solution is extracted with several quantities, each of 5 ml, of dithizone extraction solution, draining off each extract into another separating funnel, until the dithizone extraction solution retains its green colour. The combined dithizone solutions are shaken for 30 seconds with 30 ml of a 1 per cent w/v solution of nitric acid and the chloroform layer discarded. To the acid solution exactly 5 ml of standard dithizone solution and 4 ml of ammonia-cyanide solution Sp. are added and shaken for 30 seconds; the colour of the chloroform layer is of no deeper shade of violet than that of a control made with a volume of dilute standard lead solution equivalent to the amount of lead permitted in the sample under examination.

All reagents used for the test should have as low a content of lead as practicable. All reagent solutions should be stored in containers of borosilicate glass. Glassware should be rinsed thoroughly with warm dilute nitric acid, followed by water.

LIMIT TEST FOR CHLORIDES

This test involves the reaction of silver nitrate with soluble chlorides to form the precipitate of silver chloride which is insoluble in dilute nitric acid. The extent of precipitation depends upon the amount of silver chloride formed, i.e. on the amount of chloride ions present in the substance. The opalescence produced is compared with a reference opalescence obtained by a standard silver nitrate solution, under the same experimental conditions.

$$NaCl + AgNO_3 \longrightarrow AgCl\downarrow + NaNO_3$$
$$\text{Precipitate}$$

Method

The specified quantity of the substance is dissolved in water, or a solution prepared as directed in the text and transfer to a Nessler cylinder. To it 10 ml of dilute nitric acid is added, except when nitric acid is used in the preparation of the solution, diluted to 50 ml with water, and 1 ml of silver nitrate solution added. It is stirred immediately with a glass rod and allowed to stand for 5 minutes. The opalescence produced is not greater than the standard opalescence, when viewed transversely.

Standard Opalescence

1.0 ml of a 0.05845 per cent w/v solution of sodium chloride and 10 ml of dilute nitric acid are placed in a Nessler cylinder. It is diluted to 50 ml with water and 1 ml of silver nitrate solution added. It is stirred immediately with a glass rod and allowed to stand for five minutes.

LIMIT TEST FOR SULPHATES

Limit test for sulphates is based on the reaction between barium chloride and soluble sulphate in the presence of dilute hydrochloric acid. The turbidity formed by a given amount of the sample is compared with a reference turbidity obtained from an authentic amount of the sulphate under the same experimental conditions.

$$BaCl_2 + Na_2SO_4 \longrightarrow BaSO_4\downarrow + 2NaCl$$
Precipitate

Reagents

Barium Sulphate Reagent : 15 ml of 0.5 M barium chloride, 55 ml of water, and 20 ml of sulphate-free alcohol are mixed, 5 ml of a 0.0181 per cent w/v solution of potssium sulphate are added, diluted to 100 ml with water, and mixed. Barium Sulphate Reagent must be freshly prepared.

0.5 M Barium Chloride : Barium chloride dissolved in water to contain in 1000 ml 122.1 g of $BaCl_2$, $2H_2O$.

Method

The specified quantity of the substance is dissolved in water or a solution is prepared as directed in the text, transferred to a Nessler cylinder, and 2 ml of dilute hydrochloric acid are added, except where hydrochloric acid is used in the preparation of the solution. It is diluted to 45 ml with water; 5 ml of barium sulphate reagent are added, stirred immediately with a glass rod, and allowed to stand for five minutes. The turbidity produced is not greater than the standard turbidity, when viewed transversely.

Standard Turbidity : 1.0 ml of a 0.1089 per cent w/v solution of potassium sulphate and 2 ml of dilute hydrochloric acid are placed in a Nessler cylinder, diluted to 45 ml with water, 5 ml of barium sulphate reagent added, stirred immediately with a glass rod, and allowed to stand for five minutes.

LIMIT TEST FOR IRON

The limit test for iron depends on the reaction of iron in ammoniacal solution in the presence of citric acid, with thioglycollic acid to obtain a pale pink to deep reddish purple colour. Citric acid forms a complex with iron which is not precipitated by ammonia. The colour is obtained due to formation of a ferrous salt, Fe $(S.CH_2COO^-)_2$, which disappears in air due to oxidation.

Thioglycollic acid, $HS.CH_2COOH$, is a sulphur derivative of glycollic acid, $CH_2(OH)COOH$. It is a colourless liquid with unpleasant odour. The colour produced from a known amount of the substance is compared with the standard colour obtained from a known amount of iron under the same experimental conditions.

$$2HSCH_2COOH + Fe^{3+} \longrightarrow Fe(HSCH_2COO)_2 + 2H^+$$

Standard Iron Solution : Accurately 0.1726 g of ferric ammonium sulphate is weighed and dissolved in 10 ml of 0.1N sulphuric acid and sufficient water to produce 1000.0 ml. Each ml of this solution contains 0.02 mg of Fe.

Method

The specified quantity of the substance being examined is dissolved in 40 ml of water, or 10 ml of the solution prescribed in the monograph used and transfered to a Nessler cylinder. 2 ml of a 20 per cent w/v solution of iron-free citric acid and 0.1 ml of thioglycollic acid are added, mixed, made alkaline with iron-free ammonia solution, diluted to 50 ml with water and allowed to stand for five minutes. Any colour produced is not more intense than the standard colour.

Standard colour : Standard iron solution is diluted with 40 ml of water in a Nessler cylinder. 2 ml of a 20 per cent w/v solution of iron-free citric acid and 0.1 ml of thioglycollic acid are added, mixed, made alkaline with iron-free ammonia solution, diluted to 50 ml with water and allowed to stand for five minutes.

LIMIT TEST FOR HEAVY METALS

The test for heavy metals is designed to determine the content of metallic impurities that are coloured by sulphide ion, under specified conditions. The limit for heavy metals is indicated in the individual monographs in terms of the parts of lead per million parts of the substance (by weight), as determined by visual comparison of the colour produced by the substance with that of a control prepared from a standard lead solution.

The amount of heavy metals is determined by one of the following methods and as directed in the individual monograph: Mothod A is used for substances that yield clear, colourless solutions under the specified test condition. Method B is used for substances that do not yield clear, colourless solutions under the test conditions specified for Method A, or for substances which, by virtue of their complex nature, interfere with the precipitation of metals by sulphide ion. Method C is used for substances that yield clear, colourless solutions with sodium hydroxide solution.

Method A

Standard Solution : Into a 50 ml Nessler cylinder, 2 ml of standard lead solution are pipetted and diluted with water to 25 ml, adjusted with dilute acetic acid Sp. or dilute ammonia solution Sp. to a pH between 3.0 and 4.0, diluted with water to about 35 ml, and mixed.

Test Solution : Into a 50 ml Nessler cylinder, 25 ml of the solution are prepared, adjusted with dilute acetic acid Sp. or dilute ammonia solution Sp. to a pH between 3.0 and 4.0, diluted with water to about 35 ml and mixed.

Procedure : To each of the cylinders containing the standard solution and test solution respectively, 10 ml of freshly prepared hydrogen sulphide solution are added mixed, diluted with water to 50 ml, allowed to stand for five minutes, and viewed downwards over a white surface; the colour produced in the test solution is not darker than that produced in the standard solution.

Method B

Standard Solution : Proceed as directed under Method A.

Test Solution : In a suitable crucible the quantity of the substance is weighed, sufficient sulphuric acid Sp. added to wet the sample, and ignited carefully at a low temperature until thoroughly charred. To the charred mass 2 ml of nitric acid Sp.

and five drops of sulphuric acid Sp. are added; heated cautiously until white fumes are no longer evolved, ignited preferably in a muffle furnace, at 500° to 600°, until the carbon is completely burnt off. It is cool, 4 ml of hydrochloric acid Sp. are added, covered, digested on a water-bath for 15 minutes, uncovered and slowly evaporated to dryness on a water-bath. The residue is moistened with one drop of hydrochloric acid Sp., 10 ml of hot water are added and digested for two minutes. Ammonia solution Sp. is added dropwise, until the solution is just alkaline to litmus paper, diluted with water to 25 ml and adjusted with dilute acetic acid SP. to a pH between 3.0 and 4.0. It is filtered, if necessary, the crucible rinsed and filtered with 10 ml of water, the filtrate and washings combined in a 50 ml Nessler cylinder, diluted with water, to about 35 ml, and mixed.

Procedure : Proceed as directed under Method A.

Method C

Standard Solution : Into a 50-ml Nessler cylinder, 2 ml of standard lead solution are pipetted, 5 ml of dilute sodium hydroxide solution added, diluted with water to 50 ml and mixed.

Test Solution : Into a 50 ml Nessler cylinder, 25 ml of the solution prepared are placed, the specified quantity dissolved in a mixture of 20 ml of water and 5 ml of dilute sodium hydroxide solution. It is diluted to 50 ml with water and mixed.

Procedure : To each of the cylinders containing the *standard solution* and the *test solution*, respectively, 5 drops of sodium sulphide solution are added, mixed, allowed to stand for five minutes and viewed downwards over a white surface; the colour produced in the test solution is not darker than that produced in the standard solution.

17

IDENTIFICATION TESTS FOR CATIONS AND ANIONS

IDENTIFICATION REACTIONS

The following tests may be used for the identification of chemicals referred to in the Pharmacopoeia. They are not intended to be applicable to mixtures of substances unless so specified.

Acetates

1. The substance is heated with an equal quantity of *oxalic acid*. Acid vapours with the characteristic odour of acetic acid are liberated.

$$CH_3COONa + (COOH)_2 \longrightarrow CH_3COOH + Na_2CO_3$$

2. The substance (1g) is warmed with 1 ml of *sulphuric acid* and 3 ml of *alcohol*; ethyl acetate, recognisable by its odour, is evolved (estrification reaction).

$$C_2H_5OH + CH_3COOH \xrightarrow{H_2SO_4} CH_3COOC_2H_5 + H_2O$$

3. About 30 mg of the substance are dissolved in 3 ml of *water* solution, successively 0.25 ml of *lanthanum nitrate solution*, 0.1 ml of *0.1 N iodine* and 0.05 ml of *dilute ammonia solution* are added and heated carefully to boiling. Within a few minutes a blue precipitate is formed or a dark blue colour develops.

4. The substance (20 mg) is heated with 50 mg of *calcium oxide*; acetone is evolved, which may be detected by the

indigo blue colour obtained when vapours impinge on filter paper which has been moistened with a 2 per cent w/v solution of *2-nitrobenzaldehyde* in *alcohol*, dried, and moistened with *N sodium hydroxide*.

$$Ca(CH_3COO)_2 \xrightarrow{\text{heat}} CH_3COCH_3 + CaCO_3$$

Aluminium

1. The substance (20 mg) is dissolved in 2 ml *water*, 0.5 ml of *2 N hydrochloric acid* and about 0.5 ml of *thioacetamide reagent* are added, no precipitate forms. *2 N sodium hydroxide solution* is added dropwise; a gelatinous white precipitate appears that redissolves on addition of further sodium hydroxide solution. Gradually *ammonium chloride solution* is added; the gelatinous white precipitate reappears.

$$Al^{3+} + 3OH^- \longrightarrow Al(OH)_3 \downarrow$$

2. The substance (20 mg) is dissolved in 5 ml of *water*, five drops of *ammonium acetate solution* and five drops of a 0.1 per cent w/v solution of *mordant blue 3* are added; an intense purple colour is produced.

$$Al^{3+} + CH_3COONH_4 + \text{Mordant blue 3}$$
$$\longrightarrow \text{Purple coloured complex}$$

3. To a solution of the substance in *water*, *dilute ammonia solution* is added until a faint precipitate is produced, and then 0.25 ml of a freshly prepared 0.05 per cent w/v solution of *quinalizarin* in a 1 per cent w/v solution of *sodium hydroxide* is added, heated to boiling, cooled, and acidified with an excess of *acetic acid*; a reddish-violet colour is produced.

$$Al^{3+} + 3NH_3 + 3H_2O \longrightarrow Al(OH)_3 \downarrow + 3NH_4^+$$

$$Al(OH)_3 + \text{Quinalizarin} + NaOH \longrightarrow \text{Reddish-violet colour}$$

Quinalizarsin

Ammonium Salts

1. A few mg of the substance are heated with *sodium hydroxide solution*; ammonia is evolved, which is recognisable by its odour and by its action on moist *red litmus paper*.

$$NH_4^+ + {}^-OH \longrightarrow NH_3 \downarrow + H_2O$$

2. To the prescribed solution 0.2 g of *light magnesium oxide is* added. A current of air is passed through the mixture and the gas, that is evolved, directed to just beneath the surface of a mixture of 1 ml of *0.1 N hydrochloric acid* and 0.05 ml of *methyl red solution*; the colour of the solution changes to yellow. On addition of 1 ml of a freshly prepared 10 per cent w/v solution of *sodium cobaltinitrite*, a yellow precipitate forms.

$$Na_3[Co(NO_2)_6] + NH_4^+ \longrightarrow (NH_4)_3[Co(NO_2)_6]\downarrow$$
Sodium   yellow ppt
cobaltinitrite

Antimony

The substance (10 mg) is dissolved with gentle heating in a solution of 0.5 g of *sodium potassium tartrate* in 10 ml of *water* and allowed to cool; 2 ml of this solution, *sodium sulphide solution* is added dropwise, a reddish-orange precipitate is formed which dissolves on adding *dilute sodium hydroxide solution*.

$$Sb_2S_3 + 8OH^- \longrightarrow 2[Sb(OH)_4]^- + 2SbS_2^-$$
soluble   soluble

$$Sb_2S_5 + 6OH^- \longrightarrow SbS_4^{2-} + SbO_3S^{2-} + 3H_2O$$
soluble   soluble

$$2Sb^{3+} + 3S^{2-} \xrightarrow{Na_2S} Sb_2S_3\downarrow \text{ (antimony sulphide)}$$
orange red ppt

$$2Sb^{5+} + 5S^{2-} \xrightarrow{Na_2S} Sb_2S_3\downarrow$$

$$Sb_2O_3/Sb_2O_5 + 2C_4H_4O_6^{2-} \xrightarrow{Na_2S} 2[(SbO)(C_4H_4O_6)]^-$$
Sodium   reddish-
potassium   orange
tartrate   ppt.

Arsenic

The prescribed solution (5 ml) is heated on a water-bath with an equal volume of hypophosphorus reagent; a brown precipitate is formed.

Barium

1. Barium salts impart a yellowish-green colour to a nonluminous flame, appearing blue when viewed through green glass.
2. The substance (20 mg) is dissolved in 5 ml of *dilute hydrochloric acid*, 2 ml of *dilute sulphuric acid added*; a white precipitate forms which is insoluble in *nitric acid*.

$$Ba^{2+} + SO_4^{2} \xrightarrow{\text{HCl}} BaSO_4\downarrow$$

Benzoates

1. To 1 ml of a 10 per cent w/v neutral solution, 0.5 ml of *ferric chloride test solution* is added; a dull-yellow precipitate, soluble in *solvent ether*, is formed.

$$3C_6H_5COO^- + 2Fe^{3+} + 3H_2O \longrightarrow Fe(C_6H_5COO)_3. Fe(OH)_3\downarrow$$
$$\text{Dull-yellow ppt.} \qquad + H_2O$$

2. The substance (0.2 g) is moistened with *sulphuric acid* and the bottom of the tube warmed gently; a white sublimate is deposited on the inner walls of the tube and no charring occurs.

$$2C_6H_5COONa + H_2SO_4 \xrightarrow{\text{heat}} \text{White sublimate}$$

3. The substance (0.5 g) is dissolved in 10 ml of *water*, and 0.5 ml of *hydrochloric acid* added. The precipitate obtained, after crystallisation from *water* and drying under reduced pressure, melts at about 122°.

$$C_6H_5COONa + HCl \longrightarrow C_6H_5COOH + NaCl$$
$$\text{Benzoic acid}$$

Bicarbonates

1. Solutions of bicarbonates, when boiled, liberate carbon dioxide.

$$2NaHCO_3 \xrightarrow{\text{heat}} Na_2CO_3 + H_2O + CO_2\uparrow$$

2. A solution of the substance is treated with a solution of *magnesium sulphate;* no precipitate is formed (distinction from carbonates). On boiling, a white precipitate is formed.

$$2Na_2HCO_3 \xrightarrow{\text{heat}} Na_2CO_3 + H_2O + CO_2$$

$$Na_2CO_3 + H_2O \rightleftharpoons 2Na+ + 2OH^- + CO_2$$

$$MgSO_4 + OH^- \rightleftharpoons MgOH + SO_4^{2-}$$

$$2MgOH^+ + CO_2 \rightleftharpoons Mg_2(OH)_2\downarrow + CO_3^{2-}$$
$$\text{white ppt}$$

3. The substance (0.1 g) is suspended in 2 ml of *water* in a test tube; 2ml of *2 N acetic is added.* The tube is closed immediately using a stopper fitted with a glass tube bent at two right-angles, heated gently and the gas collected in 5 ml of *barium hydroxide solution;* a white precipitate forms that dissolves on addition of an excess of *dilute hydrochloric acid.*

$$NaHCO_3 + CH_3COOH \longrightarrow CH_3COONa + H_2O + \overline{\overline{CO_2}}$$

$$Ba(OH)_2 + CO_2 \longrightarrow BaCO_3\downarrow + H_2O$$

$$BaCO_3 + 2HCl \longrightarrow BaCl_2 + CO_2\uparrow + H_2O$$

Bismuth

1. To the substance, *2 N hydrochloric acid (10 ml)* is added, heated to boiling for one minute, cooled and filtered, if necessary. To 1 ml of the solution obtained, 20 ml of *water* are added; a white or slightly yellow precipitate appears which on addition of 0.05 to 0.1 ml of *sodium sulphide solution* turns brown.

$$Bi^{3+} + 3HCl \longrightarrow BiCl_3 + 3H^+$$

$$BiCl_3 + 4H_2O \longrightarrow Bi(OH)_3 + H_3O+ + 2Cl$$

$$Bi(OH)_2\ Cl \longrightarrow BiOCl + H_2O$$
$$\text{Bismuth oxychloride}$$
$$\text{(white ppt.)}$$

$$2BiO^+ + 3HS^- + H^+ \longrightarrow Bi_2S_3\downarrow + 2H_2O$$

2. To about 50 mg of the substance 10 ml of *2 N nitric acid* is added, heated to boiling for one minute, allowed to cool and filtered, if necessary. To 5 ml of the solution obtained 2 ml of a 10 per cent w/v solution of *thiourea* are added; an orange yellow colour or an orange precipitate is produced. A 2.5 per cent w/v solution of *sodium fluoride (4 ml)* is

added; the solution is not decoulourised within thirty minutes.

$$Bi^{3+} + 3HNO_3 \longrightarrow Bi(NO_3)_3 + 3H^+$$
$$Bi(NO_3)_3 + NH_2CSNH_2 \longrightarrow \text{Orange yellow ppt.}$$

Bromides

1. A quantity of the substance equivalent to about 3 mg of bromide ion is dissolved in 2 ml of *water*. It is acidified with *2 N nitric acid* and 1 ml of *0.1 N silver nitrate* added, shaked and allowed to stand; a curdy, pale-yellow precipitate forms. The precipitate is centrifuged and washed rapidly with three quantities in subdued light. The precipitate is suspended in 2 ml of *water* and 1.5 ml of *10 N ammonia* are added; the precipitate dissolves with difficulty.

$$NaBr + AgNO_3 \longrightarrow AgBr + NaNO_3$$

2. About 10 mg are dissolved in 2 ml of *water* and 1 ml of *chlorine solution added*, bromine is evolved, which is soluble in two or three drops of *chloroform*, forming a reddish solution. The addition of *phenol solution* to the aqueous solution containing liberated bromine yields a white precipitate.

$$2KBr + Cl_2 \longrightarrow 2KCl + Br_2$$
$$C_6H_5OH + 3Br_2 \longrightarrow C_6H_2(Br)_3OH + 3HBr$$
$$\text{phenol} \qquad\qquad \text{Tribromophenol}$$
$$\text{(white ppt.)}$$

Note : *In testing for bromides in the presence of iodides, all iodine must first be removed by boiling the aqueous solution with an excess of lead dioxide.*

Calcium

1. The substance (20 mg) is dissolved in 5ml of *5 M acetic acid*. *Potassium ferrocyanide solution (0.5 ml)* is added; the solution remains clear. About 50 mg of *ammonium chloride* are aded; a white, crystal line precipitate is formed.

$$Ca^{2+} + 2K^+ + [Fe(CN)_6]^{4-} \longrightarrow CaK_2[Fe(CN)]_6\downarrow$$

2. To a solution of the substance a few drops of a solution of *ammonium oxalate* are added; a white precipitate is obtained that is only sparingly soluble in *dilute acetic acid* but is soluble in *hydrochloric acid*.

$$(NH_4)_2C_2O_4 \rightleftharpoons 2NH_4^+ + C_2O_4^{2-}$$

$$Ca^{2+} + C_2O_4^{2-} \longrightarrow CaC_2O_4\downarrow$$

Calcium oxalate
white ppt

$$CaC_2O_4 + 2HCl \longrightarrow CaCl_2 + (COOH)_2$$

3   The substance (20 mg) is dissolved in the minimum quantity of *dilute hydrochloric acid* and neutralised with *dilute sodium hydroxide solution;* 5 ml of *ammonium carbonate solution* added; a white precipitate is formed which, after boiling and cooling the mixture, is only sparingly soluble in *ammonium chloride solution.*

$$CaCl_2 + (NH_4)_2CO_3 \longrightarrow 2NH_4Cl + CaCO_3\downarrow$$

Carbonates

1.   The substance (0.1 g) is suspended in a test-tube in 2 ml of *water;* 2 ml of *2 N acetic acid are added.* The tube is closed immediately using a stopper fitted with a glass tube bent at two right-angles, heated gently and collected the gas in 5 ml of *0.1 N barium hydroxide;* a white precipitate is formed that dissolves on addition of an excess of *dilute hydrochloric acid.*

$$CaCO_3 + 2CH_3COOH \longrightarrow (CH_3COO)_2 Ca + H_2O + CO_2$$

$$Ba(OH)_2 + CO_2 \longrightarrow BaCO_3\downarrow + H_2O$$

white ppt

$$BaCO_3 + 2HCl \longrightarrow BaCl_2\downarrow + CO_2\uparrow + H_2O$$

2.   A solution of the substance is treated with a solution of *magnesium sulphate;* a white precipitate is formed (distinction from bicarbonates).

$$5Mg^{2+} + 5CO_3^{2-} + 6H_2O \longrightarrow MgCO_3. \ Mg\,(OH)_2.5H_2O\downarrow$$
$$+ CO_2\uparrow \quad \text{white ppt.}$$

Chlorides

1.   A quantity of the substance equivalent to about 2 mg of chloride ion is dissolved in 2 ml of water. It is acidified with *dilute nitric acid* and 0.5 ml of *silver nitrate solution* added. The solution is shaked and allowed to stand; a curdy, white precipitate is formed, which is insoluble in *nitric acid*, but soluble, after being well washed with *water, in dilute ammonia solution, from* which it is re-precipitated by the addition of *nitric acid.*

$$NaCl + AgNO_3 \longrightarrow AgCl\downarrow + NaNO_3$$

$$AgCl + 2NH_3 \longrightarrow Ag(NH_3)_2{}^+\,Cl^-$$

Soluble complex

$$Ag(NH_3)_2^+\,Cl^- + HNO_3 \longrightarrow AgCl\downarrow + (NH_4)_2NO_3$$

2. A quantity of the substance equivalent to about 10 mg of chloride ion is introduced into a test-tube; 0.2 g of *potassium dichromate* and 1 ml of *sulphuric acid are added*. A filter-paper strip moistened with 0.1 ml of *diphenylcarbazide solution* is placed over the opening of the test-tube; the paper turns violet-red. The moistened paper is not brought into contact with the potassium dichromate solution.

$$K_2Cr_2O_7 + 4NaCl + 6H_2SO_4 \longrightarrow 2CrO_2Cl_2 + 2KHSO_4$$

Chromyl chloride

$$+\ 4NaHSO_4 + 3H_2O$$

CrO_2Cl_2 + Diphenylcarbazide + $H_2O \longrightarrow$ Violet red colour

Citrates

1. To a neutral solution of the substance a solution of *calcium chloride* is added, no precipitate is produced. The solution is boiled, a white precipitate, soluble in *acetic acid*, formed.

$$2Na_3C_6H_5O_7 + 3CaCl_2 + 4H_2O \longrightarrow Ca_3(C_6H_5O_7)_2.4H_2O\downarrow$$

$$+\ 6NaCl$$

2. A quantity of the substance is dissolved in 5 ml of water. Sulphuric acid (0.5 ml) and 3 ml of *potassium permanganate solutions* are added. It is warmed until the colour of the permanganate is discharged and 0.5 ml of a 10 per cent w/v solution of *sodium nitroprusside added in 2 N sulphuric acid and 4 g of sulphamic acid*, make alkaline with *strong ammonia solution*, further addition of *strong ammonia solution* produces a violet colour, turning to violet-blue.

$$C(CH_2COOH)_2\,(OH)\,COOH + KMnO_4 \xrightarrow{\quad O \quad} CO(CH_2COOH)_2$$

Citric acid

Acetone dicarboxylic acid

$$CO(CH_2COOH)_2 + Sodium + H_2SO_4 +$$

nitropru-sside

Sulphamic + NH_3 acid

$$\longrightarrow \text{Violet colour}$$

Ferric Salts

1. A quantity of the substance equivalent to about 10 mg of iron is dissolved in 1 ml of *water*. 1 ml of a 5 per cent w/v solution of *potassium ferrocyanide* added; an intense blue precipitate is formed that is insoluble in *dilute hydrochloric acid*.

$$4FeCl_3 + 3K_4Fe\,(CN)_6 \longrightarrow Fe_4[Fe(CN)_6]_3 \downarrow + 12\,KCl$$

   Potassium   Blue colour
   ferrocyanide

2. To 3 ml of a solution containing about 0.1 mg of iron, 1 ml of *2 N hydrochloric acid* and 1 ml of *ammonium thiocyanate solution* are added; the solution becomes blood-red in colour. Two portions, each of 1 ml of the mixture are taken. To one portion 5 ml of *solvent ether* are added, shaked and allowed to stand; the ether layer is pink. To the other portion 3 ml of *0.2 M mercuric chloride* are added; the red colour disappears.

$$FeCl_3 + 3NH_4SCN \longrightarrow Fe\,(SCN)_3 + NH_4Cl$$

   Ferric
   thiocyanate
   (Red colour)

$$2Fe(SCN)_3 + 3HgCl \longrightarrow 3Hg(SCN)_2 + 2FeCl_3$$

   Mercuric
   thiocyanate
   (Colourless)

3. To 2 ml of a solution containing about 0.1 mg of iron *acetic acid* is added until the solution is strongly acidic. A 0.2 per cent solution of 8-hydroxy-7-iodoquinoline-5-sulphonic acid (2 ml) is added. A stable green colour is produced.

Ferrous Salts

1. A quantity of the substance corresponding to about 10 mg of iron is dissolved in 2 ml of *water*. To it 2 ml of *dilute sulphuric acid* and 1 ml of a 0.1 per cent solution of *1, 10-phenanthroline* are added. An intense red colour is produced;

the colour is discharged by addition of a slight excess of *0.1 N ceric ammonium sulphate*.

Red coloured complex cation

2. To 1 ml of a solution of iron, 1 ml of *potassium ferricyanide solution* is added; a dark blue precipitate is formed that is insoluble in *dilute hydrochloric acid* and is decomposed by *sodium hydroxide solution*.

$$Fe^{++} + 2K^+ + [Fe(CN)_6]^{4-} \longrightarrow K_2Fe\,[Fe(CN)_6]\downarrow$$

3. To 1 ml of a solution containing not less than 1 mg of iron, 1 ml of *potassium ferrocyanide solution* is added; a white precipitate is formed which rapidly becomes blue and is insoluble in *dilute hydrochloric acid*.

$$2FeSO_4 + K_4Fe(CN)_6 \longrightarrow Fe_2[Fe(CN)_6]^+.\,2K_2SO_4$$

Ferrous ferocyanide
(white ppt) ↓ [O], Air

$$Fe_4[Fe(CN)_6]_3$$
Persion blue

Iodides

1. A quantity of the substance equivalent to about 4 mg of iodide ion is dissolved in 2 ml of *water*. It is acidified with *dilute nitric acid* and 0.5 ml of *silver nitrate solution added*, It is shaked and allowed to stand, a curdy, pale-yellow precipitae forms. It is centrifuged and the precipitate washed rapidly with three quantities, each of 1 ml of *water* in subdued light. The precipitate is suspended in 2 ml of *water* and 1.5 ml of *10 N ammonia are added;* the precipitate does not dissolve.

$$NaI + AgNO_3 \xrightarrow{HNO_3} AgI\downarrow + NaNO_3$$
Yellow

2. To 0.2 ml of a solution of the substance containing the equivalent of about 5 mg of iodide ion per ml, 0.5 ml of *2 N sulphuric acid*, 0.15 ml of *potassium dichromate solution*, 2 ml of *water* and 2 ml of *chloroform* are added. It is shaked for a few seconds and allowed to stand; the chloroform layer is violet or violet-red.

$$Cr_2O_7^{2-} + 6I^- + 14H^+ \longrightarrow 2Cr^{3+} + 7H_2O + 2I_2 \text{(violet)}$$

3. To 1 ml of a solution of the substance containing the equivalent of about 5 mg of iodide ion, 0.5 ml of *mercuric chloride solution* is added a dark red precipitate is formed which is slightly soluble in an excess of this reagent and very soluble in an excess of *potassium iodide solution*.

$$2KI + HgCl_2 \longrightarrow HgI_2\downarrow + 2KCl$$
Merecuric
iodide (red)

$$HgI_2 + 2KI \longrightarrow K_2HgI$$
(Potassium mercuri-iodide)

Lactates

A mixture of aqueous solution of the substance, bromine water and 2N sulphuric acid is heated on a water-bath until the colour is discharged. After addition of ammonium sulphate, sodium nitroprusside solution (10%) in 2N sulphuric acid is added. Strong ammonium solution is mixed and left for 30 minutes. A dark green ring appears at the junction of two layers.

Lead

1. The substance (0.1 g) is dissolved in 1 ml of *dilute acetic acid*. To it 2 ml of *potassium chromate solution* are added; a yellow precipitate forms that is insoluble in 2 ml of *sodium hydroxide solution*.

$$Pb^{2+} + CrO_4^{2-} \longrightarrow PbCrO_4\downarrow \text{ (Lead chromate)}$$
$$PbCl_2 + K_2CrO_4 \longrightarrow PbCrO_4\downarrow + 2KCl$$

2. The substance (50 mg) is dissolved in 1 ml of *dilute acetic acid*. To it 10 ml of *water* and 0.2 ml of *M potassium iodide* are added; a yellow precipitate forms. The mixture is heated to boiling for one or two minutes, and allowed to cool; the precipitate is reformed as glistening, yellow plates.

$$Pb^{2+} + 2I^- \longrightarrow PbI_2$$
$$Pb(NO_3)_2 + 2KI \longrightarrow PbI_2\downarrow + 2KNO_3$$
Yellow ppt.

Magnesium

1. The substance (15 mg) is dissolved in 2 ml of *water*. To it 1 ml of *dilute ammonia solution* is added; a white

precipitate forms that is redissolved by adding 1 ml of *2 M ammonium chloride*. To the solution 1 ml of 0.25 M disodium hydrogen phosphate is added; a white crystalline precipitate forms.

Ammonium chloride prevents precipitation of magnesium hydroxide due to suppression of dissociation of ammonium hydroxide caused by a common ion effect.

$$NH_4Cl \longrightarrow NH_4^+ + Cl^-$$

$$NH_4OH \longrightarrow NH_4^+ + OH^-$$

$$Mg^{2+} + OH^- \longrightarrow Mg(OH)_2 \downarrow$$

$$Mg^{2+} + NH_4^+ + PO_4^{3-} + 6H_2O \longrightarrow MgNH_4PO_4 . 6H_2O \downarrow$$
$$\text{White ppt}$$

$$MgSO_4 + NaHPO_4 + NH_4OH + 6H_2O \longrightarrow$$
$$MgNH_4PO_4 . 6H_2O \downarrow + Na_2SO_4 + H_2O$$

2. To 0.5 ml of a neutral or slightly acidic solution of the substance, 0.2 ml of a 0.1 per cent solution of *titan yellow* and 0.5 ml of *0.1 N sodium hydroxide* are added; a bright red turbidity develops which gradually settles to give a bright red precipitate.

Nitrates

1. The substance (15 mg) is dissolved in 0.5 ml of *water*, 1 ml of *sulphuric acid* added, mixed and cooled. The tube is inclined and without mixing, 0.5 ml of *ferrous sulphate solution* added. A brown colour forms at the interface of the two liquids.

$$3Fe^{2+} + 4H^+ + NO^{3-} \longrightarrow NO + 3Fe^{3+} + 2H_2O$$

$$Fe^{2+} + NO \longrightarrow [Fe(NO)]^{2+} (\text{Brown colour})$$

2. To a mixture of 0.1 ml of *nitrobenzene*, 0.2 ml of *sulphuric acid* and powdered substance is allowed to stand for five minutes and cooled in ice water whilst adding slowly with stirring 5 ml of *water* and then 5 ml of *sodium hydroxide solution*. To it 5 ml of acetone are added, shaked, and allowed to stand, the upper layer shows an intense violet colour.

Phosphates (Orthophosphates)

1. To 5 ml of the prescribed solution, neutralised to pH 7.0, *silver nitrate solution* is added; a light yellow precipitate forms, the colour of which is not changed by boiling and

which is readily soluble in *dilute ammonia solution* and in *dilute nitric acid.*

$$3Ag^+ + 2HPO_4^{2-} \longrightarrow Ag_3PO_4\downarrow + H_2PO_4^-$$

$$Ag_3PO_4 \qquad\qquad 3Ag^+ + PO_4^{3-}$$

$$Ag^+ + 2NH_3 \rightleftharpoons [Ag(NH_3)_2]^+$$

Silver diamino
complex soluble

$$PO_4^{3-} + H_2O \rightleftharpoons HPO_4^{2-} + OH^-$$

$$OH^- + H^+ \xrightarrow{\quad HNO_3 \quad} H_2O$$

2. The prescribed solution (1 ml) is mixed with 1 ml of *ammonical magnesium sulphate solution*; a white, crystalline precipitate is produced.

$$Mg^{2+} + HPO_4^{2-} + NH_3 + 6H_2O \longrightarrow MgNH_4PO_4 . 6H_2O$$

3. To 2 ml of the prescribed solution, 2 ml of *dilute nitric acid* and 4 ml of *ammonium molybdate solution* are added and the solution warmed; a bright canary-yellow precipitate is formed.

$$12MoO_4^{2-} + HPO_4^{2-} + 3NH_4^+ + 23H^+ \longrightarrow$$

$$(NH_4)_3[P(Mo_{12}O_{40})] + 12H_2O$$

ammonium
phosphomolybdate
(Canary-yellow)

Potassium

1. The substance (50 mg) is dissolved in 1 ml of *water*. To it 1 ml of *dilute acetic acid* and 1 ml of a freshly prepared 10 per cent solution of *sodium cobaltinitrite* are added; a yellow or orange-yellow precipitate forms immediately.

$$[Co(NO_2)_6]^{3-} + 3K^+ \longrightarrow K_3[Co(NO_2)_6]\downarrow$$

Potassium cobaltnitrite

2. The substance (0.1 g) is dissolved in 2 ml of *water*. The solution is heated with 1 ml of *sodium carbonate solution*; no precipitate forms. To it 0.05 ml of *sodium sulphide solution* is added; no precipitate forms. It is cooled in ice water and 2 ml of a 15 per cent w/v solution of *tartaric acid* are added and allowed to stand; a white, crystalline precipitate forms.

$$KCl + H_2C_4H_4O_6 \longrightarrow KHC_4H_4O_6 + HCl$$

Yellow ppt

3. A few mg of the substance is ignited, cooled and dissolved in the minimum quantity of *water*. To this solution 1 ml of *platinic chloride solution* is added in the presene of 1 ml of *hydrochlorice acid;* a yellow, crystalline precipitate forms, which on ignition leaves a residue of potassium chloride and platinum.

$$H_2[PtCl_6] + 2KCl \longrightarrow K_2[PtCl_6] + 2HCl$$
$$\text{Yellow ppt.}$$

Salicylates

1. To a neutral solution of the substance, ferric chloride test solution is added. A violet colour is produced which persists after the addition of dilute acetic acid.

$$3C_6H_4(OH)COONa + FeCl_3 \longrightarrow [C_6H_4(OH)COO]_3Fe + NaCl$$
$$\text{Ferric salicylate}$$
$$\text{(violet)}$$

2. To an aqueous solution of the substance, hydrochloric acid (0.5 ml) is added. The precipitate is filtered and recrystallized from hot water which melted at 159°.

$$C_6H_4(OH)COONa + HCl \longrightarrow C_6H_4(OH)COOH\downarrow + NaCl$$
$$\text{Salicylic acid}$$

3. To an aqueous solution of the substance, bromine solution is added. A cream-coloured precipitate is produced.

$$C_6H_4(OH)COONa + Br_2 \xrightarrow{\ H_2O\ } C_6H_2(OH)Br_3$$
$$\text{Tribromophenol}$$

Silver

1. The substance (10 mg) is dissolved in 10 ml of *water*. To it 0.3 ml of *dilute hydrochloric acid is added;* a curdy white precipitate is formed that is soluble in *dilute ammonia solution. Potassium iodide solution* is added; a yellow precipitate is formed.

$$Ag^+ + Cl^- \rightarrow AgCl\downarrow \longrightarrow [Ag(NH_3)_2]^+ Cl^-$$

$$Ag(NH_3)Cl + KI + 2H_2O \longrightarrow AgI\downarrow + KCl + 2NH_4OH$$

2. The substance (10 mg) is dissolved in 10 ml of *water* and 2 ml of *potassium chromate solution* added; a red precipitate is formed which is soluble in nitric acid.

$$2Ag^+ + CrO_4^{2-} \longrightarrow Ag_2CrO_4\downarrow$$

Sodium

1. The substance (0.1 g) is dissolved in 2 ml of *water*. To it 2 ml of a 15 per cent solution of *potassium carbonate* are added and heated to boiling; no precipitate forms. To it 4 ml of freshly prepared *potassium antimonate solution* are added and heated to boiling. The solution is allowed to cool in ice water and, if necessary, rubbed the inside of the test-tube with a glass rod; a dense, white precipitate is formed.

$$NaCl + KH_2SbO_4 \longrightarrow NaH_2SbO_4\downarrow + KCl$$

2. A solution of the substance is acidified with N *acetic acid* and a large excess of *magnesium uranyl acetate solution* aded; a yellow, crystalline precipitate is formed.

$$Na^+ + Mg^{2+} + 3UO_2^{2+} + 8C_2H_3O_2^- + HC_2H_3O_2 + 9H_2O \longrightarrow$$
$$NaMg(UO_2)_3 (C_2H_3O_2)_9. 9H_2O + H^+$$

Sulphates

1. The substance (50 mg) is dissolved in 5 ml of *water*. To it 1 ml of *dilute hydrochloric acid* and 1 ml of *barium chloride solution* are added; a white precipitate forms.

$$Ba^{2+} + SO_4^{2-} \longrightarrow BaSO_4\downarrow$$

2. The substance (50 mg) is dissolved in 5 ml of *water*, 2 ml of *lead acetate solution* are added; a white precipitate is formed which is soluble in *ammonium acetate solution* and in *sodium hydroxide solution*.

$$PbSO_4 + 4C_2H_3O_2^- \longrightarrow [Pb (C_2H_3O_2)_4]^{2-} + SO_4$$
$$PbSO_4 + 3OH \longrightarrow HPbO_2^- + H_2O + SO_4^{2-}$$

3. *Iodine solution* (0.1 ml) is added to the suspension obtained in Test A; the suspension remains yellow (distinction from sulphites and dithionites) but is decolourised by adding, dropwise *stannous chloride solution* (distinction from iodates). The mixture is boiled; no coloured precipitate appears (distinction from selenates and tungstates).

Tartrates

1. The substance is warmed with *sulphuric acid*; charring occurs and carbon monoxide, which burns with a blue flame when ignited, is evolved.

$$H_2C_4H_4O_6 \longrightarrow CO_2\uparrow + CO\uparrow + 2C + 3H_2O\uparrow$$

$$C + H_2SO_4 \longrightarrow 2SO_2 + CO_2\uparrow + 2H_2O$$

$$2CO + O_2 \xrightarrow{\text{Blue flame}} 2CO_2$$

2. The substance (20 mg) is dissolved in 5 ml of *water*. To it 0.05 ml of a 1 per cent solution of *ferrous sulphate* and 0.05 ml of *hydrogen peroxide solution are* added, a transient yellow colour is produced. *2N sodium hydroxide solution* is added dropwise; an intense blue colour is produced.

$$\begin{array}{c} \text{CH(OH)COOH} \\ | \\ \text{CH(OH)COOH} \end{array} + H_2O_2 \longrightarrow \begin{array}{c} \text{C(OH)COOH} \\ || \\ \text{C(OH)COOH} \end{array} + 2H_2O$$

3. A solution (0.1 ml) containing the equivalent of about 2 mg of tartaric acid is heated for five to ten minutes with 0.1 ml of a 10 per cent solution of *potassium bromide*, 0.1 ml of a 2 per cent solution of *resorcinol* and 3 ml of *sulphuric acid*; a dark-blue colour is produced that changes to red when the solution is cooled and poured into *water*.

Thiosulphates

1. The substance (0.1 g) is dissolved is in 5 ml of *water*, 2 ml of *hydrochloric acid* are added a white precipitate is formed which soon turns yellow and sulphur dioxide is evolved, recognisable by its odour.

$$S_2O_3{}^{2-} + H^+ \longrightarrow H_2S_2O_3 + S\downarrow$$
$$H_2S_2O_3 \longrightarrow H_2O + SO_2 + S\downarrow$$

2. The substance (0.1 g) is dissolved in 5 ml of *water*, 2 ml of *ferric chloride-test solution* are added, a dark violet colour is produced which quickly disappears.

$$2S_2O_3 + 3Fe^{3+} \xrightarrow{\text{Neutral}} [Fe(S_2O_3)_2]^- \longrightarrow 2Fe^+ + S_4O_6{}^{2-}$$

Ferric thiosulphate complex (violet colour)   Colour less

$$2FeCl_3 + Na_2S_2O_3 + H_2O \underset{H^+}{\overset{H^+}{\rightleftharpoons}} 2FeCl_2 + 2NaCl + H_2SO_4 + S$$

$$Na_2S_2O_3 + 2HCl \rightleftharpoons 2NaCl + H_2SO_3 + S$$

$$2H_2SO_3 + 2FeCl_3 \qquad Fe_2(SO_3)_3 + 6HCl$$

Ferric sulphate (Violet colour)

$$Fe2(SO_3)_2 \longrightarrow FeSO_3 + FeS_2O_6$$

3. Solutions of thiosulphates decolourise *iodine solution;* the decolourised solutions do not give the reactions of *sulphates.*

$$2S_2O_3^{2-} + I_2 \longrightarrow 2I^- + [S_4O_6]^{2-}$$

4. Solutions of thiosulphates decolourise *bromine solution;* the decolourised solutions give the reactions of *sulphates.*

$$S_2O_3^{2-} + 4Br_2 + 5H_2O \longrightarrow 8Br^- + 10H^+ + 2SO_2^{2-}$$

Zinc

1. The substance (0.1 g) is dissolved in 5 ml of *water.* To it 0.2 ml of *sodium hydroxide solution* is added; a white precipitate forms. A further 2 ml of *sodium hydroxide solution* is added; the precipitate dissolves. *Ammonium chloride solution* (10 ml) is added; the solution remains clear, but a flocculent, white precipitate forms on addition of 0.1 ml of *sodium sulphide solution.*

$$Zn^{2+} + 2OH^- \longrightarrow Zn\,(OH)_2\downarrow$$

$$ZnCl_2 + 2NaOH \longrightarrow Zn(OH)_2 + NaCl$$

$$Zn(OH)_2 + 2NaOH^- \longrightarrow Na_2ZnO_2 + 2H_2O$$
Sodium zincate

$$Na_2ZnO_2 + H_2S \longrightarrow ZnS\downarrow + 2NaOH$$
White ppt.

2. The substance (0.1 g) is dissolved in 5 ml of *water,* acidified with *dilute sulphuric acid,* one drop of a 0.1 per cent w/v solution of *copper sulphate* and 2 ml of *ammonium mercuri-thiocyanate solution* are added; a violet precipitate is formed.

$$Zn + [Hg(SCN)_4]^{2-} \longrightarrow Zn[Hg(SCN)_4]$$

3. The substance (0.1 g) is dissolved in 5 ml of *water,* 2 ml of *potassium ferrocyanide solution* are added; a white precipitate is formed which is insoluble in *dilute hydrochloric acid.*

$$2Zn^{2+} + 2K^+ + 2[Fe(CN)_6]^{4-} \longrightarrow K_2Zn_2\,[Fe_3(CN_6)_6]_2$$
Potassium zinc ferricyanide
(white ppt.)

Foreign Organic Matter

Foreign organic matter is the material consisting of any or all of the following :

(i) Parts of the organ or organs from which the drug is derived other than the parts named in the definition and description or for which a limit is prescribed in the individual monograph;

(ii) Any organs, other than those named in the definition and description;

(iii) Moulds, insects or other animal contamination.

Method : 100 to 500 g or the quantity of the *original sample* are weighed and spreaded it out in a thin layer. The sample is inspected with the unaided eye or with the use of a 6 x lens and the foreign organic matter separated by hand as completely as possible. It is weighed and the percentage of foreign organic matter determined, calculated from the weight of the drug taken. The maximum quantity of sample is used for coarse or bulky drugs.

Alcohol-soluble Extractive

The air-dried drug (5 g) coarsely powdered macerated with 100 ml flask for twenty-four hours. It is filtered rapidly taking precautions against loss of alcohol, 25 ml of the filtrate are evaporated to dryness in a tared flat-bottomed shallow dish, dried at 105°, and weighed. The percentage of alcohol-soluble extractive is calculated with reference to the air dried drug.

Water-soluble Extractive

Method I : As directed for the determination of **Alcohol-soluble Extractive** is proceeded using *chloroform water* instead of *alcohol.*

Method II : 5.0 g are added to 50 ml of *water* at 80°in a stoppered flask. It is shaken well and allowed to stand for ten minutes; cooled to 15° and 2 g of *kieselguhr added;* filtered. The filtrated (5 ml) is transferred to a tared evaporating basin 7.5 cm in diameter, the solvent evaporated on a water-bath, continued drying for half an hour, finally dried in steam oven for two hours and the residue weighed. The percentage of water-soluble extractive is calculated with reference to the air-dried drug.

Ash

Method I is used for crude vegetable drugs and Method II for other substances.

Method I : A quantity of the test sample is weighed equivalent to 2 to 3 g of the air-dried drug in a tared platinum or silica dish, and incinerated at a temperature not exceeding 450° until free from carbon, cooled and weighed. If a carbon-free ash cannot be obtained in this way, the charred mass is exhausted with hot *water*, the residue collected on an ashless filter paper, the residue incinerated and the filtrate evaporated to dryness, and ignited at a temperature not exceeding 450°. If a carbon-free ash cannot be obtained in this way, the crucible is cooled, 15 ml of *alcohol* are added, the ash broken up with a glass-rod, the alcohol burnt off, and again the whole heated to a dull red heat. It is cooled, ash weighed and the percentage of ash calculated with reference to the air dried drug.

Method II : About 1 g of the substance is weighed and carried out Method I. The percentage of ash is calculated.

Acid-insoluble Ash

Method I is used unless otherwise directed in the individual monograph.

Method I : The ash obtained as directed under *Ash*, above is boiled with 25 ml of *2 N hydrochloric acid*, for five minutes, the insoluble matter collected in a Gooch crucible, or on an ashless filter paper, washed with hot *water*, ignited, and weighed. The percentage of acid-insoluble ash is calculated with reference to the air dried drug.

Method II : The *ash* or the *sulphated ash* is placed in a crucible, 15 ml of *water* and 10 ml of *hydrochloric acid* are added, covered with a watch-glass, and boiled for ten minutes; allowed to cool. The insoluble matter is collected on an ashless filter paper, washed with hot *water* until the filtrate is neutral, ignited to dull redness, cooled in a desiccator and weighed until the difference between the two successive weighings is not more than 1 mg. The percentage of acid-soluble ash is calculated with reference to the air-dried drug.

Water-soluble Ash

The ash is boiled for five minutes with *25 ml of water;* the insoluble matter collected in a Gooch crucible, or on an ashless filter paper, washed with hot *water*, and ignited for fifteen minutes at a temperature not exceeding 450°. The weight of the insoluble matter is substracted from the weight of the ash; the difference in weight represents the water-soluble ash. The percentage of water-soluble ash is calculated with reference to the air-dried drug.

Sulphated Ash

A silica or platinum crucible is heated to redness for 10 minutes, allowed to cool in a desiccator and 1 to 2 g of the substance is put accurately weighed, into the crucible, ignited gently at first, until the substance is thoroughly charred. It is cooled, the residue moisten with 1 ml of *sulphuric acid,* heated gently until white fumes are no longer evolved and ignited at $800° \pm 25°$ until all black particles have disappeared. The ignition is conducted in a place protected from air currents. The crucible is cooled, a few drops of *sulphuric acid* are added and heated. As before it is allowed to cool and weighed. The operation repeated until two successive weighings do not differ by more than 0.5 mg.

Loss on Drying

Loss on drying is a measure of water content both environmental and water of crystallization and other volatile organic solvents present in an active ingredient and its dosage form. This is an important parameter in maintaining quality of pharmaceutical product as it is associated with the physiochemical stability profile of both the pharmaceutical active ingredient and the dosage form. Presence of moisture induces decomposition of many products on subsequent storage (e.g. β-lactam antibiotics), it may even cause a pack to burst as in the case of effervescent dosage forms. It alters the dissolution profile and creates a hindrance during formulating a dosage form by affecting compression of tablets, caking of material, etc. in a drug. In many instances, presence of moisture in a drug leads to bacterial growth which may either cause side effects or may even be lethal.

The following procedure determines the amount of volatile matter of any kind (including water) that can be driven off under the conditions specified.

Loss on drying is the loss in weight in per cent w/w determined by means of the procedure given below. Unless otherwise directed in the monograph, carry out the test on 1.0 g of the substance, previously mixed well. If the sample is in the form of large crystals, reduce the size by quickly crushing to a powder.

Method

A glass-stoppered is weighed along with a shallow weighing bottle that has been dried for 30 minutes under the same conditions to be employed in the determination. The sample is put in the bottle covered and the bottle and the contents are weighed accurately. The sample is distributed by gentle sidewise shaking to a depth not exceeding 10 mm. The loaded bottle is placed in the drying chamber (oven or desiccator), the stopper removed and left it also in the chamber. The sample is dried for the time specified in the monograph or to constant weight, at the prescribed temperature under one of the following conditions (Shown in brackets are the words used in the individual monograph for the drying conditions).

(a) In a desiccator over phosphorous pentoxide at atmospheric pressure and at room temperature ("desiccator").

(b) Over phosphorous pentoxide, in vacuum at a pressure not exceeding 20 Torr at room temperature ("in vacuo").

(c) Over phosphorous pentoxide, in vacuum at a pressure not exceeding 20 Torr at a higher temperature ("in vacuo with indication of temperature and time").

(d) In an oven at the temperature indicated in the monograph.

After drying is completed, the chamber is opened, the bottle closed promptly and allowed it to come to room temperature (where applicable) in a desiccator before weighing.

Note : *Where drying in a desiccator is specified, care must be taken to keep the desiccant fully effective by frequent replacement.*

Water Content

The test sample (10 g) is weighed in a tared evaporating dish and dried in an oven at 105° for five hours. It is cooled and weighed. The drying is continued and weighing one hour intervals until the difference between two successive weighings corresponds to not more than 0.25 per cent.

EXAMINATION QUESTION PAPER

UNIVERSITY OF DELHI, DELHI

DIPLOMA-1993

1. (a) Write the important Physical and Physico-Chemical Tests of purity and standards of Pharmaceuticals.

   (b) Give the principle, reactions and procedure for the limit test of arsenic in sodium chloride.

2. (a) Give the principle, reactions and procedure for the assay of the following substances :

   (i) Yellow mercuric oxide (ii) Sodium bicarbonate

   (b) Write the medicinal uses of the following substances :

   (i) Ammonium bicarbonate(ii) Ammonium chloride
   (iii) Lithium bromide   (iv) Orthophosphoric acid
   (v) Sodium hypochlorite   (vi) Copper sulphate
   (vii) Silver nitrate   (viii) Magnesium trisilicate.

3. (a) What are stabilisers ? Classify them and give suitable examples. Name at least *three* compounds used to preserve hydrogen peroxide.

   (b) Explain the use of the following :

   (i) Potassium iodide in the assay of ammoniated mercury.
   (ii) Nitric acid in the assay of mercuric oxide.
   (iii) Glycerol in the assay of boric acid.
   ·(iv) Sodium citrate in preparations of glycerites of phenol.
   (v) Stannated hydrochloric acid in the limit test of arsenic.
   (vi) Silver nitrate solution in the limit test of chloride.

(vii) Hydrochloric acid in the limit test of sulphate.

(c) Write the principle and reactions involved in the limit test of sulphate.

4. (a) Give the storage conditions and write the stability of the following substances :

(i) Iodine (ii) Potassium iodide (iii) Potassium acetate (iv) Ferrous sulphate (v) Ammonia (vi) Sodium hydroxide (vii) Sodium bicarbonate (viii) Sodium chloride.

(b) Write *True* or *False* of the following :

(i) Phenacetin is used as preservative for hydrogen peroxide.

(ii) Aqueous solution of nitrous oxide has sweetish taste.

(iii) Hydrogen peroxide is a chemical antidote for barbiturate poisoning.

(iv) Orthophosphoric acid is used in the treatment of lead poisoning.

(v) Sodium acetate is a systemic antacid.

(vi) Sodium thiosulphate is used as an antidote for cyanide poisoning.

(vii) Sodium bicarbonate is a deliquescent substance.

(viii) Boric acid is unstable in air.

5. (a) Give the general properties, stability and medicinal preparations and the applications of the following compounds :

(i) Calcium gluconate

(ii) Ferric ammonium citrate

(iii) Bismuth oxychloride.

(b) Give a brief account of the Radio-pharmaceuticals.

6. (a) Give the calculation factors and reaction involved in the assay of the following substances :

(i) Sodium chloride

(ii) Ammonium chloride

(iii) Potassium iodide.

(b) Give a brief account of the sources of impurities commonly found in Pharmaceuticals.

7. Write the general properties, stability, assay and medicinal applications of the following compounds :

(i) Bleaching powder (ii) Iodine (iii) Zinc sulphate.

DIPLOMA - 1993/SUPPLE.

1. Comment on the following :

   (i) Pharmacopoeial Monographs (ii) Limit test for Iron (iii) Inorganic antacids and Laxative compounds.

2. (a) Explain the use of the following :

   (i) Traces of free acid and acetanilide (0.3%) in Hydrogen peroxide. (ii) Oxygen (4%) in Nitrous oxide. (iii) Choloroform in the assay of Potassium iodide. (iv) Ferric ammonium sulphate solution in the assay of Sodium chloride.

   (b) Write the effect of heat on the following substances. Give reactions (if any).

   (i) Boric Acid (ii) Zinc oxide (iii) Ammoniated Mercury (iv) Bismuth subnitrate.

   (c) Give the reactions of Iodine with the following substances:

   (i) Strong Ammonia Solution (ii) Ferrous chloride

   (iii) Sodium thiosulphate (iv) Sodium metabisulphite.

3. Write the general properties, stability, storage conditions and pharmaceutical preparations with their uses of the following compounds :

   (i) Sodium thiosulphate (ii) Magnessium sulphate (iii) Zinc oxide (iv) Kaoline.

4. Write true or false against the following :

   (i) Chlorine water is a mixture of chlorine, hypochloric acid and oxygen in solution.

   (ii) Dakin's solution is the other name of chlorinated lime.

   (iii) Sodium chloride is the electrolyte of most of the Intracellular body fluids.

   (iv) Lugol's solution is the other name of aqueous solution of Iodine (5%) and Potassium iodide (10%).

   (v) Sulphur has laxative properties.

   (vi) Zinc sulphate is an ophthalmic astringent.

   (vii) Ammoniated Mercury is a skin disinfectant.

   (viii) Potassium chloride is used in sinusitis of allergic origin.

   (ix) Permissible limit of suitable preservative in Hydrogen peroxide is upto 2%.

   (x) Ammonia possesses saponifying properties.

   (xi) Sodium thiosulphate has catharitic properties.

(xii) Preston salt is the other name of Ammonium carbonate.

(xiii) Magnesium sulphate is used as an antidote for Barbiturate poisoning.

(xiv) Blue vitriol is the other name of Ferrous sulphate.

(xv) Zinc is used in the limit test of Arsenic as reducing agent.

(xvi) Silver nitrate possesses emetic properties.

5. (a) Define sequestration and give at least *three* examples of sequestering agents.

   (b) Explain with suitable examples the complexometric titrations.

   (c) Give the applications of Radio Pharmaceuticals.

6. Write the medical applications and general properties of the following substances :

   (i) Potassium bromide (ii) Ammonium chloride (iii) Talc (iv) Zinc stearate (v) Magnesium oxide (vi) Ferrous gluconate (vii) Borax (viii) Bismuth oxychloride.

7. Give the general properties, stability, pharmaceutical preparations and assay method (with reaction) of the following :

   (i) Copper sulphate (ii) Hydrogen peroxide (iii) Antimony potassium tartrate (iv) Sodium chloride.

DIPLOMA-1992

1. (a) Given the principle, reactions and procedure for limit test for lead (I.P. and B.P. method both).

   (b) Explain with suitable examples that 'storage condition of Pharmaceuticals is one of the source of impurities'.

   (c) Justify that presence of an oxidising agent interferes in the limit test for Iron.

2. Write the general properties, storage conditions, uses and pharmaceutical preparations of the following compounds :

   (i) Antimony potassium tartarate (ii) Calcium phosphate (iii) Calcium gluconate.

3. Write notes on :

   (i) Complexometric assay (ii) Indirect titration (iii) Gutget Test (iv) Applications of radiopharmaceuticals.

4. (a) Give the various pharmaceuitical preparations and their applications of zinc oxide and sodium bicarbonate.

(b) Write the properties, principle and reactions involved in the assay of boric acid and hydrogen peroxide.

5. (a) Give the chemical reactions between :
   (i) Ferric ions with thioglycolic acid (ii) Lead ions with diphenyl-thiacarbazone (iii) Ammoniated mercury and potassium iodide solution (iv) Calcium gluconate solution and E.D.T. A. solution.
   (b) Comment on the use of :
      (i) Traces of Potassium Sulphate in preparation of barium sulphate reagent (B.P.).
      (ii) burnt sugar solution in 'limit test for lead'?
      (iii) Brominated hydrochloric Acid in the limit test for arsenic.
      (iv) Sodium hydroxide solution in place of ammonia solution in the limit test for iron.
   (c) Write the effect of impurities in pharmaceutical substances.

6. (a) Give the general properties, storage, pharmaceutical preparations, uses and assay method of iodine.
   (b) What happens when :
      (i) Ammonium chloride is heated. (ii) Ammoniated mercury is kept in light (iii) Calcium gluconate is treated with sodium oxalate solution (iv) Ferrous sulphate is heated (v) Chlorinated lime is dissolved in water (vi) Copper sulphate solution comes in contact with Litmus paper (vii) Ammonia is added to potassium permanganate solution (viii) Iodine reacts with sodium-hydroxide solution.

7. Give an account of general properties, assay method and reaction involved therein and medicinal applications of the following substances :
   (i) Sodium chloride (ii) Copper-sulphate
   (iii) Potassium permangnate.

DIPLOMA-1992/SUPPLE.

1. (a) Write the precautions to be taken in preparation of the 'Solution for test' of reducing substances for their limit test for iron and sulphate.
   (b) Give the points of consideration for deciding permissible impurities in pharmaceuticals.

(c) Explain with suitable examples the auxillary and primary solution used in limit test for lead.

(d) Explain the use of the following :

(i) Nessler glass cylinders (ii) Lead acetate plug in the limit test for arsenic (iii) Ammonia Solution 'F & T' in limit test for Iron (iv) Alcohol in preparation of barium sulphate reagent (B.P.).

2. Write the properties, storage, tests for purity, assay method, uses and pharmaceutical preparations of the following compounds :

(i) Ammonium chloride (ii) Ammoniated mercury.

3. (a) What happens when :

(i) Zinc Shlphate Solution is treated with Sodium Carbonate.

(ii) Zinc oxide is treated with sodium hydroxide solution.

(iii) Ferrous Sulphate Crystals are heated.

(iv) Yellow mercuric oxide is heated to cold hot.

(v) Potassium permangnate is heated upto 240°C.

(vi) Copper sulphate is treated with excess of potassium iodide in presence of acetic acid.

(vii) Potassium permangnate solution is treated with Potassium iodide.

(viii) Precipitated sulphur is added to potassium hydroxide solution.

(b) Name at least four official compounds of sodium and write their general properties and applications.

4. Write the general properties, medical applications with pharmaceutical preparations of the following :

(i) Potassium iodide   (ii) Precepitated sulphur

(iii) Ferric ammonium citrate (iv) Boric acid.

5. Define titrimetric assay. Classify and explain with suitable examples of each type of titrimetric assay methods.

6. Write the assay method, pharmaceutical preparations and uses of the following :

(i) Zinc sulphate (ii) Sodium bicarbonate

(iii) Antimony Potassium tartrate (iv) Magnessium Sulphate.

7. (a) Comment on 'The Tests for Purity' prescribed by Pharmacopocias".

(b) Give the procedure and reaction involved in the limit tests for iron in potassium permanganate sample.

(c) Write the principle, reactions and procedure for the limit for chloride.

B. PHARMA./I-1993 (SECTION A)

1. (a) Write the significance of 'Test of Purity' and 'Limit Test'.
   (b) Give the principle and procedure for the limit Test of Arsenic.

2. Discuss the principle involved in the assay procedure of any *four* of the following :
   (a) Boric Acid (b) Calcium gluconate (c) Ferrous sulphate (d) Sodium chlorite (e) Potassium permanganate.

3. Write short notes on any *four* of the following :
   (a) Yellow mercuric oxide (b) Potassium iodide (c) Iron and ammonium citrate (d) Zinc oxide (e) Sodium phosphate (32 P) Injection.

B. PHARMA./I-1992 (SECTION A)

1. (a) Mention the sources of impurities in Pharmaceuticals.
   (b) Give the principle and procedure for limit test of arsenic.

2. Discuss the principle involved in the assay procedure of any *four* of the following :
   (a) Boric acid (b) Sodium chloride (c) Ferrous sulphate (d) Calcium gluconate (e) Sodium bicarbonate

3. Write short notes on any *four* of the following :
   (a) Heavy Kaolin (b) Pharmaceutical aids (c) Ammoniated mercury (d) Sodium benzoate (e) Bismuth oxychloride.

B. PHARMA./I-1992/SUPPLE. (SECTION A)

1. (a) Mention the general tests of purity performed according to pharmacopoeial monograph of drugs.
   (b) Give the principle and procedure for the limit test of iron.

2. Discuss the principle involved in the assay procedures of any *four* of the following :
   (a) Chlorinated lime (b) Iodine (c) Hydrogen peroxide (d) Ammonium chloride (e) Magnesium sulphate.

3. Write short notes on any *four* :
   (a) Zinc oxide (b) Radio pharmaceuticals (c) Yellow mercuric

oxide (d) Potassium permanganate (e) Iron and ammonium citrate.

DIPLOMA - 1995 (NS)

1. (a) Discuss the factors to be considered while fixing the limits of impurities in a pharmaceutical compound.
   (b) Write reactions involved in limit test for 'arsenic' and 'lead'.

2. What are antioxidants ? What is the criteria for the selection of inorganic-antioxidants ? Give the method of preparation, and uses of any *one*.

3. What are anticaries agents ? Discuss the role of fluoride as anticaries. Describe the method of preparation, uses and assay of sodium fluoride.

4. What are expectorants ? How do they act ? Write the preparation and assay of potassium iodide.

5. Give a list of official compounds of calcium and sulphur along with their official chemical formulae. Give the method of preparation, assay and uses of one compound of calcium.

6. Write notes on :
   (i) Radiopharmaceuticals (ii) Buffers.

7. (a) Explain the following giving chemical equations :
   (i) When ammonium oxalate is added to $CaCl_2$ and the ppt. is treated with HCl.
   (ii) When neutral solution of sodium citrate is boiled with calcium chloride solution and acetic acid is added to the ppt.
   (iii) Thioglycolic acid is added to preparations containing traces of iron, in the presence of ammonia.
   (b) Discuss the incompatibilities of :
   (i) Potassium permanganate (ii)   Ferrous sulphate (iii) Boric acid.

JAMIA HAMDARD (HAMDARD UNIVERSITY) DELHI

DIPLOMA IN PHARMACY I YEAR EXAM. 1995

1. Give a list of official compounds of iron and calcium along with their formulae. Write the method of preparation, properties, assay and chemical incompatibility of any one compound of iron.

2. Write a detailed account of radio plarmaceuticals and their use in medicine.

3. What are antioxidants and what is their utility in pharmaceuticals ? Give an account of the anti-oxidants studied by you. Illustrate your answer with suitable examples.

4. Write a detailed account of the major Intra and Extra cellular electrolytes which you have studied.

5. Explain :
   (a) Importance and necessity of limit tests.
   (b) Usually in limit tests the two solutions are labelled as 'Test' and 'Standard' but in the limit test for lead they are labelled as 'Primary' and 'Auxiliary' why ?
   (c) What is the role of a small hole near the narrow end of the tube in the limit test of arsenic and this narrow end is not dipped in the solution. The cotton plug of lead-acetate is kept below the mercuric-chloride paper and not above it.
   (d) Why sulphuric acid is added to the solution of ferrous sulphate during its assay.

6. Write notes on any **two** of the following :
   (a) Dentifrices containing fluorides (b) Buffer solutions (c) Protectives and adsorbensts.

7. Give the incompatibility of the following substances : (any six).
   (a) Boric acid (b) Calcium carbonate (c) Povidone-iodine (d) Silver nitrate (e) Ferrous sulphate (f) Hypophosphorous acid (g) Ammoniated mercury (h) Hydrogen peroxide.

D.P. IN PHARMACY - I YEAR, 1994

1. Explain the identification tests along with chemistry involved for the following cations and anions; (a) Acetate, (b) Phosphate (c) Calcium (d) Aluminium.

2. What are protectives and adsorbants ? Describe the method of preparation, properties, assay of any compound used in this regard.

3. What are antioxidants ? How do they act ? Give the methods of preparation of sodium metabisulphite and sodium thiosulphate. Explain the assay of sodium metabisulphite.

4. What do you know of major intra and extracellular

electrolytes ? Explain the method of preparation, properties, assay and uses of sodium chloride.

5. Describe the various sources of impurities in a pharmaceutical substance. Enumerate the various factors taken into consideration while fixing the limits of impurities.

6. What are antacids ? Explain the preparation, properties, assay and uses of a compound of calcium used as an antacid.

7. What are the various official compounds and preparations of iodine ? Describe povidone iodine, ammoniated mercury and chlorinated lime.

PHARM. CHEMISTRY-I (PART-A), 1994

1. Discuss method of preparation and uses of the following (any three).
   (a) Chlorinated lime   (b) Ammonium chloride
   (c) Calcium gluconate   (d) Hydrogen peroxide

2. (a) Describe the procedure and theory involved in carrying out the limit test for lead.
   (b) Give an account of radiopharmaceuticals.

3. Describe the procedure employed in the official assays of the following substances. Discuss chemistry involved in each care.
   (a) Magnesium sulphate (b) Sodium chloride
   (c) Hydrogen peroxide   (d) Zinc sulphate

B. PHARM. IST YEAR (PART A), 1992

1. (a) What is a limit test ? What is their importance in Pharmacy ? Enumerat the factors responsible for causing impurities in pharmaceutical substances.
   (b) Describe the procedure and chemistry of the limit test of heavy metals as given in the I.P.

2. Explain the assay method along with the chemistry involved in the following pharmaceuticals :
   (i) Copper sulphate (ii) Antimony potassium tartarate
   (iii) Chlorinated lime (iv) Boric acid

3. Describe giving chemical reactions the various steps involved in the methods of preparations of the following :
   (i) Potassium permanganate (ii) Iron and ammonium citrate
   (iii) Hydrogen peroxide (iv) Potassium iodide

UNIVERSITY OF BOMBAY, BOMBAY

B. PHARM. 2ND YEAR, NOVEMBER 1994

1. (a) Discuss the limit test in which following reagents are used.
   (i) Dithiazone
   (ii) Thioglycollic acid
   (b) Mention the reagent used in sulphate limit test. Give the composition of the reagent and explain the function of each ingredient in it.
   (c) Give the significance of "Ash Value" and "Moisture Content" in pharmaceuticals giving suitable examples.

2. (a) Outline the significance of Potassium ions in the body. Write a short account of the monograph of any **two** official compounds of potassium.
   (b) Describe the mechanism of action of inorganic antimicrobials. Explain atleast two examples of the compounds used as antimicrobials.
   (c) Explain the following terms giving suitable examples :
   (i) Emetic (ii) Expectorant (iii) Antidote (iv) Cathartic (v) Antacid.

3. Give the assay methods for the following compounds :
   (a) Bleaching powder (b) Hydrogen peroxide (c) Mercuric oxide.

4. (a) Give a brief account of Radiation Therapy.
   (b) Explain Isotopes of Iron Salts.
   (c) Discuss Gasometric methods of analysis.

5. Explain the following :
   (a) Beryllium resembles Aluminium in many respects.
   (b) Transition elements exhibit variable oxidation states.
   (c) Oxygen molecule is paramagnetic.

6. Write short notes on any **two** of the following :
   (a) Pharmaceutical aids (b) Mohr's method (c) Water for injection.

MAY 1994

1. (a) Discuss the contamination in pharmaceutical products.
   (b) Suggest some modifications for lead limit test.

(c) Explain the role of the following tests in pharmaceutical compounds :

(i) Sterility test (ii) LOD (iii) Test for pyrogens.

2. (a) Discuss the physiological role of copper in human body. Describe the official compounds of copper.

(b) Define Allotropy. Give the allotropic modifications of sulphur and outline the properties and uses of precipitated sulphur.

(c) Briefly describe protectives and adsorbents.

3. Give the assay methods for the following compounds

(a) Zinc oxide (b) Ammonium chloride (c) Titanium dioxide

4. (a) Explain the terms "Exposure dose", and "absorbed dose" of radiation. Define Rad, REM and RBE.

(b) Discuss the assay of oxygen and carbon dioxide.

(c) Briefly describe water as universal vehicle.

5. (a) Give reasons for the following

(i) Electron affinity of fluorine is less than that of chlorine.

(ii) The electronegativity of elements in a group shows a decreasing trend.

(b) Explain the main features of long form of periodic table

(c) Give a short account of α-and β-radiations.

6. Write short notes on any **two** of the following :

(a) Antidotes (b) Expectorants and Emetics (c) Saline cathartics.

MAHARSHI DAYANAND UNIVERSITY, ROHTAK

DIPLOMA IN PHARMACY (IIA) EXAMINATION, 1994

1. Describe briefly the 'Radio Pharmaceutical Aids'. How are they stored ? Comment on sodium iodide (131 I) and ferric chloride (59 Fe) solutions.

2. Discuss one each method of preparation, test for purity, storage conditions and pharmaceutical uses of any *four* of the following :

(a) Sodium oxalate (b) Boric acid (c) Ammoniated mercury

(d) Sodium bicarbonate (e) Antimony potassium tartrate.

3. Explain any *three* of the following :
   (a) What are different sources of the impurities in pharmaceutical substances ?
   (b) What are different tests which may be run to ascertian the purity of a substance ?
   (c) Describe the underlying principle and method for the limit test of lead in pharmaceutical substances.
   (d) Describe the limit test of chloride in a sample of zinc sulphate.

4. Explain the assay method along with the chemistry involved in any *four* of the following pharmaceuticals :
   (a) Copper sulphate (b) Chlorinated lime (c) Hydrogen peroxide (d) Potassium permanganate (e) Bismuth oxychloride.

5. Explain why (any *five*) of the following :
   (a) Glycerine is added in the assay of boric acid
   (b) Potassium thiocynate is not added too early in the assay of copper sulphate
   (c) Thioglycollic acid solution is added to the ammonical solution of ferrous sulphate in the limit test of iron.
   (d) Aqueous solution of calcium gluconate is treated with ferric chloride solution
   (e) HCl and H_2S gas is passed to potassium permanganate solution
   (f) Burnt sugar solution is added in the limit test of 'lead'?

6. Descibe with chemical equations (where necessary) and the uses of any *five* of the following :
   (a) Potassium iodine in the limit test of arsenic.
   (b) Trace amounts of potassium sulphate and alcohol in preparation of barium sulphate reagent for the limit test of sulphate.
   (c) Hydrochloric acid in the limit test of sulphate ions.
   (d) Brominated hydrochloric acid 'AST' in the limit test of Arsenic.
   (e) Standard ammonium thiocyanate solution in the assay of yellow mercuric oxide.
   (f) Mordant black mixture in the assay of calcium gluconate
   (g) Potassium iodide in the assay of ammoniated mercury

7. Discuss different sources of common impurities in pharmaceutical compounds. Explain how will you detect the presence of the following impurities (any *five*) :

(a) Bromates in sodium bromide (b) Chlorides in sodium bromide (c) Carbon dioxide in oxygen (d) Calcium and magnesium in sodium phosphate (e) Copper in ammonium chloride (f) Phosphate in barium sulphate (g) Oxidizable substances in purified water (h) Mercurous chloride in mercuric chloride.

8. What do you know about :

(a) Buffer solutions (b) Indicators used on assay methods (c) Bismuth oxychloride (d) Modified Volhard's method ?

DIPLOMA IN PHARMACY (II-A) SUPPL. EXAMINATION, 1994

1. Describe giving chemical reactions the various steps involved in the methods of preparations and pharmaceutical uses of the following :

(i) Potassium permanganate (ii) Hyddrogen peroxide
(iii) Potassium iodide (iv) Iodine

2. Explain the assay method along with the chemistry involved in the following pharmaceuticals :

(i) Copper sulphate (ii) Ammonium chloride
(iii) Magnesium sulphate (iv) Yellow mercuric oxide

3. Write explanatory description of the following (any *three*) :

(i) Radio pharmaceuticals (ii) Pharmaceutical aids (iii) Assay of hydrogen peroxide (iv) Pharmacopoeial monographs of drugs.

4. (i) Describe in detail the limit tests for iron, chloride and sulphate in pharmaceutical substances.

(ii) Write the theory of Arsenic limit test and describe the apparatus used for this test.

5. (i) How many official compounds of sodium are known to you ? Give the methods of preparations and official procedures for the assay of sodium chloride.

(ii) Describe pharmaceutical uses of chlorinated lime, zinc sulphate and ammoniated mercury.

6. What happens when :

(i) Ammoniated mercury is treated with water and excess of potassium iodide.

(ii) Zinc sulphate is treated with hydrochloric and ammonium oxalate.

(iii) Ammonium hydroxide is added to a solution of ferrous sulphate in the presence of citric acid.

(iv) Ammonia passes over hot copper oxide.

(v) Silver compounds are exposed to light.

(vi) Boric acid is heated to 100°C

7. (i) Give the test for absence of metallic borates and insoluble impurities in a sample of calcium gluconate.

(iii) Enlist the compounds of zinc or calcium official in I.P.

8. (i) What is difference between :

(a) Washing soda and Baking soda.

(b) Hydrochloric acid and Aqua regia.

(c) Iodine tincture and Lugol's solution.

(ii) Explain the following statements :

(a) When one substance is oxidized, another substance must be reduced.

(b) Sodium hydroxide is not used in the limit test of lead.

(c) Methyl orange is a suitable indicator in the titration of sodium carbonate.

(d) Sublimed sulphur is especially used for the preparation of ointment of sulphur.

(e) Barium sulphate reagent is recommmended in the B.P. for the limit test of sulphates.

SECOND D. PHARMACY SUPPLEMENTARY EXAMINATION, 199:

1. Give a detailed account of the method the apparatus used and the chemistry involved in the Limit Test for Arsenic by Gutzeit's method.

2. Give one economical method of preparation, tests for purity, storage conditions and uses of any *four* of the following :

(a) Precipitated sulfur; (b) Hydrogen oxide; (c) Iodine (d) Chlorinated lime; (e) Potassium bromide

3. Write short notes on the any *two* of the following :

(a) Sources of impurities in pharmaceutical compounds

(b) Modified Volhard's method; (c) Assay of Copper Sulphate

4. Write short notes on any *two* of the following :
   (a) Monograph of drug; (b) Storage of radiopharmaceuticals;
   (c) Pharmaceutical aids.

5. Give the basic principle involved in the assay of the following compounds :
   (a) Boric acid; (b) Sodium chloride; (c) Calcium chloride;
   (d) Potassium permanganate.

6. Explain with chemical equations (where necessary) why :
   (i) Acetic acid is added in the assay of chlorinated lime.
   (ii) Nitrobenzene is added in the assay of ammonium chloride.
   (iii) Glycerol is added in the assay of boric acid.
   (iv) Ammonium chloride is added in the assay of zinc oxide.
   (v) Sodium potassium tartrate is added in the assay of antimony potassium tartrate.
   (vi) Potassium permangnate is added in the the assay of ferric ammonium citrate.
   (vii) Citric acid is added in the limit test for Iron.
   (viii) Cotton wool is soaked in dry lead acetate solution before packing in the tube of Gutzeit's apparatus.

7. How would you detect the following impurities in the given compounds ?

   (i) Phosphine in oxygen; (ii) Oxidisable matter in purified water; (iii) Aluminium, iron and matter insoluble in hydrochloric acid in sodium hydroxide; (iv) Bromate in sodium bromide; (v) Copper, iron and zinc in sodium sulphate; (vi) Sodium thiosulphate in sodium metabisulfite; (vii) Phosphate in Barium sulphate. (viii) Mercurous chloride in amoniated mercury.

BOARD OF TECHNICAL EDUCATION, GOVERNMENT OF NATIONAL CAPITAL TERRITORY OF DELHI

DIP. PHARM 1ST YERAS JAN/FEB-1995 (NS)

1. Write physical and chemical properties, medicinal and pharmaceutical uses and storage conditions of any two of the followings :
   (a) Dicalcium phosphate (b) Sodium melabisulphate
   (c) Sodium potassium Tartarate.

2. (a) What are antioxidants ? What should be ideal characteristics for air autooxidant to be used in parenteral preparations ?

   (b) Describe properties, storage and chemical incompatability of any one of the following :

      (i) Hypophosphorous acid (ii) Sodium nitrite

3. Enlist the official compounds of Iron with chemical formulae. Discuss the role of Iron in metabolism. Discuss the properties and medicinal uses of Ferrous Fumerate and Iron Dextron injection.

4. Write properties, medicinal uses and official preparations of any two of the followings :

5. What do you understand by the terms 'Purity', 'limit test', 'Test for purity' and 'Assay'. Discuss the principle and procedure involved in limit test of Iron.

6. Write notes on any *two* of the following :

   (a) Isotonicity. (b) Buffer solutions and their importance in Pharmacy. (c) Oral rehydration powder and justification of ingredients added.

7. What are radioactive substances ? How radioactive substances are useful. Discuss the problems associated with handling of radioactive substances of pharmaceutical interest. Write a brief note on two pharmaceutically important isotopes used in medicinal practice.

8. Complete the following :

   (i) The pH of a $3.43 \times 10N$ solution of hydrochloric acid ————

   (ii) Magnesium sulphate is used orally as a ———— and parenterally as an ————

   (iii) Potassium Permanganate is heated to 240°C, it decomposes to ———— leaving ———— and ————.

   (iv) The chemical composition of Ammoniated mercury is ———— and is soluble in ————.

   (v) Antimony Potassium tartarate is a drug of choice in the treatment of ————.

   (vi) The mechanism of action of inorganic antimicrobial agents can be divided into three general categories ————, ———— and ————.

   (vii) Calcium zons abrorption and distribution is controlled by ———— and ———— harmones.

   (viii) The preferred antidote for cyanide poisoning is ————

AUGUST 1994 (NS)

1. Explain with chemical equation distinguish between
   (a) Carbonates and Bicarbonates (b) Nitrites and Nitrates
   (c) Sulphites and Sulphides (d) Sulphate and Thiosulphate.

2. Explain giving examples, what are acids and bases in the light of Arrhenitus Bronsted Lowry and Lewis concepts ?

3. Name the any inorganic respiratory stimulants you have studied. Explain the method of preparation propetites and assay of any one of them.

4. Describe the methods of preparation, properties, assay and uses of any one inorganic astringent you know.

5. Explain the methods to obtain iodine from sea weeds and Chile salt petre, How it is stored ? How is it assayed ? What are its uses ? Give list of various preparations of iodine.

6. Explain the characteristics of alpha particles, beta particles and gamma radiations. How are the various radiophar-maceuticals stored ? Describe what you know of a radio-opaque contrast media of barium.

7. What are the various classes of gastro-intestinal agents ? Name the inorganic compounds belonging to each class. Write what you know about bismuth sub-carbonate.

JANUARY/FEBRUARY-1995 (OS)

1. What is the importance of various purity tests in Pharmaceuticals ? Discuss the basic principle involved in any two of the limit tests.

2. What are radiopharmaceuticals ? Illustrate your answer with examples. Describe various radiopharmaceuticals used for diagnostic purposes.

3. Write down the theoretical background for the following assays :
   (a) Sodium oxalate (b) Copper sulphate (c) Ammonium chloride (d) Iodine

4. Describe the method of preparation and uses in detail for the followings :
   (a) Sodium Chloride (b) Hydrogen Peroxide (c) Potassium Iodide

5. Discuss the pharmaceutical uses, storage conditions and pharmaceutical formulations of the following compounds :
   (a) Boric acid (b) Iodine (c) Magnesium trisilicate (d) Potassium permanganate.

6. Describe the method of preparation and assay procedure for the followings :

   (a) Ammoniated mercury (b) Calcium gluconate (c) Ferrous sulphate.

7. Write notes on the followings :

   (a) Inorganic pharmaceutical aids.

   (b) Inorganic compounds as astringents and protectives.

AUGUST, 1994 (OS)

1. Write the method of preparation of sodium bicarbonate. Describe its pharmaceutical formulations and detailed uses.

2. Write the basic principle of the assay of the following compounds with chemical reactions :

   (i) Ammonium chloride   (ii) Ferrous sulphate

   (iii) Magnesium sulphate   (iv) Boric acid

3. What is the importance of purity in pharmaceuticals ? What are the various sources of impurities in pharmaceuticals ? How will you perform the quantitative test for lead as per I.P.?

4. Write the storage conditions with justification and medicinal uses of the followings :

   (i) Hydrogen peroxide solution I.P. (ii) Chlorinated lime (iii) Iodine (iv) Potassium iodide

5. Write notes on the following :

   (i) Radiopharmaceuticals as diagnostic agents

   (ii) Pharmaceutical aids.

6. Write the name of the indicator and its colour change at the end point in the assay of the following compounds :

   (i) Ammoniated mercury (ii) Iodine (iii) Sodium chloride (iv) Chlorinated lime (v) Sodium oxalate (vi) Zinc sulphate (vii) Bismuth oxychloride (viii) Yellow mercuric oxide

7. Describe the method of preparation, assay procedure and pharmaceutical uses of any one of the official calcium salts.

8. Write the method of preparation, properties, test for purity, assay procedure, storage conditions and pharmaceutical uses of Antimony Potassium Tartrate.

BOARD OF TECHNICAL EDUCATION, HARYANA (CHANDIGARH)

DIP. PHARM. IST YEAR, SEPT. 1994

1. Mention different types of impurities found in pharmaceuticals. Discuss the importance of quality control and various methods used to control the quality of drugs and pharmaceuticals.

2. Define and explain 'Limit test' and 'Test for purity'. Give the importance of limit test in pharmacy. Describe the principle and procedure for the limit test for 'Iron' and 'Chloride'.

3. Give strronge conditions and uses of any eight of the following :

   (i) Oxygen (ii) Sodium metabisulphite (iii) Silver nitrate (iv) Ammoniated mercury (v) Magnesium trisillicate (vi) Titanium dioxide (vii) Zine sulphate (viii) Iodine (ix) Potassium permanganate (x) Sodium nitrate

4. Define and explain 'Radiopharmaceuticals.' Discuss in detail about the application of radioisotopes in pharmacy, their storage conditions and precautions during handling.

5. (a) Explain why :
   - (i) Black stain results when silver nitrate comes in contact with the skin.
   - (ii) Calcium carbonate is soluble in water containing carbon dioxide.
   - (iii) Antimony compounds are treated with NaOH before the limit test for Lead.
   - (iv) Citric acid is added in the limit test for 'Iron'.

   (b) Give the general properties and uses of any Four of the following :
   - (i) Alum (ii) Hydrogen peroxide (iii) Sodium citrate (iv) Antimony potassium tartrate (v) Magnesium oxide

6. Give physical, chemical properties, medicinal and pharmaceutical uses and storage conditions of any Two inorganic official compounds of calcium.

7. Write short notes on any Three of the following :

   (i) Measurement of radioactivity (ii) I.P. Limit test for sulphate. (iii) Expectorants and Emetics (iv) Antacids.

8. (a) Give the identification tests for Calcium, Aluminium, Sodium and Chloride.

   (b) Calculate the amount of salt necessary to make a solution that contains 153 m eq/litre each of Na^+ and Cl^-.

MAY 1994

1. What are the common types of impurities found in pharmaceutical compounds. What is the basis for fixing a limit test for these impurities in the pharmacopoeia. Discuss various methods to control the quality of pharmaceutical products.

2. What do you understand by the term "Limit test". Give significance of limit test for Iron and Lead.

3. Write short notes on the following :

   (i) Scintillation Counter (ii) Geiger Muller Counter (iii) Storage of radio pharmaceuticals (iv) Precaution during handling of pharmaceutical

4. Enlist the official compounds of calcium with their formulae. Give the properties, uses and storage conditions of Calcium gluconate and calcium carbonate.

5. Complete and balance the following :

   (i) $KOH + I_2 \longrightarrow$

   (ii) $MgCO_3 + H_2SO_4 \longrightarrow$

   (iii) $HgCl_2 + NaOH \longrightarrow$

   (iv) $CH_3COOH + KHCO_3 \longrightarrow$

   (v) $KNaC_4H_4O_6 + CH_3COOH \longrightarrow$

   (vi) $Na_2CO_3 + H_3C_6H_5O_7 \longrightarrow$

   (vii) $ZnSO_4 + Na_2CO_3 \longrightarrow$

   (viii) $Al_2(SO_4)_3 + K_2SO_4 + H_2O \longrightarrow$

6. Write the physical and chemical properties, storage and pharmaceutical uses of the following :

   (i) Boric acid (ii) Potassium permanganate (iii) Iodine (iv) Magnesium oxide

7. Give storage conditions and uses of any eight of the following :

   1. Calcium hydroxide   2. Sodium bisulphite
   3. Sodium nitrite·   4. Aluminium phosphate
   5. Kaolin   6. Magnesium sulphate
   7. Mercury   8. Talc

8. Write short notes on any two of the following :
   (i) Limit test for 'sulphate' (ii) Limit test for Heavy metals
   (iii) Antioxidants

JULY 1993

1. With suitable examples, discuss sources of impurities in Pharmaceutical chemicals.

2. Explain briefly the principle underlying arsenic limit test.

   Or

   Explain how the limit test for heavy metals differ from limit test for lead.

3. Give the method of preparation and uses of any four of the following :
   (i) Sodium benzoate (ii) Ferric ammonium citrate
   (iii) Precipitated sulphur (iv) Potassium iodide (v) Calcium phospate (Diabasic).

4. Describe the properties, uses and principle of assay of any two of the following :
   (i) Calcium gluconate (ii) Bismuth oxychloride
   (iii) Chlorinated lime.

5. What are Radiopharmaceuticals ? Describe Ferric citrate (59 Fe) injection and Sodium Phosphate (32 P) injection.

6. Write an essay on the application of Pharmaceutical aids and discuss Zinc oxide and Bentonite.

7. (a) How the following compounds are stored ? Explain reasons of their specific storage conditions.

   (i) Ammoniated mercury (ii) Antimony potassium tartarate (iii) Hydrogen peroxide (iv) Sodium iodide (^{131}I) solution.

   (b) Write the I.P. preparations as uses of the following :
   (i) Heavy Kaolin (ii) Mercuric oxide (iii) Potassium iodide
   (iv) Zinc sulphate.

8. (a) Comment on the use of :
   (i) Citric acid and ammonia solution in the limit test of iron.
   (ii) Small traces of potassium sulphate and alcohol in preparation of Barium sulphate reagent of the limit test of of sulphate.
   (iii) Acetic acid in the assay of copper sulphate.
   (iv) Nitrobenzene in the assay of Ammonium chloride.

(b) Give the assay procedure with reactions of boric acid and ferrous sulphate.

JULY-1992

1. Enlist different official compounds of sodium. Describe sodium bicarbonate in detail giving methods of preparation, test for purity, assay procedure, uses and different pharmaceutical preparations.

2. Describe the pharmaceutical preparations and uses for the following :

   (a) Iodine, (b) Sodium chloride, (c) Calcium gluconate (d) Boric acid.

3. (a) Write down important tests for purity for calcium gluconate and sodium benzoate.

   (b) How will you perform the limit test for chloride in a sample of sodium bromide.

4. (a) Write a note on impurities in pharmacueticals and their control.

   (b) Describe dithizone test for lead.

5. Write the basic principle for the assay of :

   (a) Potassium permanganate. (b) Sodium chloride. (c) Magnesium sulphate. (d) Ammoniated mercury.

6. Write down the methods of preparation, storage conditions and uses of the following :

   (a) Calcium gluconate. (b) Ammoniated mercury (c) Chlorinated lime. (d) Forrous sulphate.

7. What are radiopharmaceutical ? Describe the importance of different radiopharmaceuticals in pharmacy.

8. (a) Describe the assay procedure of the following :

   (i) Copper sulphate. (ii) Iodine.

   (b) Write down the method of preparation and properties of (i) Boric acid. (ii) Zinc oxide.

BOARD OF EXAMINING AUTHORITY, GOVERNMENT OF KARNATAKA

FINAL YEAR D. PHARM. EXAMINATION, NOVEMBER 1994 (REVISED REGULATION)

1. Define the term 'Limit test' and 'Test for Purity'.

2. Write the principle involved in Iron limit test.

3. Give reasons for the following :
   (a) Nitric acid is used in chloride limit test.
   (b) Ammonia is used in Iron limit test.

4. Name one inorganic compound used for each of the following purpose.
   (a) Cathartic (b) Hypnotic and sedative (c) Emetic (d) Diuretic

5. Name any two inorganic medicinally important compounds each of Calciums and Magnisium.

6. Write the synonyms and uses of the following :
   (a) Weak Iodine solution (b) Borax (c) Sodium bicarbonate (d) Potassium Antimony tartrate

7. Mention the specific medicinal use of the following :
   (a) Yellow mercuric oxide (b) Bentonite (c) Sodium metabisulphite (d) Precipitated sulphur

8. Write the principle involved in Sulphate limit test.

9. Give balanced equations for the following and name the reactants and products.
   (a) $I_2 + Na_2 S_2 O_3$
   (b) $NH_4 SCN + Ag NO_3$

10. Mention the medicinal uses of the following :
    (a) Kaolin (b) Sodium chloride (c) Calcium Gluconate (d) Hydrogen peroxide

11. Give reasons for the following :
    (a) Chlorinated lime should be stored in well-closed containers.
    (b) Stannous chloride is used in Arsenic limit test.

12. What happens when the following are made to react. Write the balanced equation.
    (a) Copper sulphate solution is treated with Potassium Iodide.
    (b) Boric acid is dissolved in the mixture of water and glycerin.

13. Write the Stability and Storage conditions of the following:
    (a) Hydrogen peroxide (b) Ferrous sulphate

14. Discuss the principle involved in the I.P. method of Assay of the following compounds.

(a) Chlorinated lime (b) Yellow mercuric oxide (c) Ammonium Chloride (d) Magnisium sulphate

Or

Write short notes on any two of the following :

(a) Essential features of monograph of I.P. (b) Sources of Impurity (c) Pharmaceutical Aids

15. Discuss the principle, procedure and apparatus used for I.P. limit test of Arsenic.
16. Write the method of preparation, use and storage for the following :

    (a) Iodine (b) Ammoniated mercury (c) Zinc oxide
17. How are the following tests carried out :

    (a) Iodate in Potassium Iodide
    (b) Chloride in Potassium permanganate
    (c) Acid consuming capacity of Aluminium hydroxide gel
    (d) Cyanogen in Iodine

MAY 1993 (OLD SCHEME)

1. Define and classify limit tests with example. Mention the factors affecting limit tests.
2. Give the chemical composition and uses of :

   (i) Epsom salt (ii) Kaolin (iii) Bleaching powder (iv) Bentonite
3. Give stability, storage conditions and uses of :

   (i) H_2O_2 (ii) Caustic Soda (iii) Green Vitriole (iv) Ferric ammonium Citrate
4. Name two deliquescent and efflorescent and two light sensitive and two oxygen sensitive inorganic medicinal agents.
5. Name three Inorganic pharmaceuticals assayed by Gravimetry with their uses.
6. Give the composition and functions of barium sulphate reagents in sulphate limit test.
7. Give the uses of following in the limit tests.
8. (a) Why SNH_2SO_4 is added in Hydrogen peroxide assay ?

   (b) Why starch indicator is added at the near of end point?
   (c) NH_2SO_4 in H_2O_2 Assay.
9. Give the balanced Equations :
10. (a) Mention the difference between Iodimetry and Iodometry.

(b) Give two examples of pharmaceutical inorganic compounds assayed by iodimetry with their uses.

11. Give the sources of impurities in pharmacopoeia compounds.

12. Name an inorganic agent used as :
    (i) Germicide (ii) Diuretic (iii) Astringent (iv) Buffer

13. Give the chemistry of assay of ferrous sulphate by I.P. 85.

14. Discuss the principles involved in the assay of following
    (i) Calcium Gluconate (ii) Bleaching powder (iii) Ammoniated Mercury (iv) Boric acid

Or

Discribe Arsenic Limit Test :

15. Give the principle and procedure for :
    (i) Iron limit test. (ii) Lead limit test IP.

16. Outline the assay procedures for the following :
    (i) Sodium sulphate (ii) Copper Sulphate (iii) Sodium Choride Inj. (iv) Yellow Mercuric Oxide.

17. Write short notes on any two.
    (i) Radio Pharmaceuticals. (ii) Pharmaceutical Aids. (iii) Monographs in pharmacopoeia.

NOVEMBER 1992 (O.S)

1. Classify the impurities in pharmacuticals and write a note on how the limit of tolerance is fixed.

2. Write the principle involved in Arsenic Limit test.

3. Describe the uses of the following in the limit tests.
   (a) Lead Acetate cotton wool. (b) 20% w/v solution of citric acid.

4. How sulphate limit test is performed in potassium permanganate.

5. Write the chemical formula, and uses of the following.
   (a) Caustic soda (b) Common salt (c) Tartar emetic (d) Green vitreol

6. Name any **two** medicinally important compounds each of Mercury and Iron. Mention their uses.

7. Give balanced equations. Name reactants and products formed in the following :
   (a) $K_2SO_4 + BaCl_2$ (b) $KMnO_4 + H_2SO_4 + H_2O_2$

8. Name one Inorganic compound used for each of the following purpose.

   (a) Astringent (b) Expectorant (c) Analgesic (d) Local Antibacterial

9. Write a brief note on, give its uses also :

   (a) Bentonite (b) Sod. Phosphate (32^P)

10. Write on the stability and storage conditions of the following:

    (a) Chlorinated lime (b) Ferrous sulphate

11. Write the chemical composition and pharmaceutical uses of

    (a) Bleaching powder (b) Precipitated sulphur (c) Ammonium citrate (d) Iodine.

12. Draw a neat labellel diagram of Arsenic Limit test apparatus.

13. Give reasons for the following :

    (a) Hydrogen peroxide is stored in dark coloured bottles.

    (b) Ammonia is used in the iron limit test.

14. Discuss the principle involved in the assay of the following compounds. (Any three) :

    (a) Copper sulphate (b) Calcium gluconate (c) Boric Acid (d) Bismuth oxy-chloride

                              Or

    Write short notes on any **two** of the following :

    (a) Sources of impurities in pharmaceuticals.

    (b) Pharmaceutical aids. (c) Radiopharmaceuticals.

15. Discuss the principle and a brief procedure of the limit test for

    (a) Heavy metals and (b) Lead as given in I.P.

16. Describe the general properties, stability, storage conditions, uses and pharmaceutical preparations of any **two** of the following medicinal agents.

    (a) Sodium Bicarbonate (b) Potassium Iodide (c) Hydrogen peroxide

17. Outline the method of assaying the following compounds. (Attempt any **three**) :

    (a) Yellow mercuric oxide (b) Zinc sulphate (c) Chlorinated lime (d) Sodium oxalate

FINAL D. PHARM EXAMINATION, OCTOBER 1990

1. Describe the principle, general procedure and appartus for Arsenic limit test I-P.

2. (a) How the following tests for purity are carried out ?
     (i) Sulphate in potassium permanganate
     (ii) Acid consuming capacity of Aluminium Hydroxide gel
     (iii) Chloride in sodium benzoate
   (b) Write a note on sources of impurities in pharmaceutical compounds.

3. Give reasons for Seven/Eight of the following :
    (i) Glycerol is used in Boric acid assay.
    (ii) Nitric acid is used in Chloride limit test.
    (iii) Hydrogen peroxide should be stored in a well closed container.
    (iv) Lead acetate cotton is used in Arsenic limit test.
    (v) In Volhard's method of assay, nitrobenzene is used.
    (vi) Yellow mercuric oxide is prepared by precipitation method.
    (vii) In the assay of potasium Iodide, starch is added at the end point.
    (viii) Iodine solution is prepared using Potasium Iodide.

4. Discuss the principle involved in the assay of any *four* of the following :
   (i) Bleaching powder (ii) Copper Sulphate (iii) Calcium Gluconate (iv) Magnesium Sulphate (v) Ammonium Chloride (vi) Iodine

5. Describe the preparation, storage condition and uses of any *four* of the following :
   (i) Iodine (ii) Copper Sulphate (iii) Ferrous Sulphate (iv) Boric acid (v) Silver Nitrate

6. Give Chemical balanced equations for Seven/Eight the following :
    (i) Barium Peroxide + Sulphuric acid
    (ii) Ferrous Sulphate + Thioglycollic acid
    (iii) Sodium Chloride + Silver Nitrate
    (iv) Bleaching Powder + Acetic Acid
    (v) Lead Nitrate + Hydrogen Sulphide
    (vi) Potassium Iodide + Bromine
    (vii) Mercuric Chloride + Sodium Hydroxide
    (viii) Ammoniated Mercury + Potassium iodide + Water

7. (a) Name two Inorganic Compounds used for each of the following. Give their Chemical formula.

   (i) Antacids (ii) Antiseptics (iii) Emetic (iv) Preservatives (v) Sedatives

   (b) Write briefly a note on Radiopharmaceuticals.

FINAL D. PHARM EXAMINATION, APRIL 1990

1. Describe the principle, general procedure, use of various reagents and apparatus of I.P. limit test for Arsenic impurity in pharmaceuticals.

2. Write a note on the following .

   (a) Sources and Types of impurities in pharmaceuticals.

   (b) Principles involved in chloride and heavy metal limit tests.

3. Discuss the principle involved in the assay of the following compounds.

   (a) Copper sulphate (b) Calcium Gluconate (c) Ammoniated Mercury (d) Ammonium chloride

4. Write a brief note on the following :

   (a) Typical pharmacopoeial Monograph (b) Radio pharmaceuticals (c) Pharmaceutical Aids

5. Write a note on stability and storage conditions of the following compounds.

   (a) Sodium Hydroxide (b) Sodium chloride (c) Iron and ammonium citrate (d) Chlorinated Lime (e) Iodine (f) Sodium Iodide I^{131} solution (g) Bentonite (h) Hydrogen peroxide solution

6. Write the chemical formula, important general properties (one each) and the specific use of the following compounds.

   (a) Sodium Benzoate (b) Precipitated Sulphur (c) Magnesium sulphate (d) Sodium Bicarbonate (e) Yellow Mercuric oxide (f) Antimony potassium Tartarate (g) Purified Tale (h) Ferrous Sulphate.

7. (a) Give reasons for the following :

   1. Use of HCl in sulphate limit test.
   2. Use of Barium Sulphate reagent in sulphate Limit Test.
   3. Thioglycollic Acid is used in Iron Limit Test.

(b) Complete and balance the following equations. (Write chemical formula, name the products and, reactants wherever necessary).

1. $HgO + HNO_3$
2. Sod. chloride + Silver Nitrate
3. Sod. Sulphate + Barium Chloride
4. Pot. Permangnate + Sulphuric Acid + Hydrogen peroxide

FINAL D. PHARM. EXAMINATION. APRIL 1991

1. Define limit tests. Why limit tests are performed for pharmaceutical substances ? How limit tests are carried out in general ?
2. What are the sources of impurities in Pharmaceutical substances ? Explain with examples.
3. What are "tests for purity" ? Enumerate different tests for purity carried out for Pharmaceutical Substances.
4. What is a "Monograph" ? Mention the essential features of a Monograph.
5. What are "Radio Pharmaceuticals" ? What are their uses ? Give two examples for Radiopharmaceuticals with their specific uses.
6. What is an "Assay" ? Mention different types of reactions involved in titrimetric methods of assay giving their uses.
8. Give the stability and storage conditions for
   (a) Hydrogen Peroxide and (b) Ferrous sulphate
9. Give reasons for the use of
   (a) Potassium iodide and
   (b) Potassium thiocyanate in the assay of copper sulphate.
10. Give the reasons for using
    (a) Iron-free citric acid and
    (b) Iron-free ammonia solution in the limit test for Iron.
11. Mention the uses of
    (a) Sodium benzoate   (b) Potassium permanganate
    (c) Precipitated Sulphur   (d) Zinc Oxide
12. Mention the Pharmacopoeial preparations of the following compounds.
    (a) Sodium Chloride (b) Calcium gluconate (c) Heavy Kaolin
    (d) Yellow mercuric oxide
13. Why glycerol is used in the assay of Boric acid ? Whatelse can be used instead of Glycerol for the same purpose ?

14. Give the principles and official procedures for the limit tests for

    (a) Chlorides and (b) Sulphates

15. Explain the chemical principles involved in the assays of

    (a) Magnesium Sulphate (b) Ferrous Sulphate (c) Hydrogen peroxide (d) Chlorinated lime.

16. Give the procedures for the following assays :

    (a) Sodium bicarbonate (b) Ammoniated Mercury (c) Chlorinated lime (d) Ammonium Chloride (e) Antimony potassium tartrate.

17. Give the principles and procedures for the limit tests for

    (a) Lead and (b) Heavy metals

18. Give the Principles and procedures for the assays of

    (a) Yellow mercuric oxide (b) Bismuth oxychloride and (c) Iodine.

INDEX